Smart Computing and Intelligence

Series Editors

Kinshuk, Athabasca, AB, Canada

Ronghuai Huang, Beijing Normal University, Beijing, China

Chris Dede, Technology, Innovation, and Education, Harvard University, Cambridge, MA, USA

This book series aims to establish itself as a medium for the publication of new research and development of innovative paradigms, models, architectures, conceptual underpinnings and practical implementations encompassed within smart computing and intelligence.

The scope of the series includes but is not limited to smart city, smart education, health informatics, smart ecology, data and computational analytics, smart society, smart learning, complex systems-chaos, computational thinking, brain computer interaction, natural/computer interaction, humanoid behaviour, and impact of educational psychology on computing.

The cornerstone of this series' editorial policy is its unwavering commitment to report the latest results from all areas of smart computing and intelligence research, development, and practice. Our mission is to serve the global smart computing and intelligence community by providing a most valuable publication service.

Suparna Biswas · Chandreyee Chowdhury ·
Biswaranjan Acharya · Chuan-Ming Liu
Editors

Internet of Things Based Smart Healthcare

Intelligent and Secure Solutions Applying
Machine Learning Techniques

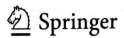

Editors

Suparna Biswas
Department of Computer Science
and Engineering
Maulana Abul Kalam Azad University
of Technology, West Bengal
Haringhata, West Bengal, India

Biswaranjan Acharya
School of Computer Engineering
KIIT University
Bhubaneswar, Odisha, India

Chandreyee Chowdhury
Department of Computer Science
and Engineering
Jadavpur University
Kolkata, West Bengal, India

Chuan-Ming Liu
Department of Computer Science
and Information Engineering
National Taipei University of Technology
Taipei, Taiwan

ISSN 2522-0888   ISSN 2522-0896 (electronic)
Smart Computing and Intelligence
ISBN 978-981-19-1410-2   ISBN 978-981-19-1408-9 (eBook)
https://doi.org/10.1007/978-981-19-1408-9

This Springer imprint is published by the registered company Springer Nature Singapore Pte Ltd.
The registered company address is: 152 Beach Road, #21-01/04 Gateway East, Singapore 189721,
Singapore

Contents

IoT Based Smart Healthcare

Wearable Sensors and Machine Intelligence for Smart Healthcare

Samaleswari Pr. Nayak, Sarat Ch. Nayak, S. C. Rai, and Bimal Pr. Kar

Abstract Continuous growth in global population and the demand of healthcare, particularly for the elderly and physically disabled people, is a challenge in the current era. The growth in ageing population led to complex health issues and rise in healthcare expenditures. Conventional health monitoring system for these people is time consuming, inconvenient, and insufficient most of the times. However, there has been a demand for developing efficient healthcare solutions for these people for an improved lifestyle. Advances in artificial intelligence (AI) technologies and Internet of Things (IoT) have opened up a new revolution in the healthcare domain. The response time in diagnosis and treatment of elderly and disabled patient can be reduced through Internet of Things and wearable body sensors. Using low-cost and lightweight body sensors placed very close to the body of the patient, the lifestyle data can be collected, and the information, in turn, could be shared with the doctors and health caretakers remotely. Machine intelligence is another aspect to remote healthcare system in analyzing the huge and heterogeneous data collected by the sensors. The promising technological area of wearable sensors, IoT, and machine intelligence seems to afford a smart and intelligent means for an automated health monitoring system for elderly and disabled patients staying remotely. The intension of this chapter is to explore the advancement, modality, specification, and applications of wearable body sensors for acumination of body symptoms from remote patients. Then, the importance and necessity of machine intelligence for analysis of healthcare data will be discussed. Finally, a conceptual model integrating wearable body sensors, IoT, and machine intelligence for remote healthcare will be presented. The model

S. Pr. Nayak (✉) · S. C. Rai
Silicon Inst. of Tech., Bhubaneswa, India
e-mail: samaleswari.nayak@silicon.ac.in

S. C. Rai
e-mail: satya@silicon.ac.in

S. Ch. Nayak
CMR College of Eng. & Tech., Hyderabad, India

B. Pr. Kar
Gandhi Institute of Tech. Adv., Bhubaneswar, India

© The Author(s), under exclusive license to Springer Nature Singapore Pte Ltd. 2022
S. Biswas et al. (eds.), *Internet of Things Based Smart Healthcare*, Smart Computing and Intelligence, https://doi.org/10.1007/978-981-19-1408-9_1

3

may be helpful in reducing the complexities and healthcare expenditure faced by aging, physical disabilities and remote population.

Keywords Internet of Things · Wearable sensors · Remote healthcare · Artificial intelligence · Machine intelligence · Smart healthcare

1 Introduction

Living with good health is the most important activity in human life. Healthcare demand has been growing with the rapid growth of world population while the resources are limited. Satisfying the high demand in healthcare resources starting from manpower to modern hospital infrastructure is creating significant challenges in the current era (Australian Institute of Health & Welfare, 2014; Perrier, 2015). Particularly, the growth in ageing population and patients staying in remote areas led to complex health issues and rise in healthcare expenditures. Conventional health monitoring system for these people is time consuming, inconvenient, and insufficient most of the times. However, there has been a demand for developing efficient healthcare solutions for these people for an improved lifestyle. Health of non-critical patients could be monitored remotely at their residence rather than in hospitals, which can reduce the pressure on hospital resources. It could be helpful in providing better access to healthcare for patients living in rural areas, aged people to live independently at home or physically disabled persons as self-assistance. More specifically, it can progress admittance to healthcare assets at the same time as dropping excess load on healthcare systems. Also, it can give people be in charge of over their own health at all times.

IoT has been emerging as an alternative to abridged pressures on the current healthcare systems in the form of remote monitoring of patients with certain criteria, aiding rehabilitation through continuous monitoring the patient's progress etc. (Fan et al., 2014; Gope & Hwang, 2016; Zhu et al., 2015). IoT has opened up a new revolution in the healthcare sphere of influence. The response time in diagnosis and treatment of elderly, remotely and disabled patient can be reduced through Internet of Things and wearable body sensors. IoT is a relatively new research area and its adequate applications in healthcare are still under exploration. Several IoT healthcare-related technologies such as accessible solutions, possible applications, as well as challenges are surveyed in literature (Baker et al., 2017; Islam et al., 2015). The possibilities and potential of IoT as a solution for remote healthcare have been identified by many researchers recently. A system to generate a rehabilitation plan using IoT based on the symptoms is suggested by different authors (Fan et al., 2014). The system is proved successful in almost 87.9% cases where IoT is used for monitoring patients suffering from Parkinson's disease (Pasluosta et al., 2015). An IoT-based system for monitoring the glucose level in blood of diabetic person is suggested in Chang et al. (2016) by researchers. The system is claimed to be practical in analyzing the abnormalities in the glucose level and notifying the healthcare personnel. The easy availability of low-cost wearable sensors improved the style of remote healthcare system. These are used to extract and measure the physiological conditions of a patient. Using low-cost and lightweight body sensors placed very close to the body of the patient, the lifestyle data can be collected and the information in turn could be shared with the doctors and health caretakers remotely. More applications of wearable sensors to identify chronic heart diseases are elaborated in Sect. 2.

Major challenges in IoT-based healthcare system are security and big data management and analysis. The volume and varieties in sensor data collected from remote patients can be huge and need to be managed and analyzed in a systematic way to extract meaningful insights, which can be then used by the healthcare experts. Cloud-based data storage models are suggested in this regard (Ghanavati et al., 2016; Xu et al., 2014). For analysis and inference drawing from these huge data stored in cloud, machine intelligence could be used (Abawajy & Hassan, 2017; Sahoo et al., 2016). Few researchers suggested and compared the performance of machine learning methods such as deep learning, multilayer perceptron, support vector machine etc. for processing and analysis of cloud-based healthcare data (Hung et al., 2017; Park et al., 2014).

The overall contributions of this chapter are as follows:

- Presents healthcare issues and challenges for remote patients, particularly elderly and physically disable people.
- The possibilities of IoT as an alternate to conventional healthcare system.
- The state of the art and advances in Wearable sensors, specifications, and applications to IoT enabled healthcare system
- The necessitate and significance of machine intelligence for analysis and extraction of noteworthy insights from large and heterogeneous data collected by sensors.
- Designing a conceptual IoT-enabled autonomous healthcare model for remotely staying elderly and physically challenged people.

The remaining of the chapter is structured into four sections. Section 2 discusses present healthcare scenarios and challenges faced by remote patients. The possibilities of IoT as a suitable solution to the current healthcare system are discussed in Sect. 3. Section 4 presents our conceptual IoT-based model for remote healthcare monitoring. Section 5 concludes the chapter.

2 Presents Healthcare Issues and Challenges for Remote Patients

For every human being, heart is considered to be the most vital organ and assumed to be most affected in human body due to surrounding parameters. Different types of heart diseases are creating panic among all human beings of the world out of which coronary heart disease named as CHD is accepted as the greatest enemy to old age patients, due to which the death rate is increasing in most of the developing countries rather in developed. "The Registrar General of India" announced that CHD has caused 17% of total mishap and 26% of mature mishaps in 2001–2003, which is now expanded to 23% of total and 32% of mature mishaps in 2010–2013 (Perrier, 2015). In US about one in every three deaths are caused by cardiovascular disease, which leads to nearly 801,000 deaths with an average of 1 death in every 40 s as per 2017 survey (Australian Institute of Health & Welfare, 2014). CHDs take more life compared to cancer and another disease related to respiratory jointly in every year. So, the monitoring of heart condition is very much essential for each and every person, especially for the old age people. But with the increasing population, it is very difficult to continuously monitor each and every patient by a medical expert. Also, there are several critical situations need to be monitored where the patient lives in a rural area or far away from the hospital and suffering from different diseases, also the aged people who are suffering from a physical disorder with some cardiac issues.

Real-time monitoring during game is necessary as few players seem as invincible due to sudden demise and unaware of their health issues during game. Balers performing phenomenal feats in the playground can sometimes make us forget that they are even mortal. Due to previous cardiovascular diseases, sudden mishap may occur for athlete. An athlete's heart is normally considered as a benevolent development in cardiac mass, with specific circulatory and cardiac morphological alterations, that defines a functional variation to procedural training, Boston Celtic.

From the history, it is found that at the age of 27 after collapsing Reggie Lewis faced death in an open session game (Naik & Sudarshan, 2019). Sudden mishap forced people to think seriously about the other star athletes those who had faced sudden mishap while performing in the sports they interested in and it is considered to be common that players will die during their game through severe cardiac stroke and other health issues. Many players had already faced the same situation and followers are losing their favorite sports down the memory lane. Thus, the great loss of all modest players had put a great challenge over healthcare communities to overcome the situation. Day by day, the medical profile of all athletes is becoming getting better due to availability of ECG, echocardiography, cardiac magnetic resonance and health training, due to which they are being recognized by a wide variety of population and are accessible by number of people (Al-Makhadmeh & Tolba, 2019). On a serious note, the cardiac change depends on the extended recognition conditioning, which is impacting on several athlete health situations. This may create some situation due to which sudden mishap or development in stages of disease may arise for athletes, which needs to be restricted but not completely avoided. So, the monitoring of real-time heart condition is very much essential for each and every person, especially for the old age people as well as sports persons during the game.

It has been considered that body temperature along with heartbeat and patient's surrounding parameters need to be monitored for providing status. 72 BPM is considered as the natural heart rate of any adult where babies have 120 BPM and others are of 90 BPM (Fan et al., 2014). Between 97°F to 99°F the body temperature ranges for a person and in average it is 98.6°F. Considering these facts about the human being,

Table 1 Normal BPM at different ages (Zhu et al., 2015)

Age	BPM values for normal heart rate
Till month 1	70 >= BPM <= 190
1 >= month <= 11	80 >= BPM <= 160
1 >= month <= 2	80 >= BPM <= 130
3 >= years <= 4	80 >= BPM <= 120
5 >= years <= 6	75 >= BPM <= 115
7 >= years <= 9	70 >= BPM <= 110
Years >= 10	60 >= BPM <= 110

the healthcare model needs to detect the patient temperature and heart rate along with the room temperature and the humidity. To accurately measure the patient's objective, different sensors need to be used with the microcontroller in every healthcare model. The model should be designed in such a way that it should accumulate the real-time patient data and can forward to the destination server for storage. So, the model has to include a major area in network of sensors and communication-enabled things in IoT to achieve remote health care (Table 1).

The standard procedure for the calculation of blood pressure and glucose along with heart beat level was carried out through physical healthcare centers with various kinds of tests. But to overcome these lengthy processes, the technological advancement in wireless connectivity along with sensors like glucometer, blood pressure, and temperature is used to get the vital symptoms on regular basis instead of going to hospital (Fan et al., 2014). Through this IoT-based mechanism, different categories of people are getting benefitted like people who are staying in remote areas and patients with physical disabilities. Lots of opportunities are being created through this technology so that people with manageable heath issues should not come to be admitted to the hospital as they can be monitored remotely by the concerned person. IoT in healthcare provides the early symbols through continuous check up and make the patient know about the deteriorating signs of health and involves other healthcare attention to get rid of it. Statistics says people used to feel more comfortable at home rather at hospital, which provides machine to human communication (Pasluosta et al., 2015). The treatment and monitoring of the patient at a hospital including shifting physically consume huge amount of money and time. Also once admitted in hospital, no one related to patient can monitor the status of the patient. With the help of remote patient monitoring, these problems can be solved and some solutions can be provided to monitor the patient from anywhere at any time by anybody no matter where the patient lies.

3 The Possibilities of IoT as an Alternate to Conventional Healthcare System

Internet of Things combines cloud computing along with wireless network using wearable sensors to revolutionize remote healthcare for different kinds of patients. IoT for healthcare is determined as HealthIoT (Chang et al., 2016), which can be differentiated into three different stages (Xu et al., 2014). Out of that in first stage hardware uses sensors and devices for communication, where as in stage 2 keeps place for data storage and uses analytical tool for data analysis. The last stage is to provide virtualization through which the user can get all relevant data to visualize the current status of the patient. Based upon the mentioned stages, patient health can be effectively monitored and handled with negligible error (Ghanavati et al., 2016). The procedure is followed to collect the patient data by using wearable devices or sensors and communication is built among the devices and sensors to communicate with themselves and lastly the transmitted data need to be kept at a place to be analyzed by some applications. With respect to context awareness, computational intelligence and data storage using IoT along with cloud computing known as CloudIoT (Sahoo et al., 2016), plays a vital role in real-time healthcare (Abawajy & Hassan, 2017). The advanced network generations make the patient monitoring easier for anyone from anywhere at any time (Hung et al., 2017). Not only the alert system but also a display device needs to be attached for logical as well as physical monitoring of patient by reading the data through sensors before communicating to the authenticated and connected users.

Transmitter and receiver are the two basic components used in the article Heartbeat and temperature Monitoring System for Remote Patients using Arduino (Park et al., 2014) by the authors. Along with ATMEGA328, a radio frequency module is attached in both sections. Transmitters like LM35 and LM358 are used to collect the relevant record from the patient in real time and transmit to the receiver using module RF. The LCD is associated with the receiver section, which is responsible to display the values collected by the RF module. In few models, ESP8266 Wi-Fi module along with Message Queuing Telemetry Transmission (MQTT) protocol (Gupta et al., 2016) is used for achieving the goal of real-time healthcare of any patient. The Raspberry pi in the model is used like a broker for establishing the connection between sensors and client. The value of BPM is collected from the patient body by pulse sensor collectively with the Arduino and forwards to the broker protocol MQTT, which transmits the same by creating new session to the client when required instead of creating new session for every data transfer. The error rate between manual and sensor module can be enhanced through the use of multiple sensors. From number of researches on these healthcare models, one model (Heart Disease & Stroke Statistics, 2017) uses PIC16F73 as an embedded system along with different sensors, filter, GSM module, LED sensor, and one IR receiver for detecting the photo. All are associated to capture the heart rate and to calculate temperature of patient body LM35 is used. In another study (Mallick & Patro, 2016), PIC16F877, A Peripheral Interface Controller RISC processor is used to monitor the heart rate and body temperature parameter. Here also a heart rate sensor with digital output along with LM35 is used to gather the real-time patient temperature and heart rate accordingly. GSM module along with LCD is also used in the embedded system to clarify the status of patient healthcare in real-time. Nagaravali et al (Yick et al., 2008) have provided some light on the heart rate and different activities to monitor using microcontroller Arduino Uno in connection with CPR and pulse sensor to control emotional activities as well as heat rate, respectively. GSM module is responsible to send the status of patient as per requirement to the respective users.

One more model on healthcare using microcontroller AT89s51 (Kevin, 2009) is being described where a photo resistance sensor along with a LED are working on behalf of heartbeat sensor to provide readings of patient heart rate. But the analog signal produced by the mentioned integration is processed through LM358 and forwards the result to the microcontroller. Also, LM35 is used to collect body temperature, and ZigBee module is attached for wireless communication between sender and receiver. Schlessinger has proposed (Logvinov, 2016) an OOP, full-time, continuous modeling for providing a vast area of clinical, technical, organizational, and economical choices related to patient health. The model consists of physiological as well as care process. The care process model is mathematically designed to provide a detailed procedure to generate a complete healthcare application. Nisha et al. uses PIC16F877 as the microcontroller for the microcontroller-based wireless temperature and heart beat read-out (Gómeza et al., 2016). LED and LDR have been placed side by side of a finger to detect the heart beat and LM35DZ is used to measure the body temperature. IEEE 802.25.4 (ZigBee) is used for wireless communication. CC2500 wireless transceiver module is integrated with the PIC controller to receive the data from the sensor nodes. A JHD162A series LCD is attached with the PIC controller to display the data locally. In a study of "Heart beat and Temperature Monitoring system per Minute rate" (Ahmed et al. 2015), ARM microcontroller-based unit is used as the controller of the system. Infrared LED, OP-AMP and photodiode sensors are combined together for supporting the working mechanism of the model to calculate the heartbeat. The most common LM35 is used as the temperature sensor. The data collected by the sensors are passed to the controller and in critical situations, the data are being sent to the concerned authority via SMS with the help of GSM module, which is integrated with the microcontroller.

4 IoT-Enabled Healthcare System

The revolution in the Internet of Things provides facility to track and monitor everything throughout the globe at any instant of time to achieve remote healthcare. The noble cause of this chapter is to provide an overall idea for the development of a real-time model to monitor the health status of every patient in different modes like offline or online. For communication between the source and destination, different network layers are necessary for end-to-end data delivery. The required layers need to be interconnected due to the composition of forwarding followed by acquisition and extraction of information from the body of the patient to the expert of healthcare.

4.1 General Architecture

To fulfill the requirements, the proposed design architecture consists of five layers like application, storage, network, data gathering with preprocessing and data acquisition layer. Figure 1 describes the layered architecture of the healthcare IoT model.

In the first layer of model, i.e. data acquisition layer, patient data are collected through the use of various wearable sensors including environmental parameters to perform various operations. Also, the patients are attached with few implant sensors

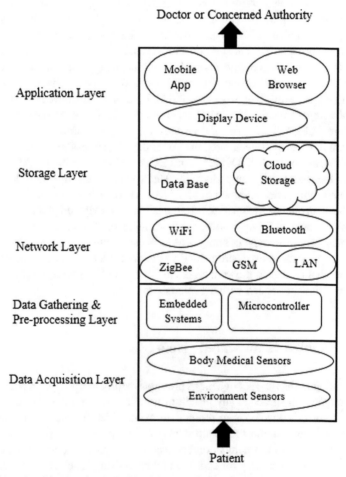

Fig. 1 General architecture for the IoT-based remote patient monitoring system

for clinical observation (Hossaina & Muhammadb, 2016) and are hidden inside the patient body whereas the surface of body is implanted with different sensors known as wearable devices. After collecting the parameters as per the characteristics of sensors, the data are forwarded to the next layer for rest of the operations. To identify a patient in a remote healthcare, RFID tag can be used (Gubb et al., 2013). To map the patient data with corresponding patient, the RFID tag plays a very vital role. Data acquisition is achieved through the first layer of the model.

For data gathering and preprocessing, several categories of embedded systems (ES) or microcontrollers are used. These devices are consisting of small memory unit with limited processing capacity along with provision for data collection and storage from the connected sensors and perform different operations on the gathered data (Liu et al. 2016). For internet connectivity and data forwarding, NODEMCU microcontroller can be used and automated to gather appropriate data for processing. The collected data processed by NODEMCU are forwarded to the application layer directly or through the storage layer passing via different wireless or wired networks. Different patient data are important in terms of monitoring and analyzing, so tracking of the same record is possible by storing these in a convenient place. To accommodate a large number of patient's data, cloud storage can be considered as the best possible option to implement any kind of healthcare application using IoT. Global as well as local servers can be used for more effectiveness of model, which provides service to online and offline users. Different users like healthcare authority, doctor, and concerned people will get an interface to be connected with the patient virtually through application layer for monitoring, analyzing, and visualizing the status of patient. Virtualization of status can be provided through web as well as mobile application to the online users and through display device near the patient will meet the objective of offline users.

4.2 Proposed Architecture for the Healthcare System

By following the common IoT architecture, the model has been designed using architecture and divided into five different layers. The patient with the wearable body sensor stays in the data acquisition layer. Sensors detect the vital signs from the body of the patients and pass it to the next layer. NODEMCU-12e is the microcontroller integrated with Wi-Fi module, used collect information from all the sensors and converts the analog data of the sensors in a human-readable format. Wi-Fi connectivity is used in the network layer to transmit the data from the microcontroller to the database. MySQL database server can be used as the database in the Storage layer. Finally, in the application layer, the view of the collected information has been displayed. A 16×2 display LCD can be directly associated to the NODEMCU-12e helps to monitor the patient locally. Different mobile applications and web applications have been designed to analyze the collected information and give the status of the patient. For mobile applications Blynk, a third-party application has been used

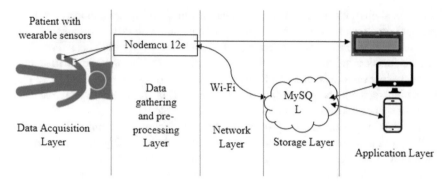

Fig. 2 Architecture for the IoT-based remote healthcare system

to display the results. Data have been sent to the Blynk server as well and the user with proper authorization to monitor the patient (Fig. 2).

4.3 Proposed Model

For monitoring the patient heart bit rate (BPM) and body temperature, Pulse Sensor and LM35 as body medical sensors can be used whereas to measure the patient's environment temperature and humidity, DHT11 is used. To keep updated records, date-wise DS3231 along with RTC modules can be attached with sensors in the ES to facilitate rigorous analysis on the collected record of the patients. The development board NODEMCU-12e is a microcontroller and can work like an interface where all the components are attached, through which it can collect all relevant data as per requirement and can able to transmit through Wi-Fi network to the storage server. MySQL server can be used as a storage device for the online users to get all the information as per their wish throughout the globe and similarly the LCD can be used to display the relevant contents like environment parameters along with patient's heart rate and temperature to the offline users all the time. Also, one buzzer can be attached to provide any kind of alert messages related to the patient during the critical situation.

4.4 Component Description

4.4.1 Pulse Sensor

For scheduling an activity, anticipating the movement or uneasiness levels, heart rate information can be extremely valuable in our day to day life (Botta et al., 2016). The problem associated with real-time model is that it is very difficult to measure heart

Fig. 3 Pulse sensor

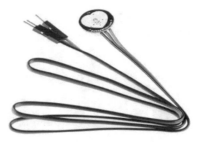

rate manually. So, the pulse sensor can be attached to solve this issue and provides solution for the patients. The use of sensor is so simple that any layman can use and get the values as per requirement effortlessly. Generally, it consists of heart rate sensor with optical output including enrichment and cancelation of noise from the hardware, used for capturing raw facts about the heart rate in a simple and efficient way. It can work with 4 mA current draw at 5 V, which is considered as efficient for portable device designing. The sensor is attached with patient fingertip and can be connected to the 3- or 5-V power supply, ground and analog pin of the ES. The wire connected to the heartbeat sensor is ended with normalized male header so there's no closure required (Fig. 3).

4.4.2   LM35

Temperature is the most common and important characteristics of the patient body measured by the doctor. These sensors basically generate some output voltage after detecting heat/cold from the object to which it is connected. These sensors are classified into two classes, non-contact temperature sensor, and contact temperature sensor. Non-contact temperature sensors are used to measure the weather temperature and the other sensors are attached with the object to collect the temperature information. The contact temperature sensors are furthermore classified into three categories, electro-mechanical, resistive resistance temperature detector, and semiconductor-based temperature sensors (Stergiou et al., 2018).

LM35 is a semiconductor-based contact temperature sensor, which is incorporated simple body temperature sensor with output as electrical signal is relative to centigrade in degree. This does not need any outside adjustment or trimming to give average accuracy. The output with low resistance, direct output, and exact natural for making the alignment as interface to get or control hardware particularly simple (Fig. 4).

For effective calculation of patient health temperature, this sensor can be utilized as body temperature wearable sensor device, which can provide output per degree Celsius as 10 mv.

Fig. 4 Pin configuration of
LM35 temperature sensor

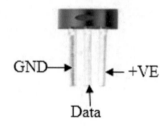

4.4.3 DS3231

This sensor is merged with temperature-compensated crystal oscillator (TCXO) along with I2C real-time clock (RTC) having a maximum accuracy and low cost to implement. This electronics sensor needs a battery input and records the exact time while this gets principle energy (Silva et al., 2015). It combines the stone resonator with the long-haul precision while decreasing piece part in assembling line. Specifically, the DS3231 is used in business and mechanical devices that provide a 16-stick, 300-mil SO bundle. The RTC looks after seconds, minutes, hours, day, date, month, and year data. The date toward the finish of the month is consequently balanced for quite a long time with less than 31 days, counting alterations for next year. The adjustment of time slot related to 12-h or 24-h can be dynamically managed with AM/PM notations. Two programmable time-of-day alerts and a programmable square-wave yield are given. Using the I2C, bidirectional transport information and addresses can be interchanged serially. Correctness of temperature-remunerated voltage orientation and comparator circuit screens the status of VCC to differentiate control dissatisfactions, to give a reorganized vintage, and to subsequently change to the strengthening supply when necessary (Fig. 5).

4.4.4 DHT11

It is a simple, extremely cost-effective digital humidity and temperature sensor (Parihar et al., 2017). It uses a generalized moistness sensor and a different thermistor to calculate the surrounding parameters and modifies an advanced flag on the data stick. It is easy to use, however, needs watchful planning to get information. The main feature of this sensor is that the user can find updated data from it every 2 s intervals (Fig. 6).

Fig. 5 DS3231 pin
configuration

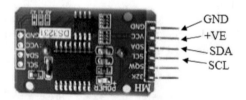

Fig. 6 DHT11 pin out

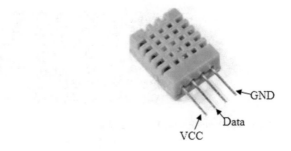

Fig. 7 16 × 2 LCD

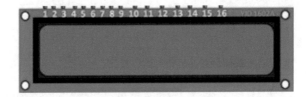

4.4.5 16 × 2 LCD

In general fluid, gem is used in the electronic device, i.e. LCD module for display purpose to provide a clear picture of the result.

As a fundamental device, the LCD with 16 × 2 usually operated in different kind of circuit designs. It is a combination of 16-character length for total number of lines, i.e. 2 to display varieties of results as per the requirements where each character occupies matrix of 5 × 7 pixel of the LCD (Chooruanga & Mangkalakeeree, 2016). Different properties are associated with the LCD to make it a convenient one like the working voltage is being set between a range of values 4.7–5.3 V and without backup it can consume electricity around 1 mA. Regardless of use, the LCD can be designed for alphanumeric values where any kind of formatted result can be displayed. Also, each line of LCD can display 16 characters using two columns of the device with 4 as well as 8 bit mode compatibility and this is accessible with green and backlight (Fig. 7).

4.4.6 I2C Adapter

This connector changes over 16 × 2 parallel display data format into serial in LCD using I2C measured by four different wires (Alam et al., 2016). Connector utilizes PCF8574 chip because it communicates with different kinds of microcontroller using the format of I2C with I/O enlargement. An aggregate of several LCD displays such as 8 can be associated with a similar 2 wires of I2C transport of respective board containing an alternate location (Kale et al., 2015). Features of I2C adapter consist of properties like each connector incorporates 16 different PIN with male header connector to fasten the display device LCD. Complexity is balanced through installed

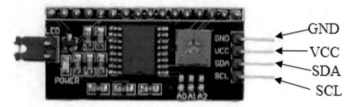

Fig. 8 Pin configuration of I2CAdapter

potentiometer. Backdrop illumination might be switched on/off by means of jumper with 5 V supply of voltage (Fig. 8).

4.4.7 CD4051B

CD4051B is a single 8-channel multiplexer with three binary control input S0, S1, and S2 and an inhibit input. One of the eight input channels is selected based on the values of the three select lines. It has an active low input circuit. So, whenever the inhibit input is low then only one of the eight input signals can work else no input channel will work. The value of the selected channel will be passed through the common output line. The working voltage for CD4051 is 4.5–20 V (Turlapati et al., xxxx) (Fig. 9 and Table 2).

4.4.8 Push Button Switch

Push button switches are two-state switches that have two states as ON and OFF. These are called push button switches as user will push to on or push to off. This mechanism is also called as push-to-make or push-to-break mechanism (Singh & Mishra, 2013; Schlessinger and Eddy, 2002; Shelar et al., 2013).

Fig. 9 Pin diagram of CD4051B

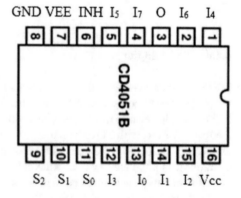

Table 2 Pin description of CD4051

Pin no.	Pin name	Description
13, 14, 15, 12, 1, 5, 2, 4	I0–I7	Independent input channels
3	O	Common output channel
6	INH	Enable input (active low)
11, 10, 9	S0, S1, S2	Select line
7	VEE	Negative supply voltage connected to ground
16	VCC	Positive supply voltage
8	GND	Ground

4.4.9   Piezo Buzzer

This is the device used for generating alarming signal as per requirement. Due to its simple characteristics like easy for deployment, lightweight and cheap in value it is used in wide spread applications like vehicles, computers and call doorbells. The prodigies of generating power during mechanical measurement are bind to particular properties and the alternative route is likewise valid. These buzzer substantial are either accessible or artificial planned. This is a group of artificial material, which carriages piezo electric influence and is approximately used to make different plates, which are considered to be the core part of buzzer (Sandeep et al., 2016). As per the recurrence of the flag for delivering sound, the substituting electric field can be extended.

4.4.10   NODEMCU

It is basically a LUA-based in-built firmware to express the utilization of Wi-Fi like ESP8266 and also it works like an open source apparatus board that needs to be connected with USB port for different programmable and troubleshooting purpose. It can be accommodated with breadboard and controlled by USB ports. This module is one of the least expensive accessible Wi-Fi modules in advertise. The most recent rendition of the discussed module that can be used for experimental purpose is V3 or Version3. This instructional exercise, however, will encourage you to interface every one of the forms of ESP8266 NODEMCU, i.e. V1, V2 or V3 (Naik & Sudarshan, 2019; Talpur, 2013; Zhao et al., 2011). Features of NODEMCU 12e are consisting of different occasion-driven API for arrange applications with 10 different GPIOs pins from D0-D10, usefulness of PWM, IIC and SPI communication, 1 for wire and ADC needs to be connected at A0 and so on across the board. The basic objective of using this to obtain Wi-Fi from different access point and from different stations along with webserver to get required information with input supply voltage ranging from is 5v to 19v (Fig. 10 and Table 3).

Fig. 10 NODEMCU 12E

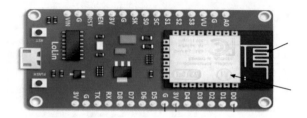

Table 3 Common pin description of NODEMCU-12e

Pin name	Pin mapping	Description
D0	GPIO16	General purpose input output pin is used to connect peripheral devices with the NODEMCU. Rx and Tx are used connect Bluetooth or other communicator devices with the NODEMCU. These pins are also known as Data Output pin
D1	GPIO05	
D2	GPIO4	
D3	GPIO0	
D4	GPIO2	
D5	GPIO14	
D6	GPIO12	
D7	GPIO12	
D8	GPIO12	
RX	GPIO3/Receiver	
TX	GPIO1/Transmitter	
A0	ADC pin	Only one analog input pin, takes analog signal as input and convert it to digital signal
Vin	–	+5 V output power supply
G	–	Ground
3 V	–	+3.3 V output power supply

4.5 Working Procedure of Healthcare Model

The desirable model can work on an open source development IoT board like NODEMCU-12e through integration of ESP8266, which will enable of using the stationary mode as well as an access point mode. This Wi-Fi module consists of a SPI controller, an ADC pin with multiple I2C and 10 GPIO pins. Each pin is capable of doing different tasks with using specified configuration of pin. Even if total pins are not required to design the healthcare model but the complete pin configuration can be proposed by connecting the required pins. But few things need to be taken care like both pulse and LM35 sensors provide output as analog signal, for which CD4501 module with 8:1 multiplexer needs to be attached to the ADC pin of NODEMCU-12e. By doing this, the output of both wearable sensors of patient healthcare can be collected in serial manner. The relevant data can be collected from the respective sensor modules using the combinations of the three selected pins of

CD4051. NODEMCU-12e can combine the data collected from the single output pin of CD4051 using ADC and forwards the same via the line of chip select conferring to the respective sensor's productivity signal. For offline users, a 16×2 LCD device can be used as a monitor for getting the status of patient locally. Although the embedded system has limited pins in it, to make compatible all 16 pins of the display device with NODEMCU-12e, I2C adapter can be used as an interface. A switch with 6-pin button push characteristics can be used as the mode selector for LCD device for display purposes. NODEMCU-12e supports the connectivity of DHT11 and DS3231 through the corresponding GPIO pins as digital output is provided by both the modules.

5 The Need and Importance of Machine Learning in Smart Healthcare

The recent development in IoT-based technologies helps in producing a large number of smart and wearable healthcare devices connected through internet. Huge amount of healthcare data are collected through these smart devices and need to be stored for future use. The amount of data may increase drastically with an increase in number of users of wearable sensors as well as kinds of sensor devices. Cloud storage is a suitable approach in this regard and has been suggested in the literature (Al-Makhadmeh & Tolba, 2019; Srivastava et al., 2019; Syed et al., 2019). These data need to be processed and analyzed in order to extract meaningful information that will be helpful for the medical practitioners. Analysis of this big data is a matter of concern. Machine learning (ML) algorithms can be adopted for the analysis of healthcare big data in the high-computing environment of the cloud. ML algorithms could be considered for.

- Mining through the healthcare big data,
- Discover the trend in previously unidentified disease, and
- Provide diagnostics and treatment strategy to the health worker.

The meaningful information thus extracted can be stored or forwarded to healthcare practitioners. ML applications can trim down human uncertainty and thus would help patients receive instant suitable care. Few ML methods such as logistic regression (LR), deep neural networks (DNN), gradient boosting decision tree (GBDT), and support vector machine (SVM) for predicting stroke is suggested in the literature where the DNN performed well. Meanwhile, ML algorithms such as generalized regression neural networks (GRNN), multi-layer perceptron (MLP), SVM, and k-nearest neighbor (kNN) were applied for determining a person's psychological wellness index, where SVM performed better. Artificial neural networks are usually data-driven model and can be considered as suitable model for fitting of large healthcare data. These studies suggested that there is still lack of best ML algorithms for healthcare and need to be explored. Hence, ML is going to play a vital role in IoT-based healthcare systems.

6   Conclusion

Health of non-critical patients could be monitored remotely at their residence rather than in hospitals, which can reduce the pressure on hospital resources. It could be helpful in providing better access to healthcare for patients living in rural areas, aged people to live independently at home or physically disabled persons as self-assistance. More specifically, it can progress admittance to healthcare assets at the same time as dropping excess load on healthcare systems. Also, it can give people be in charge of over their own health at all times. This chapter explored the advancement, modality, specification, and applications of IoT, wearable body sensors for acumination of body symptoms from remote patients. Then, the importance and necessity of machine intelligence for the analysis of healthcare data are discussed. A conceptual model integrating wearable body sensors, IoT, and machine intelligence for remote healthcare is then presented. The model may be supportive in dropping the complexities and expenditure in healthcare system faced by aging, physical disabilities and remote population.

References

Abawajy, J. H., & Hassan, M. M. (2017). Federated Internet of Things and cloud computing pervasive patient health monitoring system. *IEEE Communications Magazine, 55*(1), 48–53.

Ahmed, M. U., Bjorkman, M., Causevic, A., Fotouhi, H, Linden, M. (2015). An overview on the Internet of Things for health monitoring systems. *International Internet of Things Summit*, 429–436.

Alam, M. W., Sultana, T., Alam, M. S. (2016). A heartbeat and temperature measuring system for remote health monitoring using wireless body area network. *International Journal of Bioscience and Biotechnology, 8*, 171–190.

Al-Makhadmeh, Z., & Tolba, A. (2019). Utilizing IoT wearable medical device for heart disease prediction using higher order Boltzmann model: A classification approach. *Measurement, 147*, 106815.

Australian Institute of Health and Welfare. (2014). *Australia's Health*. [Online]. http://www.aihw.gov.au/WorkArea/DownloadAsset.aspx-?id=60129548150

Baker, S. B., Xiang, W., & Atkinson, I. (2017). Internet of things for smart healthcare: Technologies, challenges, and opportunities. *IEEE Access, 5*, 26521–26544.

Botta, A., de Donato, W., Persico, V., & Pescapé, A. (2016). Integration of cloud computing and Internet of Things: A survey. *Future Generation Computer Systems, 56*, 684–700.

Chang, S.-H., Chiang, R.-D., Wu, S.-J., & Chang, W.-T. (2016). A contextaware, interactive M-health system for diabetics. IT Professional, *18*(3), 14–22.

Chooruanga, K., & Mangkalakeeree, P. (2016). Wireless heart rate monitoring system using MQTT. *Procedia Computer Science, 86*, 160–163.

Fan, Y. J., Yin, Y. H., Xu, L. D., Zeng, Y., & Wu, F. (2014). IoT-based smart rehabilitation system. *IEEE Transactions on Industrial Informatics, 10*(2), 1568–1577.

Ghanavati, S., Abawajy, J., & Izadi, D. (2016). An alternative sensor cloud architecture for vital signs monitoring. In *Proc. Int. Joint Conf. Neural Netw. (IJCNN)* (pp. 2827–2833).

Gómeza, J., Oviedob, B., Zhumab, E. (2016) Patient monitoring system based on Internet of Things. *Procedia Computer Science, 83*, 90–97.

Gope, P. & Hwang, T. (2016). BSN-care: A secure IoT-based modern healthcare system using body sensor network. *IEEE Sensors Journal, 16*(5), 1368–1376.

Gubb, J., Buyy, R., Marusic, S., Palaniswami, M. (2013). Internet of Things (IoT): A vision, architectural elements, and future directions. *Future Generation Computer Systems, 29*, 1645–1660.

Gupta, R., Mohan, I., & Narula, J. (2016). Trends in coronary heart disease epidemiology in India— Annals of global Health (Published by Elsevier Inc.), *82*(2), ISSN 2214-9996.

Heart Disease and Stroke Statistics. (2017). American Heart Association I American Stroke Association.

Hossaina, M. S., Muhammadb, G. (2016). Cloud-assisted industrial Internet of Things (IIoT)— Enabled framework for health monitoring. *Computer Networks, 101*, 192–202.

Hung, C.-Y., Chen, W.-C., Lai, P.-T., Lin, C.-H., & Lee, C.-C. (2017). Comparing deep neural network and other machine learning algorithms for stroke prediction in a large-scale population-based electronic medical claims database. In *Proc. 39th Annu. Int. Conf. IEEE Eng. Med. Biol. Soc. (EMBC)* (pp. 3110–3113).

Islam, S. M. R., Kwak, D., Kabir, H., Hossain, M., & Kwak, K.-S. (2015). The Internet of Things for health care: A comprehensive survey. *IEEE Access, 3*, 678–708.

Kale, A. V., Gawade, S. D., Jadhav, S. Y., Patil, S. A. (2015). GSM based heart rate and temperature monitoring system. *International Journal of Engineering Research & Technology, 4*.

Kevin, A. (2009). That 'Internet of Things' Thing, in the real world things matter more than ideas. *RFID Journal*.

Liu, L., Stroulia, E., Nikolaidisc, I., Miguel-Cruza, A., & Rincon, A. R. (2016). Smart homes and home health monitoring technologies for older adults: A systematic review. *International Journal of Medical Informatics, 91*, 44–59.

Logvinov, O. IEEE, director of special assignments, industrial & power conversion division, STMicroelectronics, healthcare and the Internet of Things

Logvinov, O., Kraemer, B., Adams, C., Heiles, J., Stuebing, G., Nielsen, M., & Mancuso, B. (2016) Standard for an Architectural Framework for the Internet of Things (IOT) IEEE p2413. *IEEE-P2413 Working Group. Technical Report*.

Mallick, B., & Patro, A. K. (2016). Heart rate monitoring system using finger tip through Arduino and processing software. *International Journal of Science, Engineering and Technology Research (IJSETR), 5*, ISSN: 2278-7798.

Naik, S. & Sudarshan, E. (2019). Smart healthcare monitoring system using raspberry Pi on IoT platform. *ARPN Journal of Engineering and Applied Sciences, 14*(4), 872–876.

Parihar, V. R., Tonge, A. Y., & Ganokar, P. D. (2017). Heartbeat and temperature monitoring system for remote patients using Arduino. *International Journal of Advance Engineering Research and Science, 4*.

Park, J., Kim, K.-Y., & Kwon, O. (2014). Comparison of machine learning algorithms to predict psychological wellness indices for ubiquitous healthcare system design. In *Proc. Int. Conf. Innov. Design Manuf. (ICIDM)* (pp 263–269).

Pasluosta, C. F., Gassner, H., Winkler, J., Klucken, J., & Eskoer, B. M. (2015). An emerging era in the management of Parkinson's disease: Wearable technologies and the Internet of Things. *IEEE Journal of Biomedical and Health Informatics, 19*(6), 1873–1881.

Perrier, E. (2015). *Positive disruption: Healthcare, ageing and participation in the age of technology*. Sydney, NSW, Australia: The McKell Institute.

Sahoo, P. K., Mohapatra, S. K., & Wu, S.-L. (2016). Analyzing healthcare big data with prediction for future health condition. *IEEE Access, 4*, 9786–9799.

Sandeep, K., Rajendra, Prasad, V. V. G. S., & Rama Krishnaiah, M. (2016). Implementation of heart beat and temperature monitoring system per minute rate. *International Research Journal of Engineering and Technology (IRJET), 3*(7).

Schlessinger, L., & Eddy, D. M. (2002). Archimedes: A new model for simulating health care systems—The mathematical formulation. *Journal of Biomedical Informatics, 35*, 37–50.

Shelar, M., Singh, J., & Tiwari, M. (2013). Wireless patient health monitoring system. *International Journal of Computer Application, 62*(6)

Silva, B. M. C., Rodrigues, J. J. P. C., de la Torre Díez, I., Coronado, M. L., Saleem, K. (2015). Mobile-health: A review of current state in 2015. *Journal of Biomedical Informatics, 56*, 265–272.

Singh, N., & Mishra, R. (2013). Microcontroller based wireless temperature and heart beat read-out. *IOSR Journal of Engineering (IOSRJEN), 3*(1)

Srivastava, G., Crichigno, J., & Dhar, S. (2019). A light and secure healthcare blockchain for iot medical devices. In *2019 IEEE Canadian conference of electrical and computer engineering (CCECE)* (pp. 1–5). IEEE.

Stergiou, C., Psannis, K. E., Kim, B.-G., Gupta, B. (2018). Secure integration of IoT and cloud computing. *Future Generation Computer Systems, 78*, 964–975.

Syed, L., Jabeen, S., Manimala, S., & Elsayed, H. A. (2019). Data science algorithms and techniques for smart healthcare using IoT and big data analytics. In *Smart techniques for a smarter planet* (pp. 211–241). Cham: Springer.

Talpur, M. S. H. (2013). Application pervasive of Internet of Things in health care system. *IJCSI International Journal of Computer Science, 10*.

Turlapati, N., Srinivas, C. Heart rate and activity. *International Journal of Computer Science & Communication Networks, 5*(3), 173–176.

Xu, B., Xu, L. D., Cai, H., Xie, C., Hu, J., Bu, F. (2014). Ubiquitous data accessing method in IoT-based information system for emergency medical services. *IEEE Transactions on Industrial Informatics, 10*(2), 1578–1586.

Yick, J., Mukherjee, B., Ghosal, D. (2008). Wireless sensor network survey. *Computer Networks, 52*, 2292–2330.

Zhao, W., Wang, C., & Nakahira, Y. (2011). Medical application on Internet of Things. ICCTA

Zhu, N. et al. (2015). Bridging e-health and the Internet of Things: The SPHERE project. *IEEE Intelligent Systems, 30*(4), 39–46.

Architecture for Smart Healthcare: Cloud Versus Edge

Tumpa Pal, Ramesh Saha⬥, Sayani Sen, Sohail Saif, and Suparna Biswas⬥

Abstract Nowadays with the fast evolution of technology, smart healthcare plays a vital role to provide medical assistance to the patients from distant places, and checking large groups of people in a locale or country for detection and prevention of epidemics. Data handling of a critical patient is a challenging aspect for a smart healthcare system. Conventional healthcare systems can be divided into data collection layer, intermediate layer and analysis layer. Collected data by body sensor network are stored in the medical server through an intermediate layer and acted based on analysis. However, multi-modality of healthcare data causes failure of finding the hidden value of the collected data and increases the communication latency. Moreover, traditional smart healthcare systems are inflexible and heterogeneous network deployment in the lower layer causes degradation in Quality of Service (QoS). Hence, a more intelligent architecture is needed, with different QoS and Quality of Experience (QoE) parameters taken into account during the transmission of patient health data in order to obtain accurate information about a patient's health. Therefore, smart healthcare architecture, where sensing real-time data are accumulated in the cloud after analyzing them, feedback is sent to the caregiver. Due to emergency situations, the patient edge layer is introduced where decision taken promptly depends upon the patient's condition to reduce unwanted latency and delay. For future reference, data are sent and stored into the medical server through a network layer. In this chapter, cloud and edge-based smart healthcare architecture is described.

Keywords Healthcare · BAN · QoS · QoE · Edge · Cloud

T. Pal · S. Saif · S. Biswas
Department of Computer Science & Engineering, Maulana Abul Kalam Azad University of Technology, Kolkata, West Bengal, India

R. Saha (✉)
School of Computing Science and Engineering, VIT Bhopal University, Bhopal, Madhya Pradesh, India
e-mail: ramesh1saha@gmail.com

S. Sen
Department of Computer Application, Sarojini Naidu College for Women, Kolkata, West Bengal, India

1 Introduction

Nowadays, IoT (Chen et al., 2018; Muhammed et al., 2018), an emerging technology, has connections with many smart sensor devices as a result of which exchange of data takes place between them. Hence, data storage platforms like cloud computing are needed. Healthcare (Muhammed et al., 2018; Tuli et al., 2020) is an application in the IoT domain, which helps towards the improvement of a patient. Tracking and constant monitoring of the health of the patient are very much essential for the healthcare system, and it is a major concern. It helps to overcome the drawbacks of conventional healthcare systems. In Healthcare service, the patient is mobile and is monitored continuously by using sensors as we may need patient data anytime using wireless networks. During any kind of emergency, the medical staff can be aware of the patient's health. Hence, there will be less delay for the treatment. Here, patient data are transferred to the service provider for healthcare keeping an eye on the state of the patient. The aim of a medical physician is to reach to a conclusion by diagnosis of the medical image of the patient. Here, diagnosis becomes easy as the clinicians interact for analyzing, and reach to a diagnosis based on the patient data and symptoms.

Smart healthcare architecture is shown in Fig. 1 (Failed, 2017; Tuli et al., 2020). Here, sensing real-time data are accumulated in the cloud. Then after analyzing them,

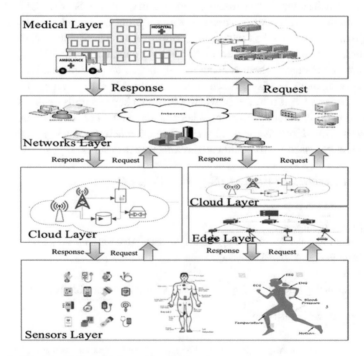

Fig. 1 Architecture of edge-cloud smart healthcare

a feedback is sent to the caregiver. Due to emergency situations, the patient edge layer is introduced as per the condition of the patient for taking decisions to reduce unwanted latency and delay. For the future utilization of data, it is sent and stored on the medical server through a network layer. Therefore, smart healthcare is an emerging issue for patient real-time health monitoring, lots of researcher developed or proposed cloud, and edge-based healthcare architecture some of them illustrated here.

2 Role of Cloud Computing in Smart Healthcare Architecture

In cloud computing, information and resources are shared, which are provided to other devices on request (Mell & Grance, 2011). Medical care industry especially has been profited because of the arrangement of universal health observing, emergency response services, electronic clinical charging, and so on. Since IoT gadgets have restricted capacity and processing power, thus, these intelligent gadgets can neither effectively give the e-health services nor it can compute and accumulate large quantities of gathered data. IoT and Cloud together create an innovation in multi-cloud structure, which fundamentally hides the restrictions of IoT by sharing resources on-request to convey successful and efficient e-health facilities.

2.1 Properties of Cloud Computing

Cloud computing has the following characteristics: as defined (Malik & Om, 2017). Users will allocate computing capabilities without any human intervention. Heterogeneous client-based platforms (e.g., tablets, mobile phones, laptops, etc.) access various potentialities, available over the network through standard mechanisms. Multiple users are served by resource pooling of different computing resources. Real-time resource management is done by client at any time. Automatic monitoring, controlling and resource utilization reporting are done by Cloud systems in a transparent manner for both the providers.

2.2 Utilities of Cloud Computing

Cloud computing performs the following services (Malik & Om, 2017; Mell & Grance, 2011).

I.   The user deploys on-premises or third-party software to the cloud infrastructure, using the tools and, as a result, the programming language offered by the platform as a service.

II.   Different client gadgets can access applications running on cloud infrastructure manipulation software as a service through the client interface.

III. Regardless of cloud infrastructure as infrastructure as a service, a customer would have access to processing power, storage, and other computing resources.

2.3   Deployment Models of Cloud Computing

Cloud deployment models can be classified into four categories (Malik & Om, 2017). A standalone company server with multiple users maintained by either the company or any outsider, known as private cloud. Users can access services within the premises of the cloud service provider called as public cloud. A selective user from the same organization having the same interest exclusively uses a cloud known as community cloud.

Hybrid Cloud configured with two or more deployment models (private, community, or public), having a singular entity for each model whether they jointly provide the benefits of multiple deployment models.

2.4   Different Architectures of Cloud Computing Used in Smart Healthcare

The greater part of the cloud-based IoT systems and applications are intended to utilize the Smartphone for observing and catching information. At whatever point, the constant network of the Smartphone gadget is faulty. In the present condition, the planned framework (Gupta et al., 2016) as appeared in Fig. 2, which shows the catching of client's actual work data from Treadmill at a health center collected data whenever moved and afterward to a different cloud worker. The created system comprises Implementation, Evaluation, Feedback, and security layers of the client as well as medical services staff.

The implementation layer separates the data's general architecture from its storage and analysis. This concept makes use of the sensors that have been implanted. It actualizes an application for observing the health of clients. Gathered information is then transferred to the necessary cloud.

Evaluation layer speaks to careful utilization of the executed application by the client. Issues announced by the client and medical services work force identified with the utilization of use or interchanges are tended to. This layer guarantees a decrease in intricacy and its selection through the improvement of the medical administrations.

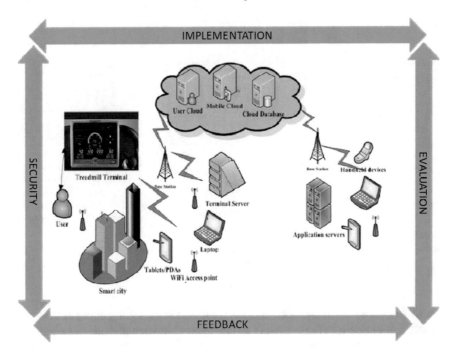

Fig. 2 IoT-based deployment architecture for cloud-centric communication

Feedback layer utilizes yields of assessment layers that are utilized to change applications.

Security layer additionally gives working to cloud-driven climate for different sorts of cloud workers like user cloud, mobile cloud constantly information base. This layer is to guarantee the security of client data for which he/she has bought in.

A cloud-driven IoT-based m-healthcare monitoring un-wellness recognition system is being developed (Verma & Sood, 2018), which predicts the magnitude of the un-wellness. The applied structure comprises three stages.

In stage 1, health-related information of the user is gained by an information securing framework, consisting of bio-sensors. They forward parameters to a Gateway framing fog layer. Procured information is sent to the associated cloud storage, utilizing wireless media, as appeared in Fig. 3.

In stage 2, the health-based tangible IoT information of every client is given in the cloud. Here, the information is universally detected and needed many times, so it is kept on the cloud server. The diagnosis and analysis decide the individual's medical issue as all the health-related data are moved to the clinical system.

In stage 3, the result based on client diagnosis is used for giving alarm to specialists as well as parental Figures. When the value of the user diagnosis result is lesser than the limit esteem at that point the individual's health state is marked as safe. Then again, the user diagnosis result is more noteworthy compared to the predetermined

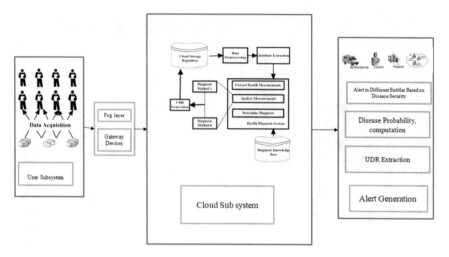

Fig. 3 m-Health monitoring framework

threshold then an alarm is produced to the guardians in the setting of the individual's health. Additionally, in the event that an emergency situation prevails, then, in order to deal with the health-related emergency, an alarm is sent to the nearby clinic.

Enormous amount of information is generated by smart healthcare system. Cloud computing is used to analysis that information and store it securely for future reference.

This method (Kumar et al., 2018) is primarily used for tracking, predicting, and diagnosing serious health issues Medical IoT devices, the UCI Repository Dataset, Medical Records, Cloud Database, Data Collection Module, Secured Storage Mechanism, Health Prediction & Diagnosing System, and Knowledge Base are the system's main components. Necessary data collection is done in the first phase and in the second phase collected medical information stored securely on cloud database. Disease prediction and diagnosis is done in third phase. The architecture is shown in Fig. 4. It is based on Fuzzy and classification algorithms using neural networks.

Smart healthcare system dealing with patient's personal data needed safest access for security of the person. So, a robust, lightweight, client authentication for continuous monitoring of the patient is created (Sharma & Kalra, 2018).The plan utilizes timestamp to deflect replay attacks. There are six unique stages: Stage 1 is *Setup stage:* where the enrollment place sets up boundaries in disconnected mode. Stage 2, *Medical expert enrollment stage:* during this stage, the clinical expert registers itself with the door hub. Stage 3, *Patient enlistment stage*: the patient gets enrolled with the enrollment place to benefit the medical care administrations. Stage 4, *Login stage*: in this stage, the clinical expert login to bring the clinical information of the patient. Stage 5, *Authentication stage*: Here, elements included, i.e., entryway hub, sensor hub and the client confirm one another. After confirmation, an irregular meeting key is produced. Stage 6, *Password change stage*: In this stage, the real client can refresh

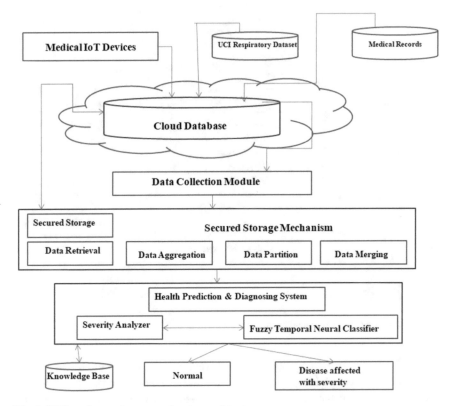

Fig. 4 UCI respiratory dataset used system architecture

his/her secret key. The legitimacy of the client is confirmed prior to refreshing the secret key.

A conventional confirmation utilizing Automated Validation of Internet Security Protocols and Applications (AVISPA) apparatus affirms security of the depicted plan.

There are semantic irregularities and absence of a thorough clinical methodology to treat a patient. To share medical records of patients between different health organizations and experts for better service to the patient, a smart healthcare system is developed based on ontology (Chen et al., 2019). Figure 5 delineates planned architecture, two fundamental actors collaborate with the framework; when the specialist or the medical services aide is distinguished, and they are allowed to consult the patient's medical records. The patient will conduct inquiries, exchange clinical directories, and communicate with their physicians once they have signed into the system.

Here, patient class contains every data identified for example, name, sex, telephone, and so on. The folder of each patient has references, which speak to the patient records and additionally reports. At long last, the medical services right-hand class speaks to the data about the medical services master (for example specialist) and every partner has one specialty. The interaction manager is the center of the

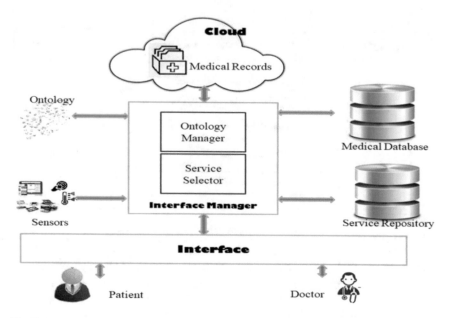

Fig. 5 Ontology-based smart healthcare architecture

design; it empowers the correspondence between various segments. It is made out of two modules; the philosophy administrator takes care of the cosmology with the crude information gathered from various sensors and provides data when required.

To counsel any report by the medical services associate or the specialist, the framework should confirm that it is as of now approved by the patient. On the off chance that they are approved, they will search for the old estimations in the clinical report and the constant information estimations in the ontology to empower the administration store to dissect all the information to produce a more point by point report on the patient's condition. In the event that the framework doesn't permit the collaborator or specialist to get to the patient's information, a solicitation should be shipped off the patient to allow them to get to their own data.

For enough computing ability and storage flexibility, a hybrid network model is created (Hassan et al., 2017) for productive continuous WBAN (Saha et al., 2019, 2021) media information transmission. The created network architecture is shown in Fig. 6.

Perception layer principally accomplishes the social affair of patient-related information, in particular imperative signs, physical activity and ecological information for medical care. In the perception layer, various sensors anticipated the human body assemble sensory data then processed locally and route it to the network layer. Network layer sends the information of a patient steadily and securely. It fundamentally comprises facilitators and different neighborhood networks which are used to accumulate sensor data and then keep it as a buffer. Cloud layer would viably and sensibly store and deal with the information getting ready for differentiated medical

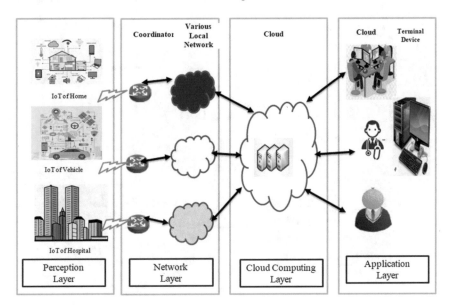

Fig. 6 Hybrid network model

services application. Application layer gives different medical care administrations. Designers build up the applications related to different medical care administrations. Clients can utilize changed terminal gadgets that convey explicit applications.

For efficient management of enormous amount of healthcare data, this model (Elhoseny et al., 2018) is created. It is for redesigning the introduction of the clinical consideration systems improving the vital accumulating of data of a patient and giving a continuous data recuperation instrument for those applications. It comprises four primary parts as appeared in Fig. 7.

Healthcare monitoring system (El Zoukaa & Hosni, 2019) targets incorporate AI in healthcare to empower the framework to function as a keen medical care model. In this model, information is collected from the patient. Logic-based algorithm converts raw data to linguistic representation using a fuzzy-based inference system that provides the status of the patient.

The block diagram of the framework appears in Fig. 8 depicts that the sensor sends all data to the microcontroller, which gives continuous monitoring by sending all data to the network. It may expand admittance to individual data leads to security and protection issues. Moreover, communicating this information to its destination safely and permitting the approved specialist to get to the patient's information. In the event of crisis circumstance, an alarm message will be shipped off to the specialist, and then the reasonable drug will be immediately endorsed.

To provide service in a secure and protected manner for Smart Medical System, a smart healthcare system "CSEF: Cloud-Based Secure and Efficient Framework for Smart Medical System Using ECC" (Kumari et al., 2020) is designed.

In Fig. 9, the proposed protocol has six phases described:

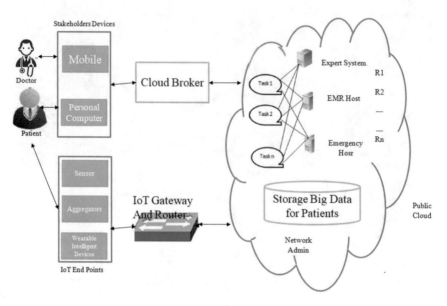

Fig. 7 A hybrid model to oversee big data in healthcare

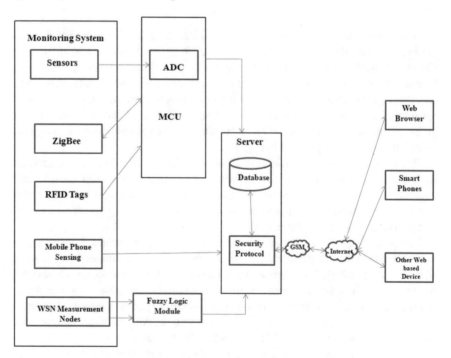

Fig. 8 Block diagram of Healthcare monitoring system

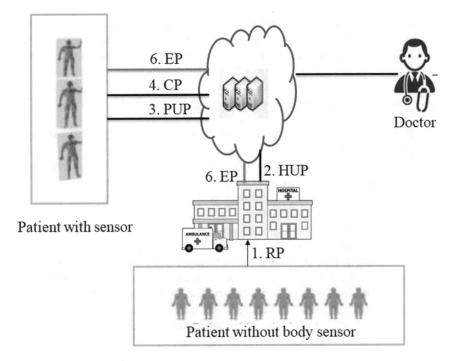

Fig. 9 Architecture of CSEF

Within the Registration section, Patient P gets registered with the assistance of Healthcare Center H. During Healthcare Center transfer section, Healthcare Center H and Cloud C manage the session key H, which sends medical information of Patient to Cloud C.

Within the Patient Information transfer section, Patient P requests for aggregating medical records from Patient P and sends to Patient P's mobile device.

In the course of the Treatment Phase, Doctor D analyzes information of Patient P from Cloud C and makes a conclusion about Patient's health.

During the medical section, patient checks its health condition from Cloud C as uploaded by the corresponding doctor.

In the Emergency section, Patient P has associated with emergency situation; body device attack informs Cloud C which in turn informs Healthcare Center H.

In this day and age, patients experiencing constant and way of life infections are considerably expanding that impacts social and financial life. Smart Patient Monitoring and Recommendation (SPMR) (Motwani et al., 2021), a completely unique structure focused on Deep Learning (DL) and Cloud-based examination, is being developed in this context. SPMR screens and predicts the real health status of patients based on their important signs and behavior background, which are produced by closed-aided Living gadgets. Both the Local Intelligent Processing (LIP) module and cloud-based analytics devised in SPMR inspire constant handling and details.

LIP is based on a novel Categorical Cross Entropy (CCE) Optimization that uses a forsightful DL. SPMR offers turning away and cares incessantly even while not internet and cloud administration. It is effective even just in case of emergencies.

2.4.1 Limitation of Cloud computing

i.   **Resources sharing**: Due to the chance of shared frameworks and foundations, the honesty of the cloud administration might be undermined.
ii. **Absence of access**: A cloud supplier may not furnish the cloud customer with satisfactory strategies and instruments for overseeing information.
iii. **Absence of data** about the handling activities of the cloud supplier expands the danger to cloud customers, which may reach out to health information subjects.
iv. **Absence of detachment**: A cloud supplier may utilize its actual authority over patient information from various medical care cloud customers to interface individual information. Where well-being managers are given restricted admittance rights, information and data could be connected from various customers.
v.   **Individual information** is moved to third nations outside the ward; these nations may not give a satisfactory degree of information insurance and moves may not be protected by proper measures and hence might be unlawful.

3 Role of Edge Computing in Smart Healthcare Architecture

Edge Computing (Zhang et al., 2018) may be a model for computation wherever resources and storage are placed at the sting of the network, which is nearer to the tip user. For providing services to patients, operations may be performed with low latency, energy potency, location awareness, which guarantees a high level of security at the sting devices and nodes with permissible process price. As outlined (Khan et al., 2019) Edge computing has the following characteristics

a.   Edge computation can run disengaged from the network, while approaching neighborhood assets. The property of isolation from different networks likewise makes it less vulnerable.
b.   Edge computing underpins versatility for communicating with mobile gadgets.
c.   Edge-circulated gadgets use low-level motioning for data sharing. It gets data for the location of the gadgets.
d.   Being conveyed at the closest area, edge computing has a preferred position to investigate and appear in big data.
e.   Edge computation is done at the nearest location of the user gadget, thus reducing the latency.

f. The period of time network info is employed to supply the context-aware services to the sting users. It improves user satisfaction and quality of experience.

g. Presence of assorted platforms, architectures, infrastructures, computation and communication technologies are referred to as heterogeneous.

3.1 Utilities of Edge Computing

i. Information from different sources is processed to filter noise prior to sending the information to the Cloud; it comprises bandwidth and storage resources.

ii. Decentralization of storage and processing enhance adaptability.

iii. Processing of information near to its data source accomplishes Proximity and low latency.

iv. The nodes of Edge models furnish every node of the network with disengagement and protection.

3.2 Different Proposed Architectures of Edge Computing Used in Smart Healthcare

To provide personalize service during patients Edge-Cognitive-Computing based (ECC) (Chen et al., 2018), keen medical care framework is developed. It is capable to screen and examine the health condition of the patient to serve promptly during emergency situation. It changes the process quality distribution of the complete edge registering network thoroughly as indicated by the upbeat hazard grade of every client.

ECC-based savvy treatment framework offers high energy proficiency, nominal price, and high client Quality of Experience (QoE) shown in Fig. 10.

It considers the multi-user resource allocation drawback within the health care surroundings, specifically, the healthcare system has a variety of patients with chronic disease whereas a standard network observes solely the switch drawback of the sting assets for every user.

i. **Data cognitive Engine**:

It collects the interior data, including all dynamic parameters from the resource network environment and accumulates the exterior data from the intellectual entreaty, including body language and habits of the user.

Furthermore, big data analysis through machine and deep learning necessitates intellectual access to exterior and interior details, as well as territorial impression cognizance and human intellect, in order to meet the demands of numerous implementations. When multi-user asset issuance is needed under an asset's combative environment, the best prioritized user is going to be serviced with the simplest network resources.

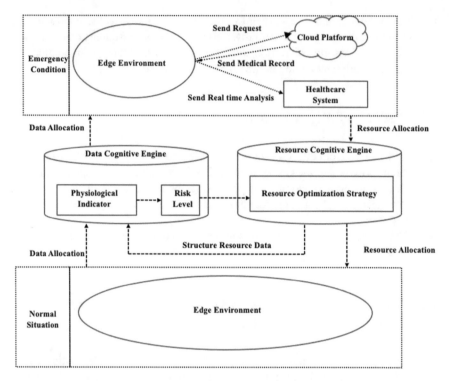

Fig. 10 ECC-based architecture

ii. **Resource cognitive engine:**

It supports the intellectual computing to take in the edge cloud processing assets, connection assets, and the network assets. After that, it sends the coherent asset information to the info cognitive engine simultaneously. In addition, it collects the study results of the info cognitive engine and perceives dynamic asset allotment and optimization simultaneously. Moreover, it draws benefit of the network technologies and provides an authentic, elastic and stretchable edge cognitive engine with minimum latency. Furthermore, it uses the cloud platform and intelligent algorithms to make asset optimized, power saver cognitive engines to improve QoE of the user for various requirements with a variety of heterogeneous entreaty.

iii. **User aspect (data-collection layer):**

The user aspect consists of sensible wear, mobile phones etc. They collect real-time physiological knowledge such as electromyography (EMG), electrocardiography (ECG), temperature, heartbeat, and blood oxygen saturation (SpO_2) of the patient and transferred to the neighboring edge computing node. Meanwhile, portable phone receives analyzed health data collected from the sting computing node.

iv. **Edge computing aspect (computing analysis layer)**:

In client network's processing, gadgets make up the portable edge computing network, which tests and dissects client health data and distributes a variety of processing assets to clients of different health levels. Within the crucial condition of the patient, it sends a caution to the emergency clinic, gets the overall client information from the cloud environment, and does an absolute and precise distant concurrent clinical resolution.

v. **Cloud platform aspect (storage management layer)**:

The clinic manages and oversees the cloud platform. It contains all necessary and clinical data, such as the client's clinical record, which includes details such as the client's age, the number of basic illnesses, and the concept of the illness. During a crisis instance of the client, the cloud platform enlists the entire data about the client and communicates that data to the edge processing node for interpretation.

To solve issues in smart healthcare like network latency, bandwidth and reliability are solved by UbeHealth (Muhammed et al., 2018) architecture. It makes use of edge computing, cloud computing, deep learning, high-performance computing (HPC), big data, and the Internet of Things (IoT), among other technologies, to maintain the Quality of Service (QoS) of next-generation portable medical care applications, especially flexible interactive media applications that will be central to smart and intelligent preventive medical services.

The structure of the architecture has four layers shown in Fig. 11. Here, the *user layer* contains healthcare professionals and gadgets that give medical services such as health surveillance and distant supervision of surgery. *The Network Traffic Analysis and Prediction (DLNTAP) Component is located in the Cloudlet layer. Following that, the Network layer is in charge of communication between the Cloud layer and*

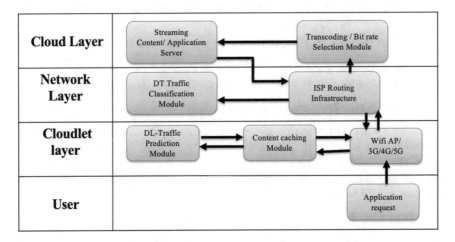

Fig. 11 Architecture of UbeHealth

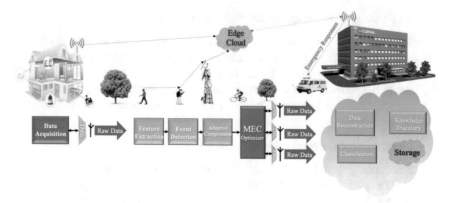

Fig. 12 MEC-based healthcare architecture

Cloudlet layer. Then *cloud layer* keeps and deals with the information that measures the information for different healthcare applications.

MEC-based healthcare architecture (Abdellatif et al., 2019) shown in Fig. 12, where data are processed and stored at the edge. The main purpose of this architecture is used data compression to minimize energy consumption for battery-driven gadgets with minimum network bandwidth consumption. Here, used feature extraction and classification data transmitted securely with low latency to predict and detect disorder.

The different subsection of the MEC-based healthcare architecture is illustrated here.

i. **Hybrid Sensing Sources**:

Sensor gadgets are attached to the patients that are utilized for knowing the state of the patient during crisis. Before sending it to the cloud, hybrid sensing nodes are processed and analyzed.

ii. **Patient Data Aggregator (PDA)**:

In WBAN collects patient data, while the Personal Digital Assistant (PDA) aggregates and transmits data by acting as a contact hub for the patient.

iii. **Mobile/Infrastructure Edge Node (MEN)**:

It handles the middle processing and storage of data from various sources, including the cloud. The MEN work in-network, handling gathered data, orders, and crisis alerts, extricates data of interest, and uploads the prepared data or data that has been removed to the cloud. Significantly, different medical services related (applications) can be executed in the MEN.

iv. **Edge Cloud**:

Here information stockpiling, refined information examination methods for design recognition, pattern revelation, and populace well-being the executives can be empowered.

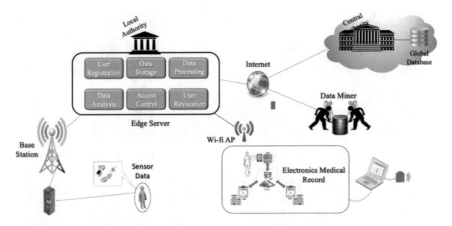

Fig. 13 Leveled architecture of edge care

v. **Monitoring and Services Supplier**:

A well-being supplier agency can be a specialist, a smart rescue vehicle, or even family members of patient who provides patients with disaster, preventive, or rehabilitative medical care administrations. For efficient and secure data management in portable medical care frameworks, Edge Care (Li et al., 2019) is developed. It accomplishes real-time framework for exchanging safe and productive information by edge processing.

The design as shown in Fig. 13 is undermined by three layers, work autonomously and together associated with advance in general framework execution.

i. **User Layer**:

Both the sensor information and electronic clinical record (EMRs) are assembled to analyze in Edge Care. They are pressed and briefly saved in convenient gadgets through remote or wired correspondence conventions.

ii. **Edge Layer**:

The entire organization is partitioned into various regions and every local authority (LA) has the overseeing extension to deal with transferred medical services information. Thus, enormous medical care information can be handled at the same time and outstanding burdens are adjusted among LAs. By this way, overall delay is reduced, especially when enormous medical service information is being handled.

iii. **Core Layer**:

The focal authority could be a public and real association utterly sure by all the organization elements. With the foremost elevated need of information the board, the focal position records and gets to personality data pretty much all the organization substances in Edge Care. The focal authority likewise records the comparing planning connections among them in portable medical care frameworks, liable for

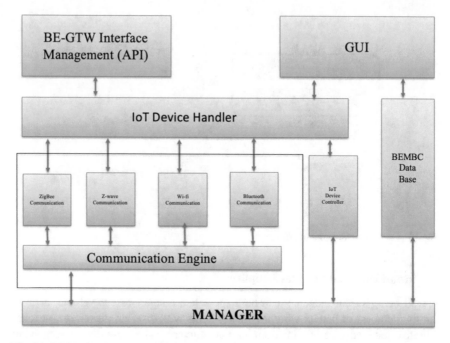

Fig. 14 BE-MBC software architecture

guaranteeing network-wide security insurance. The global data collection is being updated to keep up with an enormous amount of recording data. The geo-conveyed LAs will oversee medical services information in different areas in a deeply efficient and wise manner with the involvement of the core layer. For flexible, robust and adaptive data management in smart healthcare system Body Edge (Pace et al., 2018) is designed. It is edge-based architecture basically comprises of two reciprocal parts: a little mobile customer module, i.e. Body Edge Mobile Body Client (BE-MBC) shown in Fig. 14 and a performing Body Edge gateway *BE-GTW*, set at the edge of the network.

Administrator—it begins all product blocks by dealing with the rationale functionalities of the entreaty at a significant measure.

Communication Engine—holds the entire conceivable bound administrations (eg, ZigBee, Wi-Fi, Bluetooth and so on) by dealing with the sensible usefulness of admittance to information and computes.

IoT Device Handler—it is responsible for information translation trade, control orders execution, and dynamic connectors stacking of found gadgets. It also manages communication between the board and the GUI by prioritizing message transmission from IoT devices to the graphical interface.

IoT Device Controller—it is in charge *of dynamic gadget connector stacking by creating a unique information structure* for each new gadget and connecting it to the existing gadget module.

BE-MBC database—*it is used to save the obtained estimates on a nearby data set on the phone so that you can visualize and manage the details.*

BE-GTW Interface Management enables communication with the BE-GTW for the purposes of sending data and receiving control orders for connected IoT devices.

Graphical User Interface (GUI) it is *responsible for maintaining a simple link with clients. It is possible to view all estimations and access all product module settings using this module.*

BE-GTW uses the Body Edge Manager *(BEM) when local data processing can be performed without the use of external Cloud assets or offices.* In these circumstances, a variety of high-level data preparation and mining functionalities, such as those associated with data combination and PC vision, are made available for ongoing neighborhood handling and measurement.

All the portrayed modules are at last associated with the BEGTW Configuration that contains the overall entryway design boundaries transferred through a book record to be put away in a nearby memory.

The Window-based Rate Control Algorithm (w-RCA) (Sodhro et al., 2018) is a medical video entreaty algorithm. It improves medical quality of service (m-QoS) in mobile edge computing-based healthcare by considering a variety of network parameters. To optimize m-QoS at the foundation of the server aspect, w-RCA outperforms the standard battery smoothing algorithm (BSA) and Baseline used by MPEG-4 encoder. Here, a 5G-enabled mobile edge and QoS-aware platform for healthcare applications is presented, with three main layers at the server and client sides, each with its own set of protocols. When sending video frames over a wireless channel, a strong connection is formed between the server and the device. Three principal levels of that framework are the streaming server over priority of the network performance indicators, and therefore the streaming client noted as Level1, Level2 and Level 3 respectively.

To minimize healthcare cost, remote monitoring of patient is playing key role. In this aspect, author proposed smart healthcare framework (Zia Uddin, 2019). It predicts human movement based on wearable sensor. In this framework, a client is wearing some medical care sensors in various body parts, preparing the medical care sensor information, highlights, and activity prediction on a quick edge gadget, for example, a PC with GPU in a smart home. The gadget executes the remaining activity modeling and prognosis procedure depends on the characteristics and deep learning methods.

For different climate scenarios and health conditions, client's behavior might not be identical even with the same physiological values. So, context and private information would higher be thought about once distinguishing emergencies. Moreover, computing frameworks got to be developed to assist excellent solutions and prompt acknowledgment for abnormal state of real-time observation systems. "Context-aware emergency detection technique for edge computing-based healthcare monitoring system" (Wang et al., 2020) is suggested in this context. To solve data heterogeneity problems, the Gated Recurrent Units-based (GRU) technique is used for multi-asset data gathering. RNN (Recurrent Neural Networks) is used for its natural data processing ability to accurately detect outcomes of users in various situations and

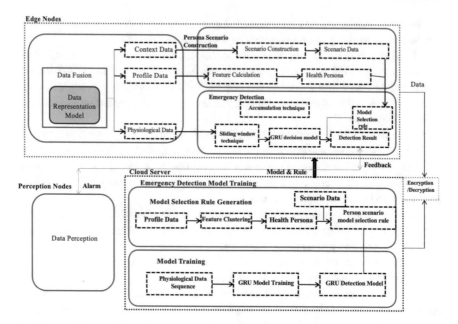

Fig. 15 Architecture for context-aware emergency detection system for edge computing-based healthcare monitoring

with varying health status. Low latency is significant. The edge computing architecture is being moved to the network extremity next to final users to compute high-speed data, network management, and depot. To protect health data and models from threats and savagery, an encoding technique is used. As shown in Fig. 15, the architecture has three layers.

In the perception layer, surrounding temperature, humidity recorded as sensor data as well as physiological information are gathered by smart wearable gadgets. Because of the confined computational capacities of IoT gadgets, the gathered information is shipped off nearest edge nodes for additional handling.

Context information, physical information, and personal information are the three types of heterogeneous IoT information that are isolated in the edge node layer. Context information portrays ecological conditions, for example, location, temperature, actual work type, etc. Physical information portrays physical records, for example, pulse, blood pressure, etc.

Personal information is utilized to infer individuals' health condition. Emergency detection models are resolved by scenario and health persona. Moreover, during the ongoing medical care checking, at times, for example, network blockage, information transmission could be deferred, with the goal that the sliding window instrument is acquainted with cradle information.

Since the processing ability of edge devices is not adequate like cloud server, emergency identification model preparing and streamlining are computed in cloud server layer as hind keeps up for edge devices. During the preparation module, the cloud server prepares fine-grained GRU recognition models using physiological data sent from the sting nodes.

Ciphertext-Policy Attribute-Based Encryption (CP-ABE) encoding calculation can be used to anticipate potential adversary who may execute collusion attack or man-in-the-middle attack, etc. to ensure security of medical services information and identification models in the conveyed checking conditions.

During the COVID-19 outbreak, while carrying different genuine dangers to the world, it advises us that we need to avoid potential risk to control the transmission of the infection. Quite probably the simplest non-drug clinical mediation measure is mask-wearing. Accordingly, there is a dire demand for a programmed continuous mask detection technique to assist forestall the pandemic. To aid public health preventive measures, an edge computing-based mask recognition structure (ECMask) (Kong et al., 2021) has been created, it is ensured that continuous performance on low-power camera gadgets used in transportation. Video reconstruction, facial recognition, and mask spotting are the three basic stages of ECMask. In the case of COVID-19 neutralization, it is a precise and effective approach.

3.3   Limitation of Edge Computing

As huge edge gadgets are connected, maintaining deployments and surveillance, the execution of the software on each gadget becomes too much challenging. It also becomes difficult when easy scalability or access to global data is required at the edge.

In this selection of Edge Computing-based IoT, the main issue is ensuring security in the information transmission measure. In Edge Computing-based IoT, huge information is produced by the multitudinous nodes and gadgets, and the entire capacity is given by various outsider providers, which will lead to information spillage and other protection issues. Another significant reliability dispute in edge computing-based IoT is to keep up reliability and quietness in transferring computational undertakings to edge computing nodes.

Currently, worldview of distant computation and storage, edge computing needs the combination of advanced communication technologies.

4   Difference Between Cloud of Edge on Smart Healthcare Perspective

Edge computing is a high-level adaptation of cloud computing, which decreases latency by initiating the administrations near the final clients. Edge computing supplements cloud computing by improving the extremity client utility for delay-aware applications. Edge computing is employed for the continual observance and analysis, whereas cloud computing is actually employed for hind data access, which may not be economical enough to supply continuous observance and analysis. As compared to edge computing, which has low latency, cloud computing has a large gap between the cloud server and mobile devices, resulting in additional latency. In cloud computing, when it comes to data retrieval, files or programs are directly accessed from the server. The Internet of Things is used to perform edge computing processing on the "edge" network (IoT). Cloud infrastructures, on the other hand, are favored over edge computing when it comes to processing resources. Unlike edge computing and cloud computing is location-aware and allows for greater mobility. However, cloud computing, which uses a centralized model for server circulation; edge computing uses an appropriated model. When data are transferred over a long distance to the server, the risk of savagery is more in edge computing compare to cloud computing. In global reach of cloud computing, the reach of edge computing is limited. Comparison of different smart healthcare systems based on either edge computing or cloud computing is summarized in Table 1.

5   Conclusion

The chapter has presented a holistic analysis of smart healthcare systems based on cloud and edge computing. These jargons are associated with cloud computing and named according to their architecture relationship. Migration of clouds and edges can be various functions more effectively. However, the review depicts a huge computation that occurred in a healthcare application and needs to be processed in a cloud-edge-based architecture. Articles that are reviewed here are architecture of a smart healthcare system based on either cloud computing or edge computing processing enormous amounts of health data. Smart healthcare system performs data handling efficiently, which is either sensor-generated or generated by medical devices.

However, data processed at edge level reduce network latency, improve quality of service but needs more energy capable, mass storage enables secure devices to process data at edge level. Whereas cloud can compute enormous amounts of data with extensible large storage and computing ability but overloads the network as all data are transferred to the central server. In addition, limitations of cloud and edge computing discussed here, and then comparing both cloud and edge computing depends upon some health care characteristics.

Table 1 Comparison of edge versus cloud computing in smart healthcare architecture

Author's proposed architecture	Computing technology	Parameters used for performance analysis									
		Efficiency		Prediction parameters			Quality of Service (QoS)			Quality of Experience (QoE)	Security
		Response time	Execution time	Accuracy	Specificity	Sensitivity	End to end delay	Throughput	PDR		
Gupta et al. (2016)	Cloud computing	Yes	Yes	NA	NA	NA	Yes	NA	NA	NA	Yes
Verma and Sood (2018)		NA	NA	Yes	Yes	Yes	NA	NA	NA	NA	NA
Kumar et al. (2018)		Yes	Yes	Yes	Yes	Yes	NA	NA	NA	NA	Yes
Sharma and Kalra (2018)		Yes	Yes	NA	NA	NA	NA	NA	NA	NA	Yes
Chen et al. (2019)		NA	NA	Yes	Yes	Yes	NA	NA	NA	NA	NA
Hassan et al. (2017)		Yes	Yes	NA	NA	NA	Yes	Yes	Yes	NA	NA
Elhoseny et al. (2018)		Yen	Yes	NA	NA	NA	NA	Yes	Yes	NA	NA
El Zoukaa and Hosni, 2019		Yes	Yes	NA	NA	NA	NA	NA	NA	NA	Yes
Kumari et al. (2020)		Yes	Yes	NA	NA	NA	NA	NA	NA	NA	Yes
Motwani et al. (2021)		Yes	Yes	Yes	Yes	Yes	NA	NA	NA	NA	NA

(continued)

Table 1 (continued)

Author's proposed architecture	Computing technology	Parameters used for performance analysis									
		Efficiency		Prediction parameters			Quality of Service (QoS)			Quality of Experience (QoE)	Security
		Response time	Execution time	Accuracy	Specificity	Sensitivity	End to end delay	Throughput	PDR		
Chen et al. (2018)	Edge computing	Yes	NA	NA	NA	NA	NA	NA	NA	Yes	Yes
Muhammed et al. (2018)		Yes	Yes	Yes	NA	NA	NA	Yes	Yes	NA	NA
Abdellatif et al. (2019)		Yes	NA	Yes	NA	NA	NA	NA	NA	NA	Yes
Li et al. (2019)		Yes	NA	NA	NA	NA	NA	NA	NA	NA	Yes
Pace et al. (2018)		Yes	Yes	NA	NA	NA	NA	Yes	Yes	NA	NA
Sodhro etal. (2018)		Yes	NA	NA	NA	NA	Yes	NA	Yes	NA	NA
Zia Uddin (2019)		Yes	Yes	Yes	NA	NA	NA	NA	NA	NA	NA
Wang et al. (2020)		Yes	Yes	NA	NA	NA	NA	NA	NA	NA	Yes
Kong et al. (2021)		NA	Yes	Yes	NA	NA	NA	NA	NA	NA	NA

Acknowledgements This work has been partially supported with the grant received in research project with sanction number CRS ID: 1-5758863831 from MHRD, Govt. of India under TEQIP III in Collaborative Research Scheme (CRS), AICTE.

References

Abdellatif, A., Mohamed, A., Chiasserini, C. F., Tlili, M., & Erbad, A. (2019). Edge computing for smart health: context-aware approaches, opportunities, and challenges. *IEEE Network, 33*(3). https://doi.org/10.1109/MNET.2019.1800083.

Chen, M., Li, W., Hao, Y., Qian, Y., & Humar, I. (2018). Edge cognitive computing based smart healthcare system. *Future Generation Computer Systems, 86*, 403–411.

Chen, L., Lu, D., Zhu, M., Muzammal, M., Samuel, O. W., Huang, G., … Wu, H. (2019). OMDP: An ontology-based model for diagnosis and treatment of diabetes patients in remote healthcare systems. *International Journal of Distributed Sensor Networks, 15*(5). https://doi.org/10.1177/1550147719847112.

El Zoukaa, H. A., & Hosni, M. M. (2019). Secure IoT communications for smart healthcare monitoring system. *Internet of Things*, Elsevier. https://doi.org/10.1016/j.iot.2019.01.003.

Elhoseny, M., Abdelaziz, A., Salama, A. S., Riad, A. M., Muhammad, K., & Sangaiah, A. K. (2018). A hybrid model of Internet of Things and cloud computing to manage big data in health services applications. *Future Generation Computer Systems, 86*, 1383–1394. https://doi.org/10.1016/j.future.2018.03.005

Gupta, P. K., Maharaj, B. T., & Malekian, R. (2016). A novel and secure IoT based cloud centric architecture to perform predictive analysis of users activities in sustainable health centres. *Multimedia Tools and Applications, 76*(18), 18489–18512. https://doi.org/10.1007/s11042-016-4050-6

Hassan, M. M., Lin, K., Yue, X., & Wan, J. (2017). A multimedia healthcare data sharing approach through cloud-based body area network. *Future Generation Computer Systems, 66*, 48–58. https://doi.org/10.1016/j.future.2015.12.016

Khan, W. Z., Ahmed, E., Hakak, S., Yaqoob, I., & Ahmed, A. (2019). Edge computing: A survey, future generation computer systems, Volume 97, PP 219–235, ISSN 0167-739X.https://doi.org/10.1016/j.future.2019.02.050.

Kong, X., Wang, K., Wang, S., Wang, X., Jiang, X., Guo, Y., Shen, G., Chen, X., & Ni, Q. (2021). Real-time Mask Identification for COVID-19: An Edge Computing-based Deep Learning Framework. *IEEE Internet of Things Journal*. https://doi.org/10.1109/JIOT.2021.3051844.

Kumar, P. M., Lokesh, S., Varatharajan, R., Chandra Babu, G., & Parthasarathy, P. (2018). Cloud and IoT based disease prediction and diagnosis system for healthcare using Fuzzy neural classifier. *Future Generation Computer Systems, 86*, 527–534. https://doi.org/10.1016/j.future.2018.04.036

Kumari, A., Kumar, V., Abbasi, M. Y., Kumari, S., Chaudhary, P., & Chen, C.-M. (2020). CSEF: Cloud-based secure and efficient framework for smart medical system using ECC. *IEEE Access, 8*, 107838–107852. https://doi.org/10.1109/access.2020.3001152

Li, X., Huang, X., Li, C., Yu, R., & Shu, L. (2019). EdgeCare: leveraging edge computing for collaborative data management in mobile healthcare systems. IEEE, Volume 7, Digital Object Identifier. https://doi.org/10.1109/ACCESS.2019.2898265.

Malik, A., & Om, H. (2017). Cloud computing and internet of things integration: Architecture, applications, issues, and challenges. *Sustainable Cloud and Energy Services*, 1–24. https://doi.org/10.1007/978-3-319-62238-5_1

Mell P., & Grance, T. (2011). The NIST definition of cloud computing.

Motwani, A., Shukla, P. K., & Pawar, M. (2021). Novel framework based on deep learning and cloud analytics for smart patient monitoring and recommendation (SPMR). *Journal of Ambient Intelligence and Humanized Computing*. https://doi.org/10.1007/s12652-020-02790-6

Muhammed, T., Mehmood, R., Albeshri, A., & Katib, I. (2018). UbeHealth: A personalized ubiquitous cloud and edge-enabled networked healthcare system for smart cities. *IEEE Access, 6*, 32258–32285.

Pace, P., Caliciuri, G., & Fortino, G. (2018). An edge-based architecture to support efficient applications for healthcare industry 4.0. *IEEE Transactions on Industrial Informatics*. https://doi.org/10.1109/TII.2018.2843169.

Saha, R., Biswas, S., & Pradhan, G. (2017). A priority based routing protocol with extensive survey and comparison of related works for healthcare applications using WBAN. In *2017 International Conference on Wireless Communications, Signal Processing and Networking (WiSPNET)*, Chennai, 2017, pp. 1424–1430. https://doi.org/10.1109/WiSPNET.2017.8299998.

Saha, R., Naskar, S., Biswas, S., et al. (2019). Performance evaluation of energy efficient routing with or without relay in medical body sensor network. *Health Technology, 9*, 805–815. https://doi.org/10.1007/s12553-019-00346-z

Saha, R., Biswas, S., Sarma, S., et al. (2021). Design and implementation of routing algorithm to enhance network lifetime in WBAN. *Wireless Personal Communications*. https://doi.org/10.1007/s11277-020-08054-y

Sharma, G., & Kalra, S. (2018). A lightweight user authentication scheme for cloud-IoT based healthcare services. *Iranian Journal of Science and Technology, Transactions of Electrical Engineering*. https://doi.org/10.1007/s40998-018-0146-5

Sodhro, A. H., Luo, Z., Sangaiah, A. K., & Baik, S. W. (2018). Mobile edge computing based QoS optimization in medical healthcare applications. *International Journal of InformationManagement, 2019*, Elsevier, https://doi.org/10.1016/j.ijinfomgt.2018.08.004.

Tuli, S., Tuli, S., Wander, G., Wander, P., Gill, S. S., Dustdar, S., ... & Rana, O. (2020). Next generation technologies for smart healthcare: Challenges, vision, model, trends and future directions. *Internet Tchnology Letters, 3*(2), e145.

Verma, P., & Sood, S. K. (2018). Cloud-centric IoT based disease diagnosis healthcare framework. *Journal of Parallel and Distributed Computing, 116*, 27–38. https://doi.org/10.1016/j.jpdc.2017.11.018

Wang, L., Xu, B., Cai, H., & Zhang, P. (2020). Context-aware emergency detection method for edge computing-based healthcare monitoring system. Willey. https://doi.org/10.1002/ett.4128.

Zhang, J., Chen, B., Zhao, Y., Cheng, X., & Hu, F. (2018). Data security and privacy preserving in edge computing paradigm: survey and open issues. *IEEE Access,* 18209–18237.

Zia Uddin, M. (2019). A wearable sensor-based activity prediction system to facilitate edge computing in smart healthcare system. *Journal of Parallel and Distributed Computing, 123*, 46–53. https://doi.org/10.1016/j.jpdc.2018.08.010.

The Medical Internet of Things: A Review of Intelligent Machine Learning and Deep Learning Applications for Leveraging Healthcare

Navod Neranjan Thilakarathne⬡ and W. D. Madhuka Priyashan

Abstract In the twenty-first century where we are witnessing full of technological miracles, the Internet of Things (IoT) appeared as an innovative technological domain that promises ubiquitous connection to the World Wide Web, turning common objects into connected devices through the connections made over the World Wide Web. This IoT has a huge potential to change the way we live, and it is being severed in many domains including healthcare, smart homes, traffic control, smart cities, agriculture, and various industries. In order to support numerous creative services and applications, it paves the way for the development of ubiquitously connected infrastructure, offering improved performance, and versatility. The emergence and the rapid evolvement of the Medical Internet of Things (MIoT), which also known as the use of IoT in healthcare have gained higher attention among the academia, industry, and researchers, for its potential to alleviate the burden on the medical sector caused by rising of pandemics like recent COVID-19, the rise of the aging population and chronic diseases and shortage of skilled medical staff. A typical IoT-based Healthcare system comprised of heterogeneous devices (miniature wearable devices, sensing devices, mobile devices, medical information systems, gateways, routers, switches, remote medical servers, and cloud databases) which continuously generates a huge amount of data that is diversified and highly sensitive. This large volume of data often demands various techniques for proper analysis to provide meaningful insights about disease diagnoses, patient condition monitoring, and security anomaly detection in the underlying systems which leads to improvement of patient care, cost reduction, rapid patient care, quick diagnosis, and securing the pervasive healthcare ecosystem. Machine learning and deep learning play a key role in the analysis of this data and generate meaningful insights. From this study, we hope to explore intelligent machine learning and deep learning applications and approaches that serve in a variety of medical domains such as disease diagnosis, medical image analysis, security, condition monitoring which have been used to leverage healthcare to the next

N. N. Thilakarathne (✉)
Department of ICT, Faculty of Technology, University of Colombo, Colombo, Sri Lanka
e-mail: navod.neranjan@ict.cmb.ac.lk

W. D. M. Priyashan
Department of Mechanical and Manufacturing Engineering, Faculty of Engineering, University of Ruhuna, Galle, Sri Lanka

© The Author(s), under exclusive license to Springer Nature Singapore Pte Ltd. 2022
S. Biswas et al. (eds.), *Internet of Things Based Smart Healthcare*, Smart Computing and Intelligence, https://doi.org/10.1007/978-981-19-1408-9_3

level. Further, in addition to providing in-depth knowledge about machine learning and deep learning-based solutions, we also provide a comprehensive overview of the architecture of MIoT and current research and the future directions through this study.

Keywords Machine Learning · Deep Learning · IoT · MIoT · Big data · Healthcare

1 Introduction

With the recent technological advancements, the IoT becomes a hype that everyone is appraised (Tarouco et al., 2012). Advances in electronics, wireless networks, wearable technologies, and the internet have nurtured the adoption of IoT powered technologies. IoT integrates a variety of technologies that allow a wide range of devices and objects to communicate and link with each other via different networking technologies (Thilakarathne et al., 2020a), allowing embedded devices and sensors to link and share information through the ubiquitous connections made over World Wide Web. Now the IoT has spread widely and used in different domains including smart homes, smart cities, health care, transportation, traffic surveillance, and various industries (Thilakarathne et al., 2020b). Day by day IoT related technologies are getting close to our lives in various forms. It is believed that IoT will become a revolutionizing technology that can change the phase of our world (Baker et al., 2017; Thilakarathne et al., 2020c, d).

In healthcare, different distributed devices aggregate, process, and communicate medical information in real-time to the cloud or to the medical data centers, allowing vast volumes of data to be processed and stored for offering various services for end-users. With the recent advancement in MIoT technologies, it is now powerful enough to mitigate most of the problems associated with rise of chronic illnesses, aging population, shortage of medical staff, and rise of pandemic situations. Modern MIoT measuring devices, such as blood pressure and blood glucose monitoring devices incorporate communication capabilities. They can create IoT networks for remote patient monitoring and allow the medical staff to monitor patient pathological details remotely (Thilakarathne et al., 2020c, d; Zhao et al., 2011), allowing ubiquitous access to the underlying medical information (Azzawi et al., 2016; Kodali et al., 2015; Rajput & Gour, 2016; Silva et al., 2019). It is noted that the healthcare reliance and dependence on IoT is rising daily to increase access to patient care, improve the quality of patient care, and eventually reduce the cost of patient care (Kodali et al., 2015).

The Internet has been the most important thing in the lives of people in recent years. In addition to this ubiquitous technology, the rapid advancement of MIoT has enhanced conventional medical systems in numerous ways (Thilakarathne et al., 2020c), such as diagnosis and examination of diseases. Researchers and medical personnel may use health data containing patient pathological information gathered through MIoT devices to diagnose and identify diseases (Catarinucci et al., 2015; Mishra & Mohapatro, 2019). The amount of data collected is also vastly increasing with the popularity and the adoption of MIoT systems in healthcare. Big data technologies have therefore been applied in MIoT to process and analyze health data in order to allow medical researchers to better assess and predict the risks of diseases, enabling them to evaluate the patient condition (Guan et al., 2019). Machine learning offers various tools and techniques in a typical MIoT environment that can help to solve various diagnosis and pattern recognition problems in different medical realms. Machine learning helps a computer to learn on its own and then make reasonable and accurate decisions afterward, and it has been used in healthcare to evaluate various clinical parameters, plan and facilitate patient care, identify diseases at early stages, and forecast disease progress. Integrating machine learning in the healthcare sector creates opportunities for improving the quality and efficacy of patient care (https://www.kdnug-gets.com/2020/05/ai-machine-learning-healthcare.html; Al-Dhief et al., 2020; Ara et al., 2017; Borthakur et al., 2017; Eddaoudy & Maalmi, 2019; Esteva et al., 2019; Hadi et al., 2019; Kumar & Gandhi, 2018; Yang et al., 2018). Deep learning, on the other hand, is used as a sub-field of machine learning to process several layers of nonlinear data and make precise decisions on complicated topics such as the outcome of clinical trials and the identification of data patterns (https://www.kdnug-gets.com/2020/05/ai-machine-learning-healthcare.html; "When to use machine learning vs deep learning in healthcare" 2018; Faggella, 2018; Thomas, 2020). Utilizing these techniques in healthcare guarantees high accuracy and high performance leading to better patient care.

Inspired by leveraging healthcare to the next level by promising better quality care we first offer an overview of the architecture of MIoT along with the use of IoT in healthcare. Then In the next section, we discuss machine learning and deep learning applications in MIoT. Next section we present a discussion about related works. Thereafter we present the challenges and future directions and finally, we conclude our paper with the conclusion.

2 The Architecture of MIoT

The aim of this section is to provide readers with a brief understanding of the underlying MIoT architecture on which the MIoT ecosystem is based on. The fundamental MIoT architecture can be apportioned into three layers. That is the physical layer which also known as the perception layer, the network layer which also known as the gateway layer, and finally the application layer (Rajput & Gour, 2016; Thilakarathne et al., 2020c). Following Fig. 1 depicts the architecture of MIoT.

The physical or the perception layer is responsible for collecting health data from a variety of devices such as wearables and various forms of sensing devices. Secondly, the gateway or the network layer, which is composed of wired and wireless systems and middleware, processes and transmits the data obtained by the perception

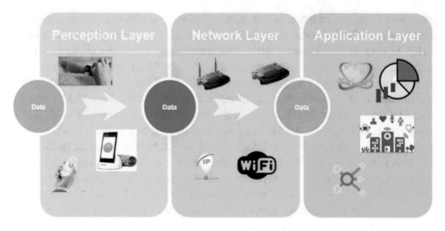

Fig. 1 The architecture of MIoT

layer with the support of underlying technological platforms. The application layer integrates all the medical information that is being processed by the network layer to provide medical services and being served for various stakeholders who need to access the information (Guan et al., 2019; Rajput & Gour, 2016; Thilakarathne et al., 2020c). This covers all aspects of the IoT life cycle that is **data acquisition, data processing, and data analytics** (https://missing-link.ai/guides/deep-learning-health care/deep-learning-healthcare/; https://www.flatworldsolutions.com/healthcare/art icles/top-10-appli-cations-of-machine-learning-in-healthcare.php; https://www.fla tworldsolutions.com/healthcare/articles/top-10-appli-cations-of-machine-learning-in-healthcare.php; https://towardsdatascience.com/ai-and-machine-learning-for-hea lthcare-7a70fb3acb67; https://healthitanalytics.com/features/what-is-deep-learning-and-how-will-it-change-healthcare; Gope & Hwang, 2015; Hassanalieragh et al., 2015; Kumari et al., 2018; Mahmud et al., 2018; Milovanovic & Bojkovic, 2017; Sebestyen et al., 2014). In the next subsections, we discuss briefly of each of the layers that the MIoT architecture is made of.

2.1 The Perception Layer

The perception layer holds the responsibility of accumulating various pathological details, body parameters from the patients. This data acquisition is performed by various physical MIoT devices such as wearable sensors, body temperature monitoring devices, blood glucose measuring, and so on. After the data acquisition is done data is sent back to the network layer. In the case of wearable sensors, they use an intermediate data aggregator to connect to the network, which usually is a smartphone placed near the patient (Guan et al., 2019; Hassanalieragh et al., 2015; Rajput & Gour, 2016; Thilakarathne et al., 2020c).

Physical MIoT devices in the perception layer include ECG monitors, Wristbands, Smartwatches, Heart rate monitors, Bio-energy patches, Ventilators, Glucometers, Pulse oximetry monitors, Fall detection monitors, Pacemakers, Defibrillators, Neurostimulators, Respiratory rate sensors, Muscle activity sensors, Embedded cardiac devices, and body temperature monitors (Guan et al., 2019; Rajput & Gour, 2016; Thilakarathne et al., 2020c).

2.2   The Network Layer

This layer is mainly responsible for communicating the gathered data with the application layer. The data transmission components in the network layer hold the responsibility for retrieving patient data and sending those to the healthcare organizations, medical data centers, or to the cloud with the assured security and privacy, ideally in near real-time (Guan et al., 2019; Rajput & Gour, 2016). The network layer is equipped with wired and wireless media for data transmission. This wireless media can be further categorized into long-range and short-range communication media.

MIoT devices use wireless (e.g.: Wi-Fi) and wired media (e.g.: Ethernet cables) to connect to the end-users, network gateways, or the medical network. It is noted that most devices that use wired connection are stationary such as medical imaging devices. Many of the wearables and miniature MIoT devices use short-range radio communication media such as Bluetooth low energy (BLE), Zigbee, Bluetooth, NFC, Wi-Fi for connecting to medical gateways and end-users. Cellular networks like 2G, 3G, 4G, and 5G are used for long-range communication. In general, once the sensor data is acquired by wearable sensing devices data is transferred to an intermediate data aggregator. This process is often happening through short-range communication media. After that, the data is relayed to medical data centers, healthcare organizations, or to the cloud using smartphone Wi-Fi connection or cellular networks (Hassanalieragh et al., 2015; Rajput & Gour, 2016; Thilakarathne et al., 2020c).

2.3   The Application Layer

The application layer act as an intermediary between MIoT devices and the end-users. It holds the responsibility for providing medical services and being served by various stakeholders who need to access information (e.g.: medical staff, insurance providers, caregivers). Also, there are various applications implemented on this layer for handling and processing the data, often to provide end-users with quality service. Nowadays, various applications hosted in the cloud are becoming an emerging trend, and performing data analytics in the cloud is also becoming a booming trend (Baker et al., 2017; Rajput & Gour, 2016; Thilakarathne et al., 2020c).

3 IoT in Healthcare

The IoT is a fast-growing technology that allows everything to be connected and communicate with each other via the internet (Azzawi et al., 2016; Baker et al., 2017; Dimitrov, 2016; Elhoseny et al., 2018; Gómez et al., 2016; Hassanalieragh et al., 2015; Joyia et al., 2017; Kodali et al., 2015; Rghioui et al., 2014; Thilakarathne et al., 2020c). It is changing and revolutionizing the healthcare industry by increasing productivity, reducing costs, and putting more focus on quality patient care (Mishra & Mohapatro, 2019; Rajput & Gour, 2016). There is no question that MIoT has now become inevitable for the healthcare sector to exist. This section aims to provide readers with a brief understanding of IoT applications and services served in healthcare and the various benefits of them.

In recent years, the IoT has received a great deal of attention for its ability to relieve the burden on medical systems (Baker et al., 2017; Catarinucci et al., 2015). The use of IoT technologies provides comfort to both doctors and patients in the modern health care setting (Elhoseny et al., 2018; Gómez et al., 2016; Gope & Hwang, 2015). An increasing interest in wearable sensors and wireless sensor network (WSN) technologies for personal health care has been drawn so much attention in recent years (Azzawi et al., 2016; Christin et al., 2009; Dridi et al., 2017; Hassanalieragh et al., 2015; Islam et al., 2015; Kumar & Gandhi, 2018; Laplante & Laplante, 2016; Li et al., 2017; Rghioui et al., 2014), where it facilitates physicians and medical staff to remotely monitor the patient condition. It is believed that these novel services and applications will strengthen the cohesion and the utilization of IoT in healthcare making it a promising technology.

3.1 IoT Services and Applications

There are many MIoT solutions present in the market. To develop applications, MIoT services are used, and are therefore services are developer-centric. On the other hand, applications are directly used by end-users who are mostly patients or physicians and are therefore user-centric (Thilakarathne et al., 2020c, d). MIoT applications can be further categorized as single condition and clustered condition applications based on the data retrieval and data collection techniques. A specific disease can be monitored through single condition applications whereas clustered condition applications facilitates to monitor a range of diseases or deals with more than one condition. The categorization of MIoT services and applications are depicted in Fig. 2.

In the following section, we present a brief review of various MIoT services.

- M-Health (Mobile Health)

M-Health is an amalgamation of mobile computing, medical sensors, and communication technologies. This includes various wireless technologies such as GPRS, 3G,

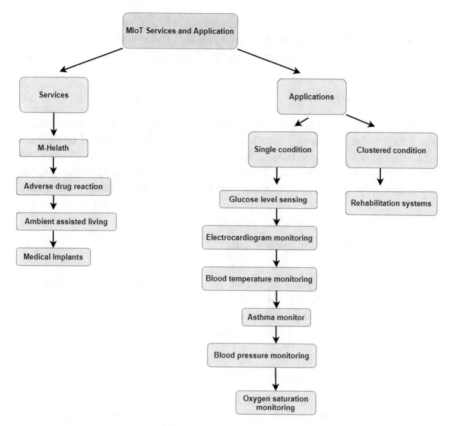

Fig. 2 Categorization of MIoT services and applications

4G, WLAN, ZigBee, and Bluetooth, and IPv6 over Low-Power Wireless Personal Area Network (6LoWPAN), used for healthcare communication. This mobile health makes it easier for patients to access their health-related data through appropriate applications at any time thus guarantee convenient access (Rajput & Gour, 2016; Thilakarathne et al., 2020c). Also, this allows for the most accurate and precise treatment as medical staff have continuous access to the patient's medical data.

- Adverse Drug Reaction

As the rate of hostile drug reaction is high in individual patients and hospitals, smart pill bottles, IoT-based knowledge-based systems, and cloud-based electronic health record management systems are used to avoid the wrong drug use.

- Ambient Assisted Living (AAL)

AAL provides technical systems based on IoT to, assist older people, and persons with special needs in their everyday routine. AAL's primary purpose is to protect and encourage the autonomy of these people and thus to improve the protection of their lifestyle and their home environment. As for that, AAL offers various services and products such as wheelchair management systems, various navigation assistants for blind people, and so on (Azzawi et al., 2016; Hassanalieragh et al., 2015; Kumar & Gandhi, 2018).

• Medical Implants

In order to strengthen and retain the basic functions in the human body such as stimulation of heart muscles, stimulating the brain functions medical implants are used. Examples include pacemakers that used to stimulate heart muscles, deep brain stimulation systems, and so on. These medical implants are used to improve patient care and improve patient life expectancy on the whole (Thilakarathne et al., 2020c).

3.2 IoT Healthcare Applications

As of now, there are currently numerous smart healthcare devices, wearables, and other pathological details monitoring devices available on the market in addition to the services aforementioned (Azzawi et al., 2016; Kumar & Gandhi, 2018). In the next section, we discuss these innovative MIoT healthcare applications (Zhao et al., 2011).

• Individual and Clustered Applications

Individual applications refer to the patient-centric applications that can be used to get data from individual patients such as blood pressure monitoring, glucose level monitoring, ECG monitoring, speech monitoring, body temperature monitoring, and so on (Azzawi et al., 2016; Tarouco et al., 2012; Thilakarathne et al., 2020c; Zhao et al., 2011), whereas clustered applications are developed to collect the data from more than one patient, such as from a community. In the following section, we discuss more on this.

• Blood Glucose Level Sensing

Diabetes is a collection of metabolic disorders in which the blood has a high level of glucose. Basically, blood glucose level sensing applications show the individual patterns of changes in glucose level in blood and assist individuals in preparing meals and diet plans by allowing them to carry their day-to-day activities normally (Rajput & Gour, 2016; Thilakarathne et al., 2020c).

• Electrocardiogram (ECG) Monitoring

This shows the electrical activity of the heart captured by electrocardiography and also it includes the measurements of heart rate (Tarouco et al., 2012).

- Body Temperature Monitoring

Body temperature monitoring assists doctors to assess the efficacy of medical therapies depending on the body temperature of the patient. The human body changes its normal temperature to support the body's own defense mechanisms and by measuring one's body temperature doctors can have a better understanding of the patient's homeostasis (Thilakarathne et al., 2020c).

- Asthma Monitor

Presently, patients use wearable smart asthma monitors that can predict the signs of an asthma attack before it starts, allowing the wearer to control it before the attack gets worse (Azzawi et al., 2016; Thilakarathne et al., 2020c).

- Blood Pressure Monitoring

As of now, miniaturized wearable's capable of measuring blood pressure such as separate blood pressure monitors, smart watches capable of monitoring blood pressure, and smart mobile application that can be used to monitor blood pressure are offered in the market, giving patients the possibility to monitor blood pressure every time (Azzawi et al., 2016; Zhao et al., 2011). These innovative devices are capable of providing high accuracy and facilitate automatically sync the gathered data with your smartphone device and enable you to share the results instantly with friends, family, or your doctor.

- Oxygen Saturation Monitoring

As blood oxygen saturation (SpO_2) being one of the vital survival parameters, which used to monitor the health of elderly patients, and new-born (Azzawi et al., 2016; Thilakarathne et al., 2020c), these applications are really important. Presently there are wearables and various wrist bands are available on the market which can monitor the SpO_2 level of patients.

- Rehabilitation Systems

In order to mitigate and aid for most of the problems associated with aging people and people with special needs, these IoT-based rehabilitation systems are used. These rehabilitations systems are capable of enhancing and restoring the functional ability and quality of life of those who are suffering from physical disabilities enabling them to engage in their day-to-day activities without any issue (Azzawi et al., 2016; Rajput & Gour, 2016).

For a better understanding of a MIoT setting, following Fig. 3 depict the structure of a general MIoT environment (Rajput & Gour, 2016).

A general MIoT setting is comprised of the following components (Rajput & Gour, 2016; Thilakarathne et al., 2020c).

- IoT sensing devices: These are ranging from implantable medical devices and wearable sensing devices to smartphones which gather vital patient body parameters.

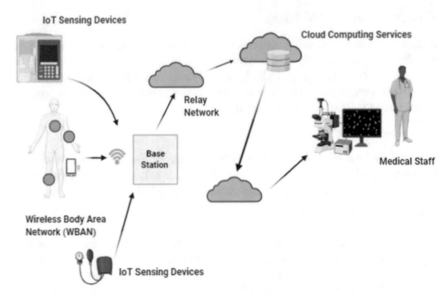

Fig. 3 Structure of a MIoT setting

- Communication networks—This includes wireless sensor networks (WSN) and wireless body sensor networks (WBAN), relaying networks, and various access networks that facilitate medical staff to access the medical data.
- Cloud servers / medical data servers—Collected medical data are often stored and processed in the cloud or in house medical data servers.
- Clinical terminals—Clinical terminals are there to provide access to the medical staff. So they can access the processed medical information and can derive more insight about the patient pathological details.

3.3   Benefits of IoT in HealthCare

MIoT provides many advantages to individuals and society. It also enables medical staff and doctors to do their work more accurately with less effort and intelligence. Following we discuss the key benefits of MIoT (Al-Dhief et al., 2020; Azzawi et al., 2016; Hassanalieragh et al., 2015; Kumar & Gandhi, 2018; Laplante & Laplante, 2016; Rajput & Gour, 2016; Thilakarathne et al., 2020c; Zhao et al., 2011).

- Continuous reporting and monitoring

In case of serious illnesses like stroke, heart failure, and asthma attacks this continuous monitoring and reporting gives immense benefits and will also help to save the lives of patients (Azzawi et al., 2016; Zhao et al., 2011).

- Faster disease diagnosis

Real time continuous patient monitoring helps to identify diseases like cancerous tumors at an early stage or even prior to symptom-based progression of the disease. Therefore this enables physicians to identify the diseases at the very early stages enabling them to save the lives of patients (Thilakarathne et al., 2020c).

- Proactive treatment

Continuous health condition monitoring opens new ways to provide proactive medical treatment under any circumstances (Thilakarathne et al., 2020c).

- Drugs and equipment management

In the healthcare industry, the management of drugs and medical devices is a big problem. These issues are often handled and solved efficiently by incorporating MIoT medical devices while minimizing needless costs and man-hours (Kumar & Gandhi, 2018).

- Tracking and notification

Healthcare IoT systems capture vital patient pathological data in the event of medical emergencies and life-threatening situations and communicate the gathered data to the medical staff while dropping alerts to relevant parties (Hassanalieragh et al., 2015; Laplante & Laplante, 2016).

- Remote medical assistance

The medics will quickly track the patients and recognize the ailments on-the-go, with innovative mobility solutions in healthcare. In the event of medical emergencies, patients can use smart mobile devices or separate smartphone applications to call a specialist who is several miles away, making the treatment process more convenient and easy (Rajput & Gour, 2016).

- Analysis of the data

In real-time, IoT devices can collect, report, and analyze data, and also it will reduce the need for raw data to be processed (Al-Dhief et al., 2020; Hassanalieragh et al., 2015; Kumar & Gandhi, 2018).

- Cost reduction

As MIoT facilitates real-time patient condition monitoring and real-time tracking of patients it drastically reduces the excessive visits to physicians, hospital stays, readmissions thus significantly reduce the cost (Azzawi et al., 2016; Thilakarathne et al., 2020c; Zhao et al., 2011).

Meantime simplicity, convenience, affordability, and ease of use are the other significant attributes that make this MIoT a promising technology.

4 Machine Learning and Deep Learning Applications for MIoT

Recent developments and advancements in IoT and machine learning and deep learning have made it possible for MIoT devices to gather healthcare data in near real-time and analyze the data in order to understand society's greater needs, thereby becoming the precursor of artificial intelligence. With the growing usage of medical IoT devices in healthcare, it is anticipated that it will lead to a huge generation of a large volume of data that is also known as Big Data that requires further study. This Big Data refers to the vast quantities of data that have to be collected, curated, handled, and analyzed in many advanced ways (). As the precursor of artificial intelligence machine learning is considered a ground-breaking method for big data analysis and is also recognized as one of the major breakthroughs of artificial intelligence, which gives pertaining systems the ability to learn and improve from experience automatically without being programmed explicitly (https://www.expert.ai/blog/machine-learning-definition/; https://www.zdnet.com/article/what-is-machine-learning-everything-you-need-to-know/; https://www.mathworks.com/discovery/deep-learning.html; Syafrudin et al., 2018).

In order to give our readers a brief understanding of what machine learning is, it is a term that refers to continuous learning and predictions from the data available. It consists of different algorithms that analyze the data to produce decisions and predictions. Deep learning, on the other hand, is a sub-field of machine learning that deals with algorithms called artificial neural networks, inspired by the human brain's structure and functioning. The data collected over a period of time is trained to build predictive models using these machine learning and deep learning algorithms to filter and prioritize the essential clinical parameters in healthcare settings with or without human supervision (Ara et al., 2017; Mishra & Mohapatro, 2019). Such examples include cluster analysis, which is an unsupervised form of machine learning that can be used towards the diagnosis of diseases (Guan et al., 2019).

Generally, machine learning is split into two main categories that are supervised and unsupervised learning (https://www.zdnet.com/article/what-is-machine-learning-everything-you-need-to-know/). Supervised machine learning techniques are applied on labeled data whereas unsupervised learning techniques are applied on unlabeled data, often to identify the patterns on data. Deep learning is also a machine learning technique that teaches computers to do what comes to humans naturally, such as learn by example (Esteva et al., 2019). The deep learning field has seen striking progress in the ability of machines to comprehend and manipulate data, including languages, images, and speech. Healthcare and medicine stand to benefit enormously from deep learning because of the sheer amount of data that can be processed and analyzed (Esteva et al., 2019). The key successor behind driverless vehicles, voice-activated applications in smartphones, smart TVs are deep learning. In deep learning, a computer model learns to perform classification tasks directly from images, text, or sound, resulting in high precision. By using a wide collection of labeled data and neural network architectures that include several layers, models are trained in deep learning. It is noted that most of the deep learning models outperform many classical machine learning approaches. It is also noted that multiple data types can be accepted as input by deep learning systems, an aspect of particular relevance for heterogeneous healthcare data (Esteva et al., 2019). For better understanding different categories of machine learning and deep learning algorithms are depicted in the following Figs. 4 and 5 respectively.

Since machine learning and deep learning are two inseparable artificial intelligence techniques, in the next section we present a brief overview of how these machine learning and deep learning applications are used in IoT-based healthcare to leverage patient care and healthcare facilities to the next level.

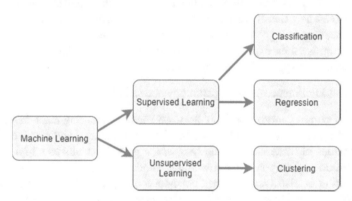

Fig. 4 Classification of machine learning algorithms

Fig. 5 Classification of deep learning algorithms

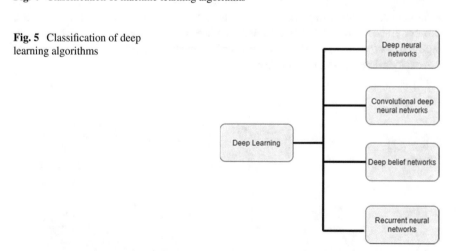

4.1 Machine Learning and Deep Learning Applications

Machine learning in healthcare is one such field that is being increasingly appraised. Recently Google developed a machine learning algorithm that could identify cancerous tumors in mammograms, and researchers at Stanford University have used deep learning to detect skin cancer which clearly shows the significance of this technology (https://www.flatworldsolutions.com/healthcare/articles/top-10-appli-cations-of-machine-learning-in-healthcare.php).

In general machine learning in MIoT helps to analyze heterogeneous data coming from various sources and recommend conclusions based on the analyzed data and provides timely risk scores, effective allocation of resources, and also has many other applications. The general workflow of a machine learning-based data processing model in healthcare is presented in Fig. 6 for better understanding.

Following, we then explore different facets of healthcare that machine learning and deep learning applications are applied.

- Artificial Intelligence assisted pathology and radiology

As it is becoming more common to store medical imaging data in electronic formats, deep learning algorithms are being used to identify and discover patterns and anomalies of these kinds of datasets which provide results as a highly trained radiologist does. Computer vision which is another technological breakthrough of deep learning is also used for medical image analysis (https://www.kdnug-gets.com/2020/05/ai-machine-learning-healthcare.html; Esteva et al., 2019). Examples include InnerEye, a Microsoft project that segments and classifies tumors using 3D radiological images using machine learning techniques (https://www.flatworldsoluti ons.com/healthcare/articles/top-10-appli-cations-of-machine-learning-in-healthcar e.php; https://www.flatworldsolutions.com/healthcare/articles/top-10-appli-cations-of-machine-learning-in-healthcare.php).

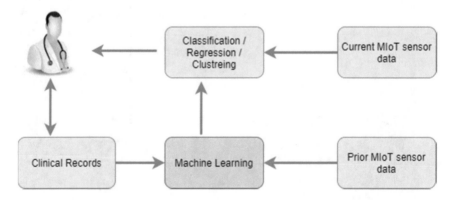

Fig. 6 General workflow of a machine learning based data analysis model in healthcare

- Robots for surgery assistance

Artificial intelligence-guided robotics may provide unique assistance to human surgeons. By enhancing the ability to see and maneuver in surgical operations, making accurate and minimally intrusive incisions, and causing less discomfort with optimal stitch geometry and wound during surgeries (https://www.kdnug-gets.com/2020/05/ai-machine-learning-healthcare.html; https://www.builtin.com/artificial-int elligence/machine-learning-healthcare; https://www.flatworldsolutions.com/health care/articles/top-10-appli-cations-of-machine-learning-in-healthcare.php; https://missing-link.ai/guides/deep-learning-healthcare/deep-learning-healthcare/), they support human surgeons.

- Identifying diseases and diagnosis

The detection and evaluation of diseases and conditions that are otherwise consid-ered difficult for diagnosis are one of the key fields of machine learning tech-nology of healthcare. This can involve everything from tumors that, in the early stages, are impossible to identify. Machine learning systems also provide signif-icant value by augmenting the display of the surgeon with informa-tion such as cancer localization during robotic procedures and other image-guided treatments during disease diagnosis (https://www.kdnug-gets.com/2020/05/ai-machine-learning-healthcare.html; https://www.builtin.com/artificial-intellige nce/machine-learning-healthcare; https://www.flatworldsolutions.com/healthcare/articles/top-10-appli-cations-of-machine-learning-in-healthcare.php;).

- Drug discovery and manufacturing

In the pharmaceutical industry, machine learning approaches based on artificial intelligence are increasingly being used to solve the hellishly complex chal-lenge of successful drug production. This also encompasses advances in research and development such as next generation sequencing and precision medicine that can help to identify alternate pathways for multifactorial disease therapy (Azzawi et al., 2016; Thilakarathne et al., 2020c; https://www.kdnug-gets.com/2020/05/ai-machine-learning-healthcare.html; https://www.builtin.com/artificial-int elligence/machine-learning-healthcare; https://www.flatworldsolutions.com/health care/articles/top-10-appli-cations-of-machine-learning-in-healthcare.php).

- Precision Medicine

Based on their personal medical history, dietary habits, genetic data, lifestyle pref-erences and pathological testings, the precision medicine tries to discover precise therapeutic choices for patients (https://www.kdnug-gets.com/2020/05/ai-machine-learning-healthcare.html; https://www.builtin.com/artificial-intelligence/machine-learning-healthcare; https://www.flatworldsolutions.com/healthcare/articles/top-10-appli-cations-of-machine-learning-in-healthcare.php; Hassanalieragh et al., 2015; Li et al., 2017).

- Outbreak Prediction

Machine and deep learning methods are currently widely used in tracking and predicting epidemics around the world. As of now, scientists around the world have access to satellite data, social media notifications in real-time, and website information for gathering the required data. Deep learning-based artificial neural networks are used to collate this information together and predict outbreaks (https://www.kdnug-gets.com/2020/05/ai-machine-learning-healthcare.html; https://www.builtin.com/artificial-intellige nce/machine-learning-healthcare; https://www.flatworldsolutions.com/healthcare/articles/top-10-appli-cations-of-machine-learning-in-healthcare.php; https://ai-med. io/ai-med-news/machine-learning-deep-learning-healthcare/; Kumar & Gandhi, 2018), before them become worsen or spread all-around the world.

- Smart health records

Documentation of patient data such as records of personal medical histories, demographic statistics, and laboratory reports are frequently inserted as health records and it is an exhaustive method for keeping up-to-date health records (https://missing-link.ai/guides/deep-learning-healthcare/deep-learning-hea lthcare/), and although technology has played a role in facilitating the data entry process, it takes a lot of time to complete most procedures. For the moment, in these medical health record systems (https://www.kdnug-gets.com/2020/05/ai-machine-learning-healthcare.html; https://www.builtin.com/artificial-int elligence/machine-learning-healthcare; https://www.flatworldsolutions.com/health care/articles/top-10-appli-cations-of-machine-learning-in-healthcare.php), text classification techniques using support vector machines and OCR recognition techniques based on machine learning are highly used to ease this time consuming processes. In order to analyze text and speech and derive meaning from words, natural language processing (NLP) methods are also used. Deep learning based recurrent neural networks (RNN) are also used at processing sequential inputs such as language, speech, and time-series data (https://missing-link.ai/guides/deep-learning-healthcare/deep-learning-healthcare/).

- Clinical trial and research

Machine learning has many potential uses in the world of clinical trials and research. It normally takes a lot of time and money for clinical trials to be performed and can take years to complete the process (https://ai-med.io/ai-med-news/machine-learning-deep-learning-healthcare/; https://missing-link.ai/guides/deep-lea rning-healthcare/deep-learning-healthcare/). Applying predictive analytics focused on machine learning to classify potential applicants for clinical trials will help researchers derive a pool from a large spectrum of data points, such as prior doctor visits. In real-time analysis and access, machine learning has also been used to track the data of clinical trial patients and to find the best sample size to be tested for those trials (https://www.kdnug-gets.com/

2020/05/ai-machine-learning-healthcare.html; https://www.builtin.com/artificial-int
elligence/machine-learning-healthcare; https://www.flatworldsolutions.com/health
care/articles/top-10-appli-cations-of-machine-learning-in-healthcare.php).

• Operation and theater management

Machine learning and deep learning-based approaches are used to solve many of the
operation and medical theater management issues (https://missing-link.ai/guides/
deep-learning-healthcare/deep-learning-healthcare/; Hassanalieragh et al., 2015; Li
et al., 2017; Thilakarathne et al., 2020c), such as long queues, bill generation, etc.

• Crowdsourcing

Today crowdsourcing is becoming so widespread in the medical sector that a
vast volume of data sent by people based on their approval can be obtained by
researchers and clinicians (https://www.flatworldsolutions.com/healthcare/articles/
top-10-appli-cations-of-machine-learning-in-healthcare.php; https://missing-link.
ai/guides/deep-learning-healthcare/deeplearning-healthcare/). (e.g.: ResearchKit
made by Apple allows users to access interactive apps which apply machine
learning-based facial recognition to try and treat Parkinson's disease).

• Security

Most MIoT devices generate vast quantities of highly sensitive and diversified data.
The amount of profit that can be gained by exploiting the devices and underlying
medical data, makes this MIoT ecosystem a sound target for attackers which has led to
a spike in MIoT based cyber-attacks. To alleviate this security challenge machine and
deep learning techniques are being devised to detect and mitigate such attacks that
target MIoT devices. Such kinds of attacks include denial of service, ransomware,
spying, probing, eavesdropping, and malicious control, and so on. Machine and deep
learning-based logistic regression, support vector machine, decision trees, random
forest, and artificial neural networks are highly used for security anomaly detection
in a typical MIoT setting (https://missing-link.ai/guides/deep-learning-healthcare/
deep-learning-healthcare/; Asharf et al., 2020; Hasan et al., 2019; Susilo & Sari,
2020).

5 Related Work and Discussion

The objective of this section is to provide readers with a brief understanding of what
are the existing approaches, solutions, studies, experiments that have done by others
with regards to this subject, which we highlighted in the Table 1.

Table 1 Related work

Reference	Year	Description / Findings
Mishra & Mohapatro, (2019)	2019	A real time health monitoring system capable of collecting data from body area networks and then feed on to a predictive model is introduced. This predictive model is trained on historical clinical data that uses a random forest classifier
Guan et al., (2019)	2019	A novel schema for medical data analysis and disease diagnosis based on K-means machine learning algorithm for cluster analysis is introduced
Ed-daoudy & Maalmi, (2019)	2019	In this study, the authors propose a new architecture that is based on big data technologies for real-time health status prediction and analytics system. It applies distributed machine learning model to streaming health data events
Kumar & Gandhi, (2018)	2018	Here a three-tier IoT architecture for the early detection of heart diseases is introduced. For the detection of such events, it uses a logistic regression machine learning algorithm
Al-Dhief et al., (2020)	2020	This study analyses and reviews machine learning algorithms used in medical care in general and in voice pathology surveillance systems in particular
Ara et al., (2017)	2017	In this study, the authors present a brief analysis of machine learning-based diabetes management applications
Yang et al., (2018)	2018	IoT-enabled stroke rehabilitation system is introduced. It consists of a smart wearable armband (SWA), and a 3-D printed dexterous robot hand, and machine learning algorithms to identify the movement patterns
Hadi et al., (2019)	2019	A novel machine learning approach for prioritizing outpatients according to their current health state is introduced. It uses a naive bayesian classifier to analyze data acquired from outpatient medical records
Borthakur et al., (2017)	2017	This study evaluates the use of low resource machine learning techniques on fog computing enabled wearables in smart healthcare
Syafrudin et al., (2018)	2018	A brief analysis and review of using scalable NoSQL (non-structured query language) databases in healthcare are provided
Thilakaratahne, (2021)	2021	Provides a comprehensive review of how artificial based techniques and other information and communication technology-based solutions can be used towards managing global pandemics
Jiang et al., (2017)	2017	A comprehensive survey is provided, about the current status of artificial intelligence in healthcare and the future

(continued)

Table 1 (continued)

Reference	Year	Description / Findings
Davenport & Kalakota, (2019)	2019	The potential for artificial intelligence techniques can be applied to healthcare is discussed with the pertaining ethical issues that will arise
Rong et al., (2020)	2020	Provides a comprehensive review about how artificial intelligence techniques can be used in healthcare with current status, challenges, and future directions
Reddy, (2018)	2018	How to use artificial intelligence in healthcare is introduced with the theories behind it
Rigby, (2019)	2019	A brief discussion provided about ethical issues pertaining to the use of artificial intelligence in healthcare
Macrae, (2019)	2019	The trust and safety of using artificial intelligence is healthcare is disused

5.1 Summary

Based on our review and the work that has been done by others, we have noted that machine learning and deep learning are becoming a major technological break-through and progressively it is becoming an integral part of pervasive IoT-based healthcare. For the time being those technologies are being used in many areas like medical image analysis, disease diagnosis, clinical trials, outbreak prediction, theater management, and so on. Also, these approaches are being used to do tasks that are difficult to do for normal medical staff such as identifying cancerous tumors at early stages. It is clear that even though, these machine learning and deep learning technologies are still in their infancy, they already brought many advantages to the pervasive IoT-based healthcare guaranteeing better quality patient care.

6 Challenges

Healthcare in recent years has been rapidly evolving with the integrated IoT tech-nologies facilitating for many people. With the years of advancement, the association of artificial intelligence-based techniques in healthcare has become more stable, and however, there are several potential challenges in healthcare in terms of data analysis that have to be addressed with an urge. Following we discuss the main associated challenges in terms of medical data analysis.

- Data privacy and security

When it comes to patient data it includes details about medical history, sexual orien-tation which are highly confidential and private. Thereby the safety of medical data becomes one of the key focal challenges in healthcare. Also, the interconnected

IoT networks bring many more vulnerabilities to exploiting this medical data. Poor privacy and security practices used in data analysis will heighten the vulnerabilities, therefore security needs to be prioritized among many other challenges (Dridi et al., 2017). Device manufacturers, researchers, and medical staff needs to put more effort towards devising solid security solutions for securing MIoT ecosystem.

- Data visualization and interaction

The variety of possible patient profiles makes the design of data visualization more complicated and tedious for medical staff and data analysts (Dridi et al., 2017).

- Heterogeneous data integration

Owing to the interoperability of medical instruments and the interoperability of these devices with medical recording systems and their records, the incorporation of heterogeneous medical data poses several difficulties. These data integration technologies have to be designed in a way to integrate with streaming and unstructured data, so more complex analytics can be performed (Dridi et al., 2017; Rghioui et al., 2014; Syafrudin et al., 2018).

- The exhaustiveness of the patient health information

The incompleteness of clinical information can have a detrimental impact on the decision-making process and on the efficacy of the services rendered and may be a risk to the patient's life as well. Thereby patient health information must be exhaustive. All potential sources of clinical data should be considered and integrated in order to maintain a complete patient history (Dridi et al., 2017; Rajput & Gour, 2016).

- Data accuracy

Typically MIoT devices collect data in bulk and it needs to be separated into chunks of data without overloading with accurate precision, for better performance and for proper analysis of data. This data overloading could have an effect on the medical care decision-making process in the longer term (Rghioui et al., 2014; Thilakarathne et al., 2020c).

- Insufficient device memory and processing power

Due to the miniaturized nature of most MIoT devices, most devices only are capable of performing small computing operations due to the small inbuilt memory, storage and processing power. But the important thing is most of these devices are generating a large volume of data that are deemed important to be further analyzed. Due to this low storage and memory of devices, it poses a question about how to hold this data for indefinite time and devices that can perform real time one demand analytics without depending much on the underlying processing power and the memory (Christin et al., 2009; Li et al., 2017; Rghioui et al., 2014; Thilakarathne et al., 2020c).

7 Future Directions

This section intends to provide readers with a brief understanding of future developments of this machine learning and deep learning in MIoT, that we can anticipate in the coming years.

- Medical image analysis using deep learning technologies likely to be the focal point for disease diagnostic in near future. (e.g.: based on the recent researches, most of the researches have recommended convolutional neural networks (CNNs), which is particularly well-suited for analyzing MRI results or x-rays) (https://healthitanalytics.com/features/what-is-deep-learning-and-how-will-it-change-healthcare). Also, computer vision will act as the main enabler of the interpretation of medical images in the forthcoming time (Rghioui et al., 2014).
- Deep learning-based NLP tools may integrate with medical documentation and translating speech-to-text and this will be an integral part of smart health records (https://www.flatworldsolutions.com/healthcare/articles/top-10-appli-cations-of-machine-learning-in-healthcare.php; https://healthitanalytics.com/features/what-is-deep-learning-and-how-will-it-change-healthcare; Rghioui et al., 2014).
- As the attacks that target MIoT ecosystem grows exponentially with the time, machine learning and deep learning-based model and techniques will be used for real-time security anomaly detection and stop the attacks before they are onset (https://healthitanalytics.com/features/what-is-deep-learning-and-how-will-it-change-healthcare; Thilakarathne et al., 2020c).
- Soon surgeries performed by robots will be a common reality. The precision and the accuracy of robotic surgery seemed to be more accurate and higher than human surgeons, based on the latest research. The accuracy that can be attained by guided robots with artificial intelligence is believed to outperform the skills of the most skilled human surgeons in the future (Thilakarathne et al., 2020c).
- Incorporation of Cloud computing, Fog computing, and Edge computing will drastically increase the performance of real-time medical data analysis (Borthakur et al., 2017; https://healthitanalytics.com/features/what-is-deep-learning-and-how-will-it-change-healthcare; Rghioui et al., 2014; Thilakarathne et al., 2020c), as the amalgamation of these technologies can be used towards performing data analysis near to the medical data sources and edge devices on the medical network.

8 Conclusion

The twenty-first century is only two decades old, and it is obvious that one of the biggest disruptive technologies and enablers in this century will be artificial intelligence. Advances in information and communication technology have contributed to the emergence of the IoT, and it provides greater versatility and convenience for physicians and patients in the healthcare setting, such as facilitating real-time patient condition monitoring, patient records management, and healthcare management. For the time being, we are in the midst of a technical revolution that uses computers to assist patients. The cloud connects people, and healthcare is supported by data and data analytics for generating valuable insights and providing medical staff with high-quality results. More focus is being placed on improving the quality of health in this new digital age. On the basis of our study, it is evident that the future of smart patient-centered medicine will be this machine learning and deep learning due to the immense benefits they offer. This paper provides a holistic 360-degree view about machine learning and deep learning approaches used in healthcare and we believe this study will assist researchers, academics, students, and medical personals who are interested in this subject area.

References

Al-Dhief, F. T., Latiff, N. M. A. A., Malik, N. N. N. A., Salim, N. S., Baki, M. M., Albadr, M. A. A., & Mohammed, M. A. (2020). A Survey of Voice Pathology Surveillance Systems Based on Internet of Things and Machine Learning Algorithms. *IEEE Access, 8*, 64514–64533.

AI and Machine Learning for Healthcare. Retrieved December 18, 2020, from https://www.kdnugg ets.com/2020/05/ai-machine-learning-healthcare.html.

Ara, A., & Ara, A. (2017). Case study: Integrating IoT, streaming analytics and machine learning to improve intelligent diabetes management system. In 2017 International Conference on Energy, Communication, Data Analytics and Soft Computing (ICECDS) (pp. 3179–3182). IEEE, August.

Asharf, J., Moustafa, N., Khurshid, H., Debie, E., Haider, W., & Wahab, A. (2020). A Review of Intrusion Detection Systems Using Machine and Deep Learning in Internet of Things: Challenges. *Solutions and Future Directions. Electronics, 9*(7), 1177.

Azzawi, M. A., Hassan, R., & Bakar, K. A. A. (2016). A review on Internet of Things (IoT) in healthcare. *International Journal of Applied Engineering Research, 11*(20), 10216–10221.

Baker, S. B., Xiang, W., & Atkinson, I. (2017). Internet of things for smart healthcare: Technologies, challenges, and opportunities. *IEEE Access, 5*, 26521–26544.

Borthakur, D., Dubey, H., Constant, N., Mahler, L., & Mankodiya, K. (2017, November). Smart fog: Fog computing framework for unsupervised clustering analytics in wearable internet of things. In 2017 IEEE Global Conference on Signal and Information Processing (GlobalSIP) (pp. 472–476). IEEE.

Bresnick, J. What Is Deep Learning and How Will It Change Healthcare?, HealthITAnalytics, 18-Dec-2019. Retrieved December 18, 2020, from https://healthitanalytics.com/features/what-is-deep-learning-and-how-will-it-change-healthcare.

Catarinucci, L., De Donno, D., Mainetti, L., Palano, L., Patrono, L., Stefanizzi, M. L., & Tarricone, L. (2015). An IoT-aware architecture for smart healthcare systems. *IEEE Internet of Things Journal, 2*(6), 515–526.

Christin, D., Reinhardt, A., Mogre, P. S., & Steinmetz, R. (2009). Wireless sensor networks and the internet of things: selected challenges. Proceedings of the 8th GI/ITG KuVS Fachgespräch Drahtlose sensornetze, 31–34.

Davenport, T., & Kalakota, R. (2019). The potential for artificial intelligence in healthcare. *Future Healthcare Journal, 6*(2), 94.

Deep Learning in Healthcare, MissingLink.ai. Retrieved December 18, 2020, from https://missin glink.ai/guides/deep-learning-healthcare/deep-learning-healthcare/.

Dimitrov, D. V. (2016). Medical internet of things and big data in healthcare. *Healthcare Informatics Research, 22*(3), 156–163.

Dridi, A., Sassi, S., & Faiz, S. (2017). Towards a semantic medical internet of things. In 2017 IEEE/ACS 14th International Conference on Computer Systems and Applications (AICCSA) (pp. 1421–1428). IEEE, October.

Ed-daoudy, A., & Maalmi, K. (2019). A new Internet of Things architecture for real-time prediction of various diseases using machine learning on big data environment. *Journal of Big Data, 6*(1), 104.

Elhoseny, M., Ramírez-González, G., Abu-Elnasr, O. M., Shawkat, S. A., Arunkumar, N., & Farouk, A. (2018). Secure medical data transmission model for IoT-based healthcare systems. *IEEE Access, 6*, 20596–20608.

Esteva, A., Robicquet, A., Ramsundar, B., Kuleshov, V., DePristo, M., Chou, K., & Dean, J. (2019). A guide to deep learning in healthcare. *Nature Medicine, 25*(1), 24–29.

Faggella, D. "Machine Learning Healthcare Applications—2018 and Beyond," Emerj, 19-May-2019. Retrieved December 18, 2020, from https://emerj.com/ai-sector-overviews/machine-learning-healthcare-applications/.

Gope, P., & Hwang, T. (2015). BSN-Care: A secure IoT-based modern healthcare system using body sensor network. *IEEE Sensors Journal, 16*(5), 1368–1376.

Guan, Z., Lv, Z., Du, X., Wu, L., & Guizani, M. (2019). Achieving data utility-privacy tradeoff in Internet of medical things: A machine learning approach. *Future Generation Computer Systems, 98*, 60–68.

Gómez, J., Oviedo, B., & Zhuma, E. (2016). Patient monitoring system based on internet of things. *Procedia Computer Science, 83*, 90–97.

Hadi, M., Lawey, A., El-Gorashi, T., & Elmirghani, J. (2019). Using machine learning and big data analytics to prioritize outpatients in HetNets. In IEEE INFOCOM 2019-IEEE Conference on Computer Communications Workshops (INFOCOM WKSHPS) (pp. 726–731). IEEE, April.

Hasan, M., Islam, M. M., Zarif, M. I. I., & Hashem, M. M. A. (2019). Attack and anomaly detection in IoT sensors in IoT sites using machine learning approaches. *Internet of Things, 7*, 100059.

Hassanalieragh, M., Page, A., Soyata, T., Sharma, G., Aktas, M., Mateos, G & Andreescu, S. (2015). Health monitoring and management using Internet-of-Things (IoT) sensing with cloud-based processing: Opportunities and challenges. In 2015 IEEE International Conference on Services Computing (pp. 285–292). IEEE, June.

Heath, N. "What is machine learning? Everything you need to know," ZDNet, 16-Dec-2020. Retrieved December 18, 2020, from https://www.zdnet.com/article/what-is-machine-learning-everything-you-need-to-know/.

Islam, S. R., Kwak, D., Kabir, M. H., Hossain, M., & Kwak, K. S. (2015). The internet of things for health care: A comprehensive survey. *IEEE Access, 3*, 678–708.

Jiang, F., Jiang, Y., Zhi, H., Dong, Y., Li, H., Ma, S., & Wang, Y. (2017). Artificial intelligence in healthcare: Past, present and future. Stroke and vascular neurology, 2(4).

Joyia, G. J., Liaqat, R. M., Farooq, A., & Rehman, S. (2017). Internet of Medical Things (IOMT): Applications, benefits and future challenges in healthcare domain. *The Journal of Communication, 12*(4), 240–247.

Kodali, R. K., Swamy, G., & Lakshmi, B. (2015). An implementation of IoT for healthcare. In 2015 IEEE Recent Advances in Intelligent Computational Systems (RAICS) (pp. 411–416). IEEE, December.

Kumar, P. M., & Gandhi, U. D. (2018). A novel three-tier Internet of Things architecture with machine learning algorithm for early detection of heart diseases. *Computers & Electrical Engineering, 65*, 222–235.

Kumari, A., Tanwar, S., Tyagi, S., & Kumar, N. (2018). Fog computing for Healthcare 4.0 environment: Opportunities and challenges. *Computers & Electrical Engineering, 72*, 1–13.

Laplante, P. A., & Laplante, N. (2016). The internet of things in healthcare: Potential applications and challenges. *It Professional, 18*(3), 2–4.

Li, C., Hu, X., & Zhang, L. (2017). The IoT-based heart disease monitoring system for pervasive healthcare service. *Procedia Computer Science, 112*, 2328–2334.

Macrae, C. (2019). Governing the safety of artificial intelligence in healthcare. *BMJ Quality & Safety, 28*(6), 495–498.

Mahmud, R., Koch, F. L., & Buyya, R. (2018). Cloud-fog interoperability in IoT-enabled healthcare solutions, January. In Proceedings of the 19th international conference on distributed computing and networking (pp. 1–10).

Milovanovic, D., & Bojkovic, Z. (2017). Cloud-based IoT healthcare applications: Requirements and recommendations. *International Journal of Internet of Things and Web Services, 2*, 60–65.

Mishra, A., & Mohapatro, M. (2019). An IoT framework for bio-medical sensor data acquisition and machine learning for early detection. *International Journal of Advanced Technology and Engineering Exploration, 6*(54), 112–125.

Rajput, D. S., & Gour, R. (2016). An IoT framework for healthcare monitoring systems. *International Journal of Computer Science and Information Security, 14*(5), 451.

Reddy, S. (2018). Use of artificial intelligence in healthcare delivery. In eHealth-Making Health Care Smarter. IntechOpen.

Rghioui, A., L'aarje, A., Elouaai, F., & Bouhorma, M. (2014). The internet of things for healthcare monitoring: security review and proposed solution. In 2014 Third IEEE International Colloquium in Information Science and Technology (CIST) (pp. 384–389). IEEE, October.

Rigby, M. J. (2019). Ethical dimensions of using artificial intelligence in health care. *AMA Journal of Ethics, 21*(2), 121–124.

Rong, G., Mendez, A., Assi, E. B., Zhao, B., & Sawan, M. (2020). Artificial intelligence in healthcare: Review and prediction case studies. *Engineering, 6*(3), 291–301.

Sarkar, T. "AI and machine learning for healthcare," Medium, 30-Apr-2020. Retrieved December 18, 2020, from https://towardsdatascience.com/ai-and-machine-learning-for-healthcare-7a70fb 3acb67.

Sebestyen, G., Hangan, A., Oniga, S., & Gál, Z. (2014). eHealth solutions in the context of Internet of Things. In 2014 IEEE International Conference on Automation, Quality and Testing, Robotics (pp. 1–6). IEEE, May.

Silva, C. A., Aquino, G. S., Melo, S. R., & Egídio, D. J. (2019). A fog computing-based architecture for medical records management. *Wireless Communications and Mobile Computing, 2019*.

Susilo, B., & Sari, R. F. (2020). Intrusion Detection in IoT Networks Using Deep Learning Algorithm. *Information, 11*(5), 279.

Syafrudin, M., Alfian, G., Fitriyani, N. L., & Rhee, J. (2018). Performance analysis of IoT-based sensor, big data processing, and machine learning model for real-time monitoring system in automotive manufacturing. *Sensors, 18*(9), 2946.

Tarouco, L. M. R., Bertholdo, L. M., Granville, L. Z., Arbiza, L. M. R., Carbone, F., Marotta, M., & De Santanna, J. J. C. (2012). Internet of Things in healthcare: Interoperatibility and security issues. In 2012 IEEE international conference on communications (ICC) (pp. 6121–6125). IEEE, June.

Thilakaratahne, N. (2021). Review on the Use of ICT Driven Solutions Towards Managing Global Pandemics. *Journal of ICT Research and Applications., 14*, 207. https://doi.org/10.5614/itbj.ict. res.appl.2021.14.3.1.

Thilakarathne, N. N., Kagita, M. K., Lanka, D., & Ahmad, H. (2020a). Smart Grid: A Survey of Architectural Elements, Machine Learning and Deep Learning Applications and Future Directions. arXiv preprint arXiv:2010.08094.

Thilakarathne, N. N., Kagita, M. K., & Priyashan, W. M. (2020b). Green Internet of Things for a Better World. arXiv preprint arXiv:2012.01325.

Thilakarathne, N. N., Kagita, M. K., & Gadekallu, D. T. R. (2020c). The Role of the Internet of Things in Health Care: A Systematic and Comprehensive Study. *International Journal of Engineering and Management Research, 10*(4), 145–159.

Thilakarathne, N. N., Kagita, M. K., Gadekallu, T. R., & Maddikunta, P. K. R. (2020d). The Adoption of ICT Powered Healthcare Technologies towards Managing Global Pandemics. arXiv preprint arXiv:2009.05716.

Thomas, M. (2020). 15 Examples of Machine Learning in Healthcare that are Revolutionizing Medicine, Built In. Retrieved December 18, 2020, from https://www.builtin.com/artificial-intell igence/machine-learning-healthcare.

Top 10 Applications of Machine Learning in Healthcare—FWS," Flatworld Solutions. Retrieved December 18, 2020, from https://www.flatworldsolutions.com/healthcare/articles/top-10-applic ations-of-machine-learning-in-healthcare.php.

Yang, G., Deng, J., Pang, G., Zhang, H., Li, J., Deng, B., & Xie, H. (2018). An IoT-enabled stroke rehabilitation system based on smart wearable armband and machine learning. *IEEE Journal of Translational Engineering in Health and Medicine, 6*, 1–10.

Zhao, W., Wang, C., & Nakahira, Y. (2011). Medical application on internet of things.

What is Machine Learning? A definition—Expert System, Expert.ai, 19-Oct-2020. Retrieved December 18, 2020, from https://www.expert.ai/blog/machine-learning-definition/.

What is Deep Learning?: How it Works, Techniques & Applications, How It Works, Techniques & Applications—MATLAB & Simulink. Retrieved December 18, 2020, from https://www.mathwo rks.com/discovery/deep-learning.html.

When to use machine learning vs deep learning in healthcare?, AIMed, 07-Nov-2018. Retrieved December 18, 2020, from https://ai-med.io/ai-med-news/machine-learning-deep-learning-health care/.

Main Challenges and Concerns of IoT Healthcare

Anindita Saha

Abstract In the last decade, there has been tremendous development in Information and Communication Technology which revolutionized the different aspects of human life, especially healthcare. With the rapid growth of the Internet-of-Things ecosystem, which conglomerates physical objects, computing devices, hardware as well as software, it is now possible to present a seamless platform that connects human beings with digitally enhanced objects or "things". They can interact, collect, exchange, and communicate among themselves to enrich the experience from a computer-based centralized approach to an application-based distributed environment. This technological advancement with Internet-of-Things (IoT) has promised great potential in health monitoring and propagating information with accuracy in time with other benefits like providing appropriate medical support to a patient, especially in remote places, enhancing the quality of living as well as saving lives during medical emergencies. IoT ecosystem renders time-saving services through technologies, provides expert diagnosis to critical ailments remotely, increases the timeliness of treatments, and also eases financial pressure on a patient. The IoT-based healthcare system also benefits the medical experts to cover more cases with less staff which improves their coordination with patients with more administrative efficiency The system is also beneficial for preventive health hazards, proactive health monitoring, follow-up, and management of patients suffering from chronic diseases. However, the IoT healthcare system is not devoid of challenges and they need to be addressed for making the ecosystem more stable and ubiquitous. This chapter provides a precise overview of several benefits of IoT and its potential applications in healthcare along with the main concerns/challenges faced by stakeholders of the ecosystem to implement the same seamlessly. The chapter also focuses on the importance of technologies like cloud computing and edge computing to empower IoT in healthcare to provide a quality life to the patient and ensure a healthy life throughout the patient's lifetime.

Keywords IoT · Benefits · Applications · IoT challenges · IoT security

A. Saha (✉)
Department of Information Technology, Techno India Group, Techno Main Salt Lake, Kolkata, West Bengal, India
e-mail: anindita_saha03@yahoo.co.in

© The Author(s), under exclusive license to Springer Nature Singapore Pte Ltd. 2022
S. Biswas et al. (eds.), *Internet of Things Based Smart Healthcare*, Smart Computing and Intelligence, https://doi.org/10.1007/978-981-19-1408-9_4

1 Introduction

In the last two decades, human life has witnessed an overall drastic change in living standards after the development of Information and Communication Technologies. It is observed that technologies like cloud computing and edge computing have significantly contributed to empower IoT in healthcare to provide a quality life to the patient and ensure a healthy life throughout the patient's lifetime. IoT is an emerging technology under Information and Communication Technologies (ICT) which is a sophisticated network of uniquely identifiable "things" and each of these objects connects to a server via the Internet to provide some predefined services. These things are "smart" Things because they can communicate with each other either physically or even virtually through RFID, Bluetooth, Wi-Fi, Zigbee, NFC, Barcode, etc. With IoT, people and things can be connected anywhere, anytime, and without minimal or no human intervention using underlying network services (Tan et al., 2010). Healthcare is one of the most important areas where IoT can be effectively utilized by diverse distributed devices that can compile, interpret, and efficiently communicate real-time medical information from patients to medical practitioners and vice versa. The integration of IoT has completely changed the traditional methods of providing healthcare services and enables healthcare providers to reach their patients at ease. A vast amount of data may be obtained through a wide number of sensors, processed and may be analyzed for providing better solutions to ailments (Baker et al., 2017). In a typical IoT-based healthcare ecosystem, a set of interconnected devices equipped with low-cost sensors create a network comprising of major stakeholders like patients, doctors, medical staff, hospital admin, and others to evaluate healthcare solutions, monitor patients remotely, and automatically detect situations where medical interventions become essential. With the increase in the population of elders all across the globe, it is becoming increasingly difficult to monitor chronic diseases and provide timely solutions. Popularly known as E-Health Monitoring, architectural frameworks may be developed under the IoT ecosystem that can monitor the daily activities of an elderly patient and provide effective solutions for several common health-related issues like diabetes, pulse rate monitoring, kidney functioning, etc. The data may be accessed through smartphones and uploaded to the cloud for further analysis by medical staff at their end (Rajput and Gour, 2016). These approaches not only reduce the massive burden on the healthcare industry, but also provide quality regular care to patients at different levels of medical problems.

As depicted in Fig. 1, IoT-based healthcare allows real-time monitoring of patient's health conditions under critical or emergencies and also provides medications for chronic diseases. Medical servers and cloud databases play a major role in the ecosystem which are used to store vital medical data and create health records for EHR which will be further analyzed by the doctors or medical staff. Such IoT-based healthcare system, as a whole reduces diagnosis time and cost, enhances patient care, and enriches user experience apart from improving the quality of life for a patient.

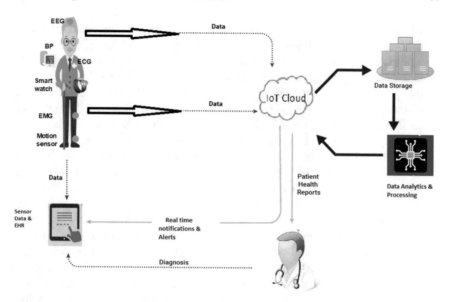

Fig. 1 IoT in healthcare

2 Applications of IoT in Healthcare

In near future, IoT will be applied in the healthcare sector to a great extent which will eventually improve the quality of healthcare with reduced cost and increased patient satisfaction. The application of IoT in this particular sector is diverse and benefits patients in several ways for a better clinical experience. Applications are targeted toward patients and clients at an individual level making them more user-centric and user-friendly for providing improved healthcare solutions. Some of the applications are mentioned in the following sections:

- **Glucose Monitoring**: Diabetes is a common metabolic disease that makes the patient suffers from a high level of blood sugar over a long period. There is a need to monitor the increased level of glucose in the blood regularly so that medications may be provided along with proper meals and activities to keep it under control. Real-time sensing of glucose levels in a noninvasive manner is demonstrated in Istepanian et al. (2011) and methods of diabetes management using concepts of m-IoT are addressed along with its potential benefits. Here the patients are provided with noninvasive, opto-physiological sensors for glucose monitoring, and with the help of IPV6 and 6LoWPAN, health data packets (both periodic and data-driven) are transmitted over the IEEE 802.15.4 protocol. In (Al-Taee et al., 2015), the system can support multiple care dimensions of diabetes through mobile apps including self-management allowing real-time clinical interactions with doctors, and providing feedback to the patients.

- **ECG monitoring**: ECG monitors the activities of the heart recorded by electro-cardiography that includes measuring basic heart rate and basic rhythm pattern with other patterns of a full cardiac cycle displayed through waveforms. It also diagnoses arrhythmia, arterial fibrillation, bradycardia, myocardial ischemia and many other diseases as well as prolonged QT intervals. Few ECG monitoring methods have been proposed by authors like (Yang et al., 2016), which are based on IoT techniques where ECG data is gathered with the help of a wearable, and directly transmitted to the cloud by Wi-Fi. All smart terminals using standard web browsers can access the data conveniently as both MQTT and HTTP protocols are applicable in the IoT cloud without any cross-platform issues. It has been proved experimentally that the system can reliably collect real-time ECG data from patients which can be further analyzed by medical practitioners for detecting heart-related diseases at an early stage. The authors of Mohammed et al. (2014) have designed an application called ECG Android App that allows the patients to see the ECG waves, log the data, and upload it to a private centralized cloud which can be retrieved by medical professionals for further analysis. As depicted in Spanò et al. (2016), a complete vertical solution for novice users has been designed, with energy-efficient low-cost sensors, for seamless integration with a smart home system in a single IoT infrastructure.
- **Medication Management**: The noncompliance issue with medication is a serious threat to the healthcare industry and also incurs substantial financial losses all across the globe. Hence, IoT can offer a pervasive, preventive, and promising medication management solution as depicted in Pang et al. (2014). The solution is based on intelligent and interactive packing (I2Pack) and intelligent medicine box (iMedBox), and this intelligent pharmaceutical packaging is controlled by wireless communication with proper sealing by CDM (Controlled Delamination Material) for extra safety. The wearable sensors can collect other vital parameters through the wireless link and high-performance architecture can perform on-site quick diagnosis with a user-friendly interface for ease of use, especially by the elders. A suitable medical control system with RFID tags is presented in Laranjo et al. (2013), along with Electronic Product Codes [EPC] standards. This application majorly focuses on AAL and integrates IoT, RFID, EPC, etc., under a suitable system for better patient–doctor interactions.
- **Body Temperature Monitoring**: Being one of the most vital monitoring activities in healthcare, body temperature can be a decisive factor in the diagnosis of several diseases and adverse health conditions of a patient. To maintain a condition of equilibrium with the internal environment, the patient's homeostasis must be understood by the doctors, by monitoring the temperature of the body. IoT-based temperature tracking is popularly designed in literature by researchers, through several applications as depicted in ElSaadany et al. (2017). The smartphone can play an essential role in collecting body temperature in a constant manner as the patients can carry it in their pockets. This helps us to classify the normal or abnormal conditions of the patients based on previously fed data. Few works in literature like (Zakaria et al., 2018) have also helped medical practitioners to measure the body temperature of infants using wearable sensors, interfacing

through a mobile phone and wireless network. Child monitoring is essential as babies cannot communicate like adults, and through such systems, it becomes easier for parents to understand whether the child is suffering from abnormal body temperature or not.

- **Blood pressure Monitoring**: Blood pressure is a common medical issue that affects almost everyone, however it is crucial for people suffering from adverse medical conditions. An increase or decrease in pressure may cause fatal injuries to the patients, hence monitoring the blood pressure of a patient on a regular basis is important. As depicted in Lamonaca et al. (2019), wearable devices under the IoT ecosystem possibly monitor BP anytime anywhere and these devices are encompassed with high precision, auto-sync capabilities with wireless communication through smartphones. Further, they are compatible with multi-OS smartphone platforms, and results can be shared with physicians or even others instantly for immediate response. An IoT-based healthcare monitoring system is proposed in Vippalapalli and Ananthula (2016) where doctors can detect vital parameters like the Blood Pressure of a patient in real time, with the help of Arduino Board, different sensors, and LabView software which allows the doctors to dynamically view vital parameters of the patient at home. In (Kario et al., 2017), the authors have designed and developed a multisensor BP monitoring system, for 24 h service that can also detect the location of the patient (like a toilet) apart from other ambient sensors. With the classic combination of both, the system can identify several details of BP variability and reduce the risk of cardiovascular diseases to a great extent.
- **Blood oxygen saturation Monitoring or (SpO2)**: Considered to be one of the most vital parameters for patients of all medical conditions, Sp02 measurement may be done through pulse oximetry which is a noninvasive device to detect oxygen saturation in the blood. Several wearable devices can be used in the IoT ecosystem for healthcare to accomplish the task. The integration of sensors measuring oxygen can be easily done and they can be connected to the clinics or hospitals via wireless communication or Bluetooth technology to monitor the accurate level of blood oxygen in patients for immediate actions if required. In (Larson et al., 2013), the authors have proposed a smartphone-based approach to measure common functions of lungs without any need for additional hardware or adapter and it has been proved to be effective to diagnose common lung ailments. It is a telemedicine-related application where the users can call the server and record exhalation data for medical staff to comprehend the irregularities if any. As depicted in Fu and Liu (2015), a portable tissue Oximeter using an STM32 microprocessor is designed, and with the help of near-infrared technology, SpO2 measurements can be obtained along with the heart rate of the patient. Then IoT-based networks like Wi-Fi or ZigBee may be used to pass the data to medical staff remotely, and it is processed in an expert decision-making system for further medications. The study in Son et al. (2017), focuses on developing a wearable device for measuring SpO2, for real-time monitoring and predicting the actual

health condition of the patient, especially elders through the Internet. This wearable device is a low power consuming as well as a low cost device which can be used in providing a comprehensive AAL or Ambient Assisted Living environment.

- **Rehabilitation**: There is a dearth of health experts globally who possess enough expertise to provide treatment to patients with functional disabilities. Patients with psychological disabilities, as well as physical impairments, need rehabilitation to lead their normal life again. IoT can be helpful to create a smart rehabilitation system as depicted in Fan et al. (2014) which is an ontology-based automatic design methodology. Through this, a smart rehabilitation may be formulated to understand the symptoms of such patients and reconfigure resources as per their requirements automatically. IoT plays an important role to interconnect all medical resources for immediate interactions among doctors and patients and makes seamless transactions possible among stakeholders. The authors of Jiang et al. (2017) have introduced an IoT-based rehabilitation assessment system for the upper limb of stroke survivors. The system can perform adequate assessments of objectives automatically with the help of wireless sensing subsystems, cloud computing, and an Android platform.

- **Drug Identification and ADR Monitoring**: Drugs given to patients in form of medication can often hurt their health which needs immediate actions to be taken for causing fatal injuries. The adverse reaction is possible due to prolonged use or even after a single dose of the drug or even due to several combinations of drugs taken in due course. It is important to arrest the cause and control the situation before it causes loss of life for a patient. A study by Jara et al. (2010) shows that an ADR or Adverse Drug Reaction service may be designed based on IoT to detect allergy interactions of the patients from his/her medical history accessed from EHR online. The patient's terminal detects the drug through NFC-enabled devices or barcodes, and the information collected is matched with Pharmaceutical Intelligent Information. This information is matched and it is decided whether the drug is compatible with the allergy profile mentioned in the EGR of the patient or not. Especially for the elderly population, a tight follow-up of drug compliance is recommended as per (Jara et al., 2014) where the authors have proposed an innovative system based on IoT to identify the compatibility of the drug and medication monitoring. IoT can detect harmful side effects of a particular drug, allergies, and other medical conditions of a patient before prescribing the medication to the patient.

Figure 2, gives a comprehensive idea about the several applications that are discussed above for ready reference of the reader.

There may be other applications of IoT in healthcare as well such as *asthma monitoring, voice monitoring,* and overall *patient monitoring* which also form an essential factor for the growing popularity of IoT implementations in this sector.

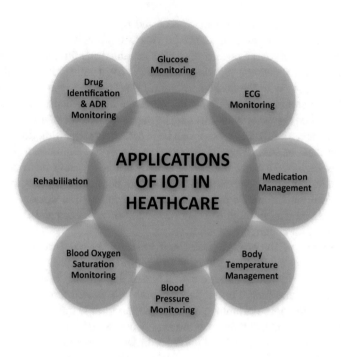

Fig. 2 Applications of IoT in healthcare

3 Benefits of IoT in Healthcare

With IoT, it is possible to facilitate seamless communication and interaction of devices with each other as well as with various stakeholders of healthcare in a medical environment. Hence, it would be imperative to embrace the benefits of IoT technology to save lives and improve quality of life with the help of smart connected devices. Several types of researches have figured out the numerous benefits of the system for consumers, businesses, individuals, and society. IoT has brought revolutionary changes in Internet communication and has been additionally beneficial for the healthcare industry by closing the gap between medical practitioners and their patients, on-site, or even in remote locations. Some of them are enlisted:

- **Accessibility to the patients for monitoring**: The development and availability of several health applications have paved the way to revolutionize the healthcare industry as they provide convenient ways for medical practitioners to keep a constant watch on their patients from anywhere and anytime. During medical emergencies, real-time continuous monitoring can save patients from severe conditions like stroke, heart failure, asthma attack, etc., which can be determined through sensors mounted on the patient body. The collected data is stored in the cloud or remote servers and can be accessed by medical practitioners, health-care organizations, or even insurance providers. Especially patients with chronic diseases are benefitted since their emergency medical conditions may be immedi-ately diagnosed for instant support through GPS. Even patients have the flexibility to communicate with the doctors through instant messaging for quick support. Facilities to communicate with doctors via social media are also allowed so that unprecedented medical conditions may be discussed and decided for better diag-nosis. Further, all medical records can be accessed as supporting documents for decision-making, irrespective of their locations or device anytime. In (Kumar and Venkateswarlu, 2016), the authors have shown that by using microcontrollers, pulse oximeters, and temperature sensors, it is possible to alert doctors about the medical condition of a patient at a remote location. The doctors can access patient-related data through web interfaces and IP addresses and automatically receive data for continuous monitoring.

- **Maintenance of Records digitally and healthcare analytics**: IoT healthcare system enables medical practitioners to keep medical records of thousands of patients across the globe through digital means that give better accessibility and reduce turnaround time. Further data can also be accessed through mobile apps that enable doctors to examine and diagnose the disease quickly for the fastest treatments. Also, medical manuals are readily available in apps that help medical practitioners to access all kinds of information needed before starting the treatment (Joyia et al., 2017). The large amount of data collected by the IoT devices also helps medical staff to progress in healthcare analytics. The Electronic Health Record or EHR can give necessary information about the patient's previous medications and their effect on his/her health.
- **Self-management through wearable devices**: The increasing popularity of wear-able devices among patients has transformed the entire mechanism of medical treatments today. Patients can use user-friendly interfaces provided by these wear-able devices (accelerometer on the wrist resembling a watch) and communicate with their caregivers beyond the physical confinements of the hospital (Nausheen and Begum, 2018). Especially in the case of chronic diseases, these wearable devices keep a track of regular visits and medications for easy record-keeping for both the doctors as well as the patients. Further, they can also act as a reminder to take medicines regularly, especially for older patients with severe diseases like Alzheimer's or others.
- **Automation**: IoT is designed to automate patient care and the related workflow which will be immensely beneficial for the healthcare industry. Facilities like machine-to-machine communication, sharing of knowledge, and flexible data movement across stakeholders with smooth delivery of services are provided by the automated systems deployed in IoT.
- **Cost reduction**: IoT devices and their network have significantly reduced the overall cost of the system. With the appropriate use of IoT devices, real-time patient monitoring is possible by physicians and it also eliminates the need of visting a doctor, prolonged stay in the hospital, or readmissions. This significantly reduces the cost to a great extent than otherwise (Farahani et al., 2018).

- **Inventory Management**: In the healthcare industry, it is imperative to have a supply of medical equipment and medicines and for easy procurement and replenishment of that inventory, IoT devices may be quite beneficial. The connected devices can easily estimate the requirement and procure them at the earliest to avoid contingency situations. This also significantly reduces man-hours, manpower, and cost.
- **Exchange of alerts and notifications**: With IoT-based healthcare, doctors can constantly monitor the condition of the patients by accessing real-time data from the sensors. If situations go beyond control, with the help of healthcare applications, caregivers can send important notifications or alerts to the patients, which can help them save lives (Zanjal and Talmale, 2016).
- **Improving quality of life**: The convenience of accessing medical data of a patient from the doctor's perspective and also the ease of accessing the medical practitioner anytime anywhere by the patient is certainly an advantage for both parties. This allows the patients to lead a healthy life and the doctors to keep a track of the same. Hence, the IoT ecosystem for healthcare has a profound influence on improving the quality of life for an individual (Nausheen and Begum, 2018).

4 Role of Cloud and Edge Computing in IoT Healthcare Services

IoT-based healthcare ecosystem relies heavily upon data collected from several sensors, which needs to be stored for future access by the medical staff. At this point, there is a need for the storage of such huge data safely and securely for maintaining patient's security and privacy and also to combat other challenges in the system. The following section describes how cloud computing and edge computing play a vital role in IoT healthcare services to serve this purpose.

4.1 Role of Cloud Computing in IoT Healthcare Services

The IoT is a system of devices, which can be a computing device, a mechanical device, or even simple things across daily lives, that can be provided with a unique identifier like an IP address and can transfer data across a network without human intervention. The sensors embedded in these mundane "Things" are inexpensive and produce a huge amount of data to be processed and sent across the network. To pave the way for the data to travel, cloud computing has a substantial role in IoT which is crucial, especially in healthcare services. The huge amount of data generated by IoT devices put a lot of strain on Internet infrastructures, and cloud services provide the required connectivity for information sharing between these devices. Further, IoT devices need to store this huge data and cloud services can provide adequate storage capacity and virtual resource utilization, with proper scalability as per the requirement of the users. Moreover, data can be accessed through the cloud which reduces the delay and thus increases the performance of the system. If cloud access remains unavailable for some technical issues, it becomes extremely difficult for these devices to store, as well as manage, such huge amount of data for a longer time.

Cloud computing allows users to maximize resources apart from sharing, and as in IoT, data can be accessed anywhere anytime using cloud services with the multitenancy feature of sharing multiple resources and costs across a large pool of users over time and spatial distribution enabling centralization of infrastructure. Both cloud and IoT have complementary characteristics and despite that their integration leads to Cloud of Things that has innumerable benefits in specific scenarios of applications. Cloud has virtually unlimited computational and processing capability which enables IoT devices to compensate for its technical constraints. Further, the cloud can provide an intermediary layer between applications and Things to abstract the complexity and functionalities that impact future application development to a greater extent. Cloud computing offers ubiquitous accessibility, throughout the connectivity of heterogeneous things, and also facilitates maximum accessibility of varied volumes of users (Biswas et al., 2014). Especially in pervasive healthcare, the vast amount of data generated by IoT devices need to be managed for further processing and analysis. Hence, the authors of Doukas and Maglogiannis (2012) have developed a cloud-based system that collects bio-signals, motion data, and contextual data from wearable sensors, to forward it directly to a cloud infrastructure. The system uses a lightweight API that is REST-based and allows direct communication of sensors to the cloud. Cloud computing not only provides rental space for the huge amount of data, but also adds processing and computational capabilities to the lightweight and low-cost sensors.

As per the authors of Cai et al. (2016), the integration of IoT and Cloud computing gives rise to the Cloud of Things or CoT, which would enrich the capabilities of the IoT devices to become more interoperable and interactive to patronize smart applications in the future. The system would require smart gateways, to perform preprocessing of such huge data and would pay more attention to business insight. The role of the cloud in CoT is similar to a central processing unit for the systematic processing of raw data collected from sensors. IoT is characterized by heterogeneous devices, protocols, and technologies, and deficits in few important attributes like flexibility, interoperability, scalability, reliability, availability, and efficiency. Cloud computing compensates for the majority of them and allows the IoT paradigm to be more robust and dynamic. Data is collected at the sensors present in the IoT devices and processed in the Cloud. As per (Botta et al., 2016), few drivers motivate the integration of IoT and Cloud computing. For example *communication* between devices is highly facilitated by cloud computing that allows them to connect, track, as well as manage the devices from anywhere, through customized web portals and in-built apps. It is possible to monitor effectively, control, co-ordinate, and communicate with remote things, apart from accessing real-time access to data produced by IoT sensors through effective high-speed networks of cloud computing. Further, *Storage* is another important area where cloud computing facilitates IoT as the latter produces a huge amount of semi-structured and non-structured data that possesses the three characteristics of Big data—volume, variety, and veracity.

As the cloud provides unlimited, large-scale, long-lived, low-cost, and on-demand storage capacity for specific needs, IoT devices can benefit significantly from that by generating new options for data aggregation, integration, and data sharing with third parties. Once data is there in the cloud, it may be treated as homogeneous, can be well defined by APIs, and remains protected with top-notch security. Cloud computing provides *Computation* facilities to IoT devices with restricted processing power and energy efficiency and significantly lacks complex, on-site processing of data. In a cloud, the computational facilities are enormous and unlimited, which helps in real-time data analysis of sensor-centric applications in case of complex events. With the adoption of the Cloud of Things, the *Scope* of the IoT paradigm multiplies many-fold enabling them to deal with unknown and complex real-life scenarios.

The role of cloud computing in IoT doubles when it comes to catering to healthcare which demands access to the latest technologies at an increasing rate. Especially with the inception of CoT, it is possible to improve the treatment process comprehensively. As per the authors of Tyagi et al. (2016), they have created a network consisting of stakeholders involved in the healthcare system like patients, doctors, nurses, attendants, pharmacists, along with infrastructures like medical labs, hospitals, legal authorities, as well and family members, of the patients. The proposed framework consists of applications like Electronic Health Records, personal health records, decision systems, etc., and each stakeholder can avail these services at different levels after proper validation and authentications. For example, patients can use this framework to assess themselves for health monitoring, find suitable hospitals that are also a part of the network, and even the physicians can use the same system for improved diagnosis and clinical results of the patients. This is accomplished by the cloud service provider through PaaS and IaaS to host these Cloud-IoT applications, especially designed for healthcare.

The cloud provides seamless communication and collaboration among the stakeholders with huge storage and ensures the safe transfer of crucial medical data for better and enhanced services to the patients. The authors of Kumar et al. (2018) have developed a novel Cloud-IoT-based Mobile Health care application, for the general public, to monitor, predict, and diagnose severe diseases. The authors have proposed a new classification algorithm and named it a Fuzzy Rule-based neural classifier, to diagnose the seriousness of a disease like diabetes. There are three phases to the system, where the first phase collects data from the IoT devices, medical records of the patients, as well as from the UCI repository. The second phase involves storing the data with ample security in cloud storage. The third phase is complex in comparison as it consists of a sub-module called a severity analyzer that detects the severity of the disease based on medical records with the help of fuzzy rules. As per (Kodali et al., 2015), IoT-based healthcare system can be implemented using ZigBee mesh protocol, which can regularly monitor the physiological parameters of a patient inside a hospital, enhancing the quality of care exhibited for a patient at a reduced cost, with simultaneous collection and analysis of data in a periodic manner. The samples are collected, and the required calibrations are performed, to be processed in the cloud.

Cloud computing thus with its massive network of unlimited storage and computational power has resolved many issues of IoT by providing a robust and flexible environment for the dynamic integration of data from various sources.

4.2 Role of Edge Computing in IoT Healthcare

As per Gartner (https://www.gartner.com/en/information-technology/glossary/edge-computing), edge computing may be defined as "a part of a distributed computing topology in which information processing is located close to the edge—where things and people produce or consume that information." Due to the exponential growth of IoT in the last decade, edge computing has developed substantially as well and this new paradigm allows seamless integration of several core capabilities like Network, Computing, and Storage closer to the end equipment. IoT devices generate a lot of data while being operational and edge computing allows such data to be analyzed directly on edge nodes that are physically closer (like Gateways) or attached (like smartphones or smartwatches) to the sensors or even at ad-hoc embedded systems like portable microcontrollers and single-board computers, before being sent to the cloud. The role of edge computing in IoT healthcare has increased substantially in the past decade as it enables end-users to monitor and take appropriate actions on health-related data generated by different edge gateways immediately, giving rise to a new paradigm called collaborative computing. Data Acquisition and Analysis are one of the major roles played by Edge computing for IoT in healthcare as the sensors can capture streaming data rapidly from the healthcare stakeholders and take immediate appropriate actions as well as process the data. This is crucial for a critical situation for a patient in need of immediate response. Through Edge Computing, Data analysis is performed at the place where data is generated and this helps to reduce the latency to generate information from data collected. This also helps to reduce network bandwidth as the analysis is done locally apart from reducing the cost of data transfer. Edge devices can also make strategic and critical decisions which are crucial since IoT devices generate a large amount of data requiring real-time processing, especially for healthcare. However, such data is not suitable to be sent to the Cloud as the response time would be too long. So edge devices can take necessary decisions locally to avoid such delays and prevent unprecedented situations for patients. Ensuring data security is another important role that edge computing plays in IoT healthcare systems as data being locally processed, identifying suspicious activities is easier, and implementing actions before severe damages may be taken at ease. Patient data is kept locally and safe from unintended recipients (Hassan et al., 2018). Several kinds of researches have proved that cloud and edge computing are becoming increasingly important day by day, especially in ensuring efficient healthcare systems. For example, in Oueida et al. (2018), the authors have proposed a resource preservation net framework using PetriNet, and well-integrated with cloud and edge computing, especially for Emergency Departments (ED) which are real-time, complex, and dynamic systems requiring tailored techniques to simulate system resources. RPN is a math-based framework that is used to model the proposed system with non-consumable resources (resources that have an expiry date), which are always preserved ensuring the safety and soundness of the system that is supported through some theorems. Here RPN is integrated with edge computing, with every resource having its smart device to communicate with the cloud. The status of the resource is informed to the cloud, and as the resource is assigned, the assignment request is sent to the edge. If the resource remains idle, the edge informs the following assignment to the cloud. This seamless integration of edge computing with RPN ensures high reliability and better performance. When applied to real life, with average patient waiting time, length of stay of the patient, and resource utilization as the KPI or Key Performance Indicator which may be modeled and optimized. Using edge technology, the first layer of storage, processing, and computation of healthcare data collected from edge nodes is accomplished which ensures better performances in the KPI. In a traditional IoT, the collected data is sent from the sensor device to the cloud directly for storage and processing. However, edge computing forms a layer between Cloud and IoT and may be personalized with the help of applications for data privacy. The authors of Dupont et al. (2017) have come up with a platform called Cloud4IoT, which can containerize IoT functions with horizontal migration (from One gateway to the other) and vertical migration (from the cloud to the gateway or vice versa). Cloud4IoT, being able to support various IoT gateways, can be used to deploy E-Health data processing containers dynamically and directly to that particular gateway where the data is being collected. As in Pace et al. (2018), a software framework called BodyEdge is proposed, which consists of a miniature mobile client module, and an Edge gateway, to collect and process data coming from several places locally. It supports multi-technology communication and guarantees robustness and high flexibility. The framework is being implemented on several hardwarenplatforms in real life and has been proved to be inexpensive, fast, and reliable. It is also observed that majority of them reduced data traffic for the Internet. Deep Learning approaches may be adopted to develop a voice disorder assessment system along with treatment as shown in Muhammad et al. (2018). Here, smart sensors are used to capture voice samples of the patients which are sent to the edge devices for processing at the initial stage, and the data is sent to the core cloud by the edge devices for next-level processing. An automatic assessment is done by the cloud manager and then the specialists capture the decision for appropriate treatment for patients. Here the authors have used CNN as the Deep Learning model that is experimentally successful in image processing applications.

From the above discussion, it is understood that cloud computing and edge computing are the inevitable components of the IoT healthcare ecosystem and their interrelation is well described as shown in Fig. 3.

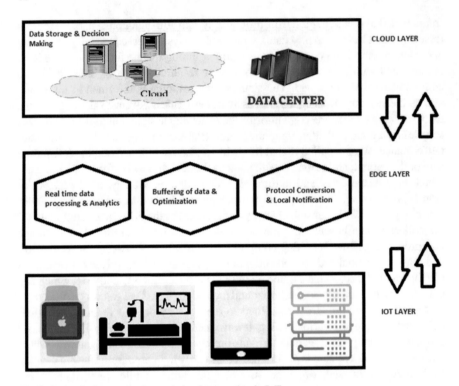

Fig. 3 Role of edge computing and cloud computing in IoT

5 Challenges and Concerns of Healthcare IoT Ecosystem

Healthcare may be considered one of the major application domains of the IoT and its dependence on the latter is increasing rapidly to enhance access and quality of care for patients and to reduce the cost of care drastically. Despite such advantages, IoT faces some severe challenges which need to be addressed for seamless integration of the IoT technologies with the essentials of healthcare.

5.1 Security and Privacy

Being one of the major challenges of IoT in healthcare, ensuring security is crucial as the data generated by IoT devices is sensitive and flows across the network without being encrypted. So it is susceptible to several types of network attacks like eavesdropping, identity theft, and even blackmailing. Unintended recipients can alter the data content and that could prove to be fatal for a patient's life. IoT sensors collect personal information from the patients as health information, communicate with cloud servers (public and private) from mobile applications, which are a major security risk since these cloud servers can be located anywhere in the world and is a part of the distributed system and can cause IP obstructions. Further, several issues like network misconfiguration, lack of proper encryption, and the inability of the devices to handle encryption cause major security threats to the system. The identification of vulnerabilities is as difficult to identify as to mitigate. Hence, management of credentials and controlled access to patients' confidential information is a major security challenge for IoT healthcare applications as they are always susceptible to cryptographic attacks. Prevalent, well-known, and high-profile cryptographic attacks have depicted the vulnerability of IoT technologies in healthcare. The major reason for this security and privacy issue is that the control of individual devices is not under one organization but shared among all co-operating stakeholders and collating such distributed information for drawing substantial contribution is surely a complex task for developers at all levels. As per (Zhang et al., 2014), object identification, authentication and authorizations, lightweight cryptosystems, security protocols, software vulnerability, backdoor analysis, Malware in IoT, etc., are some common security issues in IoT healthcare. Research has revealed cloning, jamming, Spoofing, cloud polling, etc., as the common attacks on IoT devices which is not desirable for ensuring security in healthcare. Hence, deploying appropriate cryptographic protocols that possess quick and real-time response is also essential with proper management of keys (public and private) since IoT is pervasive and continuously assesses real-time data. At the cloud level, security can also be threatened by attacks like Denial of Services, SQL injection, Phishing attacks, malicious code injections, path traversals, sniffing, trojan horses, viruses, worms, and also common ones like brute force attacks (Farahani et al., 2018). Several authentication techniques are implemented, but during emergencies, runtime delay in such techniques might prove to be crucial for a patient's life. In (Patel and Doshi, 2019), authors have demonstrated some common security parameters essential for complete protection from malicious users and they have termed it as IoT Security Octagon.

5.2 Device Vulnerability

IoT healthcare systems also suffer from acute device and memory vulnerability and deployment of firmware patches as most applications are vulnerable to code injections by malicious users, to undertake full control over the system. Memory corruption which occurs due to writable and executable code in memory and redirecting the processor to execute it might end up being a devastating challenge where the system may be compromised using vulnerabilities like buffer overflow (Alasmari and Anwar, 2016). It is very difficult for the medical staff to detect these computer-based discrepancies affecting the devices, and finding solutions for debugging such issues can be time-consuming and complex(Williams and Woodward, 2015). This could prove crucial for a patient in healthcare as the staff would unknowingly access their credentials through common web-based interfaces.

5.3 Interoperability

By basic definition, it is the ability of several homogeneous or heterogeneous systems, services, and applications to communicate and work with each other, reliably in a predicted manner. Each sensor in IoT has different processing and communication capabilities and has different bandwidth requirements with energy availability. Data should be able to get transferred across multiple interfaces, with different security protocols, underlying technologies used by the devices, the standards, and their compliance in between. In healthcare, there are various sensors used to monitor patient's health, either in the hospital or even remotely, which can be supplied by different vendors. A patient might need to use several such differently manufactured devices with varied communication protocols at a time and hence, this is considered to be a bigger challenge. IoT implementation on a large scale requires the sensors from a single vendor to achieve seamless communication among each other which undoubtedly creates a potential bottleneck in the real-time data processing. IoT vendors need to reach a common consensus on uniform standards and communication protocols, otherwise, integration would be a cumbersome task. These discrepancies also slow down the communication process and generate the need for scalability reduction in the IoT healthcare sector. The authors of Elkhodr et al. (2016) have shown several methods of integration of heterogeneous IoT devices with different communication protocols at different levels which may be a key game-changer for IoT. However, few researchers have revealed methods to communicate among these heterogeneous devices (Jabbar et al., 2017). Doctors can communicate with their patients to review their current status of health and this information can be semantically annotated through a lightweight model with multiple heterogeneous devices. In (Mavrogiorgou et al., 2019), the authors have shown that it is possible to ensure data interoperability between heterogeneous devices and to extract high-quality data from them. Apart from heterogeneity, there are few more concerns of interoperability in IoT healthcare which are a lack of open standards to follow and non-uniformity of communication protocols. To date, there are no such open standards for IoT devices for communication; however, there are few efforts made such as IoT-A and IoTivity which may be used for the purpose. Also, ETSI and IETF communities are constantly working on developing a uniform standard for IoT and soon might land up with some uniformity for a wider market.

5.4 Connectivity

IoT consists of several low-power, heterogeneous devices with lower power backup and computational capabilities. However, they need to remain connected continuously which is essential for crucial application areas like healthcare. The connectivity is mostly dynamic and has no fixed endpoints which imply that several standard communication mechanisms might not work. Hence, such communicating sensor networks require a uniform, effective addressing policy, and integration of IP standards. This would also require a secure and efficient identifier management system that can be applied to all devices across the world. With this emerges one more issue of traffic characterization and management which affects the quality of service provided by IoT, especially in healthcare. Patients need constant care from medical practitioners, and compromise in quality due to connectivity issues can be fatal for their lives. IoT uses several routing protocols in both standard wireless networks or ad-hoc and optimizing the best routing protocol is another issue that often has a great impact during large-scale implementation of IoT. Few types of researches like (Qiu et al., 2016) have been found to have formulated routing protocols, for emergency response IoT and claim improved performance, reliability of data transmission, efficient and quick response particularly designed for the healthcare industry. Another issue that poses real challenges in the connectivity of IoT devices is the reliability of signals (bidirectional) that collects and routes data across devices (Samuel, 2016). Especially in a server-client model, data must reach its destination accurately every time which is a crucial requirement in the healthcare IoT ecosystem. ZigBee, having no signal loss due to low bandwidth, is a popular choice in comparison to Wi-Fi. Another big challenge is Bandwidth consumption which increases many-fold with an increase of devices getting connected to the network. Especially during video streaming, there is a huge requirement of Bandwidth that might often increase the load on the server for handling such a huge amount of data. Hence, establishing a lightweight network is a huge challenge in IoT healthcare that can transfer data seamlessly between devices and put less burden on the servers.

5.5 Volume of Data and Its Analytics

IoT devices generate a huge amount of data from a wide variety of sensors, both wearable and implantable, all across, within a controlled environment like a hospital or even from a remote location, to ensure quality care to the patients. Interestingly, all IoT applications are data-centric and that is another major challenge for the general-purpose implementation of it on a large scale. With the increase in scalability of the network, data needs to be collected from a wide range of heterogeneous physical sensors, and storing, processing, and analyzing the same is no less than a challenge. Data hence plays a vital role in IoT, especially in healthcare synchronized execution within time becomes crucial in the case of patients with severe health conditions. The data collected from IoT devices is huge in volume and hence have compelled the healthcare stakeholders to direct their attention toward big data analysis. It is imperative from the security point of view as real-time data obtained from the devices run on open source technologies with vulnerable security schemes. (Bhatt et al., 2017). Data processing is expected to be done as per application-specific algorithms designed by developers and each application has a specific time criticality factor associated with it. For instance, remote patient monitoring needs extremely low processing and response time and typical examples include cardiac arrests, post-surgery monitoring, etc. At the same time, inventory management in a hospital is moderately critical with respect to time , since a smaller delay won't cause any fatal outcomes. The workflow in a hospital—like recording patient's data from his/her IoT device, registration at the hospital, and beginning of treatment after diagnosis must be handled on time because the patient's life might be at stake. An optimized workflow can improve the quality of patient care by reducing diagnosis time and bypassing trivial paperwork needed before the treatment. Data collected by IoT devices is mainly unstructured which, if not passed through a high- performance computing system, might take a longer time to process, which might add to the time criticality factor. But a high-performance system adds to the infrastructure cost which is also a major setback for IoT implementations. Further, interpretation of data collected from local sensors accurately is another big challenge as the service providers have to have to draw generalizable and standard conclusions from the data, especially with the aged population with wearable sensors as mentioned in Baig et al. (2019). Minor errors in interpretation might end up resulting in fatal outputs for a patient in dire condition. Noise is another major challenging factor that might incorporate in collecting data from different sensors as the data travels from the device to the control center which will significantly affect the quality. When collected in bulk, it is imperative to separate the data into manageable chunks without being overloaded, which will help in accurate precision for proper data analysis. Controlling overloading is essential as it might affect the decision-making process by medical practitioners, especially in remote monitoring. Sensor data reliability and quality are also a challenge since they are procured from multiple vendors as described in Banerjee and Sheth (2017).

5.6 Energy Efficiency

In IoT, the network of strong sensor nodes needs to be ubiquitous and pervasive that implies data to be sent round the clock across the globe. This makes them drained out of power quite often and that might compromise their quality of performance. It is a challenge to make the IoT network energy efficient as these sensors are low-power devices with limited computational capabilities. While transmitting data, they consume significant power from the battery source within and that can be a challenging scenario during an emergency in the healthcare industry. Implementation of protocol stacks in the software also needs a significant amount of power for every single transmission. Powering these devices is a challenging task itself as the wiring is impossible due to the sheer expense, infeasibility, and inconvenience that it causes, and hence they are mostly battery-powered or energy harvested. However, battery-based IoT systems have high post-deployment maintenance cost which includes the cost of acquiring new batteries, disposing of depleted batteries, labor, and even the cost incurred while the system is down. Energy harvesting is a viable option but it is not always reliable, and is mostly insufficient for many

IoT applications like healthcare that need constant monitoring of patients to avoid severity. There have been researches that have tried to exhibit the role of software to impart energy efficiency in IoT devices through programs and tool-chains which can exploit the hardware energy-saving capabilities (Georgiou et al., 2017). One of the significant challenges that also exist in IoT sensors is that different devices can retain power for different periods, for instance, smartwatches and fitness monitors have more longevity spanning for weeks before being recharged. On the other hand, automation gadgets need to be recharged after years of usage. Hence, authors like (Jayakumar et al., 2016) have proposed a new concept called approximate computing which is a new emerging design paradigm that executes computations approximately and efficiently and improves energy efficiency in IoT devices.

5.7 Trust Issues and Government Policies

Trust, an abstract factor, may be defined as the specific policies of security and crucial credentials that permit access to resources in general, especially in the IoT ecosystem. It is imperative to deploy trust mechanisms in IoT to provide "Things" a dynamic, collaborative trust environment for interacting with each other, and decrease the level of uncertainty to achieve their goals. Users must be able to control the devices, especially in healthcare, and the tools being used with simple credential policies and specifications effectively and efficiently. As described in Daubert et al. (2015), trust may be of several kinds such as *Device Trust* which allows interaction among trusted devices only and needs trusted schemes and software for proper implementation. One more type can be a *Connection Trust* that refers to exchanging the right data with the right person with all security measures like data authentication, integrity, and confidentiality. Several other types pertain to *Processing Trust* that refers to deal with only meaningful and right data and finally *System Trust* that refers to providing an overall trustworthy system of IoT with well defined and transparent system workflows, technology and processes. These are real challenges in implementing an IoT ecosystem as that needs complete control of the system and operations. Few trust management protocols are being proposed in the literature as described in Bao et al. (2012) that consider several trust attributes and nodes, nodes interact only with other devices of interest. This is crucial in healthcare as the data exchanged between patients and their healthcare is prone to security loopholes that compromise the privacy of the same. This event-driven protocol is designed in such a way that if a malicious or unwanted interaction occurs between nodes, then the trust policies are updated immediately to nullify the effect. In (Chen et al., 2011), a fuzzy reputation-based model of trust management has been proposed, that allows only specific devices to interact based on certain trust metrics like packet delivery ratio, energy consumption, and packet forwarding ratios. Governance support is also a challenging issue in IoT implementation as proper management of policies must be reinforced for the appropriate deployment of the IoT ecosystem. The Government must punish the malicious users at the earliest and support trust-related policies and decisions taken by inter-acting devices and provide enforcement mechanisms for smooth interoperability of devices across the globe. Government should also be responsible for continuous funding, spreading health awareness among people and supporting healthcare-related services, implementing standards, and protecting security and privacy rights in the IoT ecosystem.

5.8   Other Challenges

Few other challenges have made the large-scale integration of IoT a gruesome task. For instance, *stakeholder collaboration* is crucial for creating value for the patients when it comes to applying IoT in healthcare. The medical professionals, patients, their family members, nonmedical staff, labs, research areas, businesses, medical insurance providers, and government-all are considered to be the stakeholders in the IoT healthcare system. Each of them needs to be trained to be well equipped with an IoT ecosystem for large-scale integration (Mosadeghrad, 2014). Unfortunately, the system being still in the development phase, it is a challenge to collate all stakeholders to implement it professionally. Especially for the lower level of staff, coaching them properly to integrate with the system is a cumbersome job. Patients, who are the regular consumers of the services, also need to be trained to use the IoT devices in collaboration with the hospital staff. Further, different stakeholders may visualize data differently, for example, doctors might have trust issues with data presented to them by the sensors, and the patients also might raise similar comprehension issues with IoT sensor data as depicted in Jaigirdar et al. (2019). *Scalability* may be considered a real challenge for IoT devices as with each passing day, the number and heterogeneity of IoT devices will be increasing so developing a highly scalable, secured, IoT system for healthcare in adherence to all security rules may be tough to achieve as a target. The *Cost* must be considered before designing and implementing an IoT system for healthcare since deploying the devices and their maintenance require huge investments from the business point of view. A substantial amount of research is also required for creating low-cost prototypes of IoT applications for general-purpose implementation. *Self-Management* of sensor devices is essential but no less than a challenge in real transmission. The IoT devices are completely or mostly independent of human intervention so should be able to configure and adapt themselves to contingency situations, especially in case of connection failures which is not expected in the healthcare system. Hospitals and healthcare organizations have to deal with a huge number of patients with multiple ailments, as well as multiple staff rendering several kinds of services to them. Accurate identification of patients, their ailments, and the right treatment needs proper *Data Management* which is another big challenge in IoT healthcare. As per (Maksimović and Vujović, 2017), *Training and Education* of stakeholders (patients, healthcare professionals as well as family members of the patients) are essential to spread awareness of the E-Health solutions. Training them to understand the usage of the healthcare application would

Fig. 4 Challenges and
concerns of IoT in healthcare

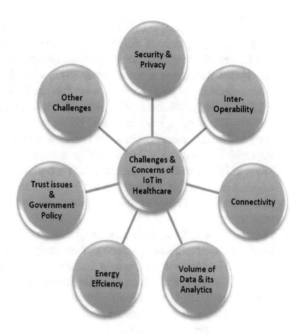

result in better deployment of the IoT healthcare services, especially for the older
population. Figure 4, accumulates the challenges mentioned above under one roof
for easy comprehension of the readers.

6 Open Issues

IoT has been widely accepted today by several medical organizations and hospitals
but still, several gaps need to be fulfilled by researchers in near future. In the following
section, some insights are provided that point out a few specific emerging open issues
and ideas for IoT in healthcare:

- Integration of IoT with cloud computing and edge computing separately has been
  successfully ongoing recently but the integration of the same with upcoming
  technologies like hybrid cloud platforms, nanotechnologies, mobile computing,
  cloudlets, etc., will be crucial and a challenging task for the researchers. With the
  emergence of concepts like the Web of Things, IoT will get a wider spectrum of
  functionalities and capabilities.
- Developing a general model of privacy with innovative enforcement techniques,
  and defining specific privacy policies that can identify a smart object accessing
  private data without legal issues, etc., are also a few areas where researchers need
  to concentrate on a holistic acceptance of the IoT in healthcare. Security issues
  in healthcare applications to restrict unauthorized access and protection of data

transmitted from patient to the hospital also needs to be addressed appropriately for a wider acceptance of the IoT ecosystem globally.

- The energy efficiency and complexity involved in wearable devices with complete accuracy is a research area that needs to be catered, especially in the case of the elder population of patients. Improving the quality of sensors for higher accuracy, reliability, and precision is also essential. For example, researchers are looking for wearable devices that can record blood pressure, especially for patients with chronic diseases related to blood pressure, and gives accurate data.
- Research is going on with NB-IoT or narrowband IoT which is a low-power WAN technology and its implementation in healthcare. Its suitability in healthcare, capabilities, and functionalities must be considered well before implementing it as a foundation communication standard for improving the quality of patient monitoring.
- Data processing is an area that needs more attention from researchers in near future as extraction and processing of meaningful data from complex sensors are of utmost importance for accurate diagnosis and medications.
- Machine Learning (ML) is an emerging field that can prove to be extremely crucial in IoT healthcare. Given a high computing power environment, ML can provide faster and more accurate diagnoses of ailments, can recognize patterns of disease trends, and help in developing newer treatment solutions. Few works like (Nandy et al., 2019) proposes a framework that gives a detailed identification of static and dynamic activities of elders at home with the help of an ensemble of ML classifiers, or as in Saha et al. (2020) that designs MIML (Multi-Instance Multi-Label learning-based ensemble model to compare and contrast spatial activity patterns with spatial activity patterns for improved performance of the system as a whole, but still the scope to incorporate ML into IoT healthcare ecosystem is still wide open for researchers.

7 Conclusion

Internet and technologies related to it have always been an essential part of human life for few decades. IoT may be considered to be a technological revolution that has immense potential to change the current living standards of human beings by providing them optimum quality healthcare services at a reasonable cost. The continuous monitoring of patients remotely with early diagnosis of their ailments can not only cure them better, but can also reduce the mortality rate considerably. However, the comprehensive implementation of IoT in healthcare faces several challenges which must be arrested beforehand for seamless integration of the same with the healthcare industry. This chapter reviews the entire IoT ecosystem with its potential benefits and possible applications and focuses on the main challenges/concerns that remain as major issues for the holistic adoption of IoT in healthcare across the globe. It also depicts the role of IoT-enabled technologies like cloud computing and edge computing in empowering modern healthcare facilities and providing quality treatment to people suffering from various ailments. There are also wide scopes for researchers to explore the challenges discussed in this chapter and find out feasible and optimum solutions to accredit IoT for a healthy future ahead.

References

Al-Taee, M. A., Al-Nuaimy, W., Al-Ataby, A., Muhsin, Z. J., & Abood, S. N. (2015). Mobile health platform for diabetes management based on the Internet-of-Things. In *2015 IEEE Jordan Conference on Applied Electrical Engineering and Computing Technologies (AEECT)* (pp. 1–5). IEEE, November.

Alasmari, S., & Anwar, M. (2016). Security & privacy challenges in IoT-based health cloud. In *2016 International Conference on Computational Science and Computational Intelligence (CSCI)* (pp. 198–201). IEEE, December.

Baig, M. M., Afifi, S., GholamHosseini, H., & Mirza, F. (2019). A systematic review of wearable sensors and IoT-based monitoring applications for older adults—a focus on ageing population and independent living. *Journal of Medical Systems, 43*(8), 233.

Baker, S. B., Xiang, W., & Atkinson, I. (2017). Internet of things for smart healthcare: Technologies, challenges, and opportunities. *IEEE Access, 5*, 26521–26544.

Banerjee, T., & Sheth, A. (2017). Iot quality control for data and application needs. *IEEE Intelligent Systems, 32*(2), 68–73.

Bao, F., & Chen, R. (2012). Trust management for the internet of things and its application to service composition. In *2012 IEEE international symposium on a world of wireless, mobile and multimedia networks (WoWMoM)* (pp. 1–6). IEEE, June.

Bhatt, C., Dey, N., & Ashour, A. S. (eds.) (2017). Internet of things and big data technologies for next generation healthcare.

Biswas, A.R., & Giaffreda, R. (2014). IoT and cloud convergence: Opportunities and challenges. In *2014 IEEE World Forum on Internet of Things (WF-IoT)* (pp. 375–376). IEEE, March.

Botta, A., De Donato, W., Persico, V., & Pescapé, A. (2016). Integration of cloud computing and internet of things: A survey. *Future Generation Computer Systems, 56*, 684–700.

Cai, H., Xu, B., Jiang, L., & Vasilakos, A. V. (2016). IoT-based big data storage systems in cloud computing: Perspectives and challenges. *IEEE Internet of Things Journal, 4*(1), 75–87.

Chen, D., Chang, G., Sun, D., Li, J., Jia, J., & Wang, X. (2011). TRM-IoT: A trust management model based on fuzzy reputation for internet of things. *Computer Science and Information Systems, 8*(4), 1207–1228.

Daubert, J., Wiesmaier, A., & Kikiras, P. (2015). A view on privacy & trust in IoT. In *2015 IEEE International Conference on Communication Workshop (ICCW)* (pp. 2665–2670). IEEE, June.

Doukas, C., & Maglogiannis, I. (2012). Bringing IoT and cloud computing towards pervasive healthcare. In *2012 Sixth International Conference on Innovative Mobile and Internet Services in Ubiquitous Computing* (pp. 922–926). IEEE, July.

Dupont, C., Giaffreda, R., & Capra, L. (2017). Edge computing in IoT context: Horizontal and vertical Linux container migration. In *2017 Global Internet of Things Summit (GIoTS)* (pp. 1–4). IEEE, June.

ElSaadany, Y., Majumder, A. J. A., & Ucci, D. R. (2017). A wireless early prediction system of cardiac arrest through IoT. In *2017 IEEE 41st Annual Computer Software and Applications Conference (COMPSAC)* (Vol. 2, pp. 690–695). IEEE, July.

Elkhodr, M., Shahrestani, S., & Cheung, H. (2016). The internet of things: new interoperability, management and security challenges. *arXiv preprint* arXiv:1604.04824.

Fan, Y. J., Yin, Y. H., Da Xu, L., Zeng, Y., & Wu, F. (2014). IoT-based smart rehabilitation system. *IEEE Transactions on Industrial Informatics, 10*(2), 1568–1577.

Farahani, B., Firouzi, F., Chang, V., Badaroglu, M., Constant, N., & Mankodiya, K. (2018). Towards fog-driven IoT eHealth: Promises and challenges of IoT in medicine and healthcare. *Future Generation Computer Systems, 78*, 659–676.

Fu, Y., & Liu, J. (2015). System design for wearable blood oxygen saturation and pulse measurement device. *Procedia Manufacturing, 3*, 1187–1194.

Georgiou, K., Xavier-de-Souza, S., & Eder, K. (2017). The IoT energy challenge: A software perspective. *IEEE Embedded Systems Letters, 10*(3), 53–56.

Hassan, N., Gillani, S., Ahmed, E., Yaqoob, I., & Imran, M. (2018). The role of edge computing in internet of things. *IEEE Communications Magazine, 56*(11), 110–115.

https://www.gartner.com/en/information-technology/glossary/edge-computing..

Istepanian, R. S., Hu, S., Philip, N. Y., & Sungoor, A. (2011). The potential of Internet of m-health Things "m-IoT" for non-invasive glucose level sensing. In *2011 Annual International Conference of the IEEE Engineering in Medicine and Biology Society* (pp. 5264–5266). IEEE, August.

Jabbar, S., Ullah, F., Khalid, S., Khan, M., & Han, K. (2017). Semantic interoperability in heterogeneous IoT infrastructure for healthcare. *Wireless Communications and Mobile Computing, 2017*.

Jaigirdar, F. T., Rudolph, C., & Bain, C. (2019). Can I Trust the Data I See? A Physician's Concern on Medical Data in IoT Health Architectures. In *Proceedings of the Australasian Computer Science Week Multiconference* (pp. 1–10), January.

Jara, A. J., Zamora, M. A., & Skarmeta, A. F. (2014). Drug identification and interaction checker based on IoT to minimize adverse drug reactions and improve drug compliance. *Personal and Ubiquitous Computing, 18*(1), 5–17.

Jara, A. J., Belchi, F. J., Alcolea, A. F., Santa, J., Zamora-Izquierdo, M. A., & Gómez-Skarmeta, A. F. (2010). A Pharmaceutical Intelligent Information System to detect allergies and Adverse Drugs Reactions based on internet of things. In *2010 8th IEEE International Conference on Pervasive Computing and Communications Workshops (PERCOM Workshops)* (pp. 809–812). IEEE, March.

Jayakumar, H., Raha, A., Kim, Y., Sutar, S., Lee, W. S., & Raghunathan, V. (2016). Energy-efficient system design for IoT devices. In *2016 21st Asia and South Pacific Design Automation Conference (ASP-DAC)* (pp. 298–301). IEEE, January.

Jiang, Y., Qin, Y., Kim, I., & Wang, Y. (2017). Towards an IoT-based upper limb rehabilitation assessment system. In *2017 39th Annual International Conference of the IEEE Engineering in Medicine and Biology Society (EMBC)* (pp. 2414–2417). IEEE, July.

Joyia, G. J., Liaqat, R. M., Farooq, A., & Rehman, S. (2017). Internet of Medical Things (IOMT): Applications, benefits and future challenges in healthcare domain. *The Journal of Communication, 12*(4), 240–247.

Kario, K., Tomitani, N., Kanegae, H., Yasui, N., Nishizawa, M., Fujiwara, T., Shigezumi, T., Nagai, R., & Harada, H. (2017). Development of a new ICT-based multisensor blood pressure monitoring system for use in hemodynamic biomarker-initiated anticipation medicine for cardiovascular disease: The national IMPACT program project. *Progress in Cardiovascular Diseases, 60*(3), 435–449.

Kodali, R.K., Swamy, G., & Lakshmi, B. (2015). An implementation of IoT for healthcare. In *2015 IEEE Recent Advances in Intelligent Computational Systems (RAICS)* (pp. 411–416). IEEE, December.

Kumar, D. D., & Venkateswarlu, P. (2016). Secured smart healthcare monitoring system based on iot. *Imperial Journal of Interdisciplinary Research, 2*(10).

Kumar, P. M., Lokesh, S., Varatharajan, R., Babu, G. C., & Parthasarathy, P. (2018). Cloud and IoT based disease prediction and diagnosis system for healthcare using Fuzzy neural classifier. *Future Generation Computer Systems, 86*, 527–534.

Lamonaca, F., Balestrieri, E., Tudosa, I., Picariello, F., Carnì, D. L., Scuro, C., Bonavolontà, F., Spagnuolo, V., Grimaldi, G., & Colaprico, A. (2019). An overview on Internet of medical things in blood pressure monitoring. In *2019 IEEE International Symposium on Medical Measurements and Applications (MeMeA)* (pp. 1–6). IEEE, June.

Laranjo, I., Macedo, J., & Santos, A. (2013). Internet of Things for medication control: E-health architecture and service implementation. *International Journal of Reliable and Quality E-Healthcare (IJRQEH)*, *2*(3), 1–15.

Larson, E. C., Goel, M., Redfield, M., Boriello, G., Rosenfeld, M., & Patel, S. N. (2013). Tracking lung function on any phone. In *Proceedings of the 3rd ACM Symposium on Computing for Development* (pp. 1–2), January.

Maksimović, M., & Vujović, V. (2017). Internet of Things based e-health systems: Ideas, expectations and concerns. In *Handbook of Large-Scale Distributed Computing in Smart Healthcare* (pp. 241–280). Springer, Cham.

Mavrogiorgou, A., Kiourtis, A., Perakis, K., Pitsios, S., & Kyriazis, D. (2019). IoT in healthcare: Achieving interoperability of high-quality data acquired by IoT medical devices. *Sensors, 19*(9), 1978.

Mohammed, J., Lung, C. H., Ocneanu, A., Thakral, A., Jones, C., & Adler, A. (2014). Internet of Things: Remote patient monitoring using web services and cloud computing. In *2014 IEEE International Conference on Internet of Things (iThings), and IEEE Green Computing and Communications (GreenCom) and IEEE Cyber, Physical and Social Computing (CPSCom)* (pp. 256–263). IEEE, September.

Mosadeghrad, A. M. (2014). Factors influencing healthcare service quality. *International Journal of Health Policy and Management, 3*(2), 77.

Muhammad, G., Alhamid, M. F., Alsulaiman, M., & Gupta, B. (2018). Edge computing with cloud for voice disorder assessment and treatment. *IEEE Communications Magazine, 56*(4), 60–65.

Nandy, A., Saha, J., Chowdhury, C., & Singh, K. P. (2019). Detailed human activity recognition using wearable sensor and smartphones. In *2019 International Conference on Opto-Electronics and Applied Optics (Optronix)* (pp. 1–6). IEEE, March.

Nausheen, F., & Begum, S. H. (2018). Healthcare IoT: benefits, vulnerabilities and solutions. In *2018 2nd International Conference on Inventive Systems and Control (ICISC)* (pp. 517–522). IEEE, January.

Oueida, S., Kotb, Y., Aloqaily, M., Jararweh, Y., & Baker, T. (2018). An edge computing based smart healthcare framework for resource management. *Sensors, 18*(12), 4307.

Pace, P., Aloi, G., Gravina, R., Caliciuri, G., Fortino, G., & Liotta, A. (2018). An edge-based architecture to support efficient applications for healthcare industry 4.0. *IEEE Transactions on Industrial Informatics, 15*(1), pp.481–489.

Pang, Z., Tian, J., & Chen, Q. (2014). Intelligent packaging and intelligent medicine box for medication management towards the Internet-of-Things. In *16th International Conference on Advanced Communication Technology* (pp. 352–360). IEEE, February.

Patel, C., & Doshi, N. (2019). Security challenges in IoT cyber world. In *Security in Smart Cities: Models, Applications, and Challenges* (pp. 171–191). Springer, Cham.

Qiu, T., Lv, Y., Xia, F., Chen, N., Wan, J., & Tolba, A. (2016). ERGID: An efficient routing protocol for emergency response Internet of Things. *Journal of Network and Computer Applications, 72*, 104–112.

Rajput, D. S., & Gour, R. (2016). An IoT framework for healthcare monitoring systems. *International Journal of Computer Science and Information Security, 14*(5), 451.

Saha, J., Chowdhury, C., Ghosh, D., & Bandyopadhyay, S. (2020). A detailed human activity transition recognition framework for grossly labeled data from smartphone accelerometer. *Multimedia Tools and Applications*, pp. 1–22.

Samuel, S. S. I. (2016). A review of connectivity challenges in IoT-smart home. In *2016 3rd MEC International conference on big data and smart city (ICBDSC)* (pp. 1–4). IEEE, March.

Son, L. P., Thu, N. T. A., & Kien, N. T. (2017). Design an IoT wrist-device for SpO2 measurement. In *2017 international conference on advanced technologies for communications (ATC)* (pp. 144–149). IEEE, October.

Spanò, E., Di Pascoli, S., & Iannaccone, G. (2016). Low-power wearable ECG monitoring system for multiple-patient remote monitoring. *IEEE Sensors Journal, 16*(13), 5452–5462.

Tan, L., & Wang, N. (2010). Future internet: The internet of things. In *2010 3rd international conference on advanced computer theory and engineering (ICACTE)* (Vol. 5, pp. V5–376). IEEE, August.

Tyagi, S., Agarwal, A., & Maheshwari, P. (2016). A conceptual framework for IoT-based healthcare system using cloud computing. In *2016 6th International Conference-Cloud System and Big Data Engineering (Confluence)* (pp. 503–507). IEEE, January.

Vippalapalli, V., & Ananthula, S. (2016). Internet of things (IoT) based smart health care system. In *2016 International Conference on Signal Processing, Communication, Power and Embedded System (SCOPES)* (pp. 1229–1233). IEEE, October.

Williams, P. A., & Woodward, A. J. (2015). Cybersecurity vulnerabilities in medical devices: A complex environment and multifaceted problem. *Medical Devices (auckland, NZ), 8*, 305.

Yang, Z., Zhou, Q., Lei, L., Zheng, K., & Xiang, W. (2016). An IoT-cloud based wearable ECG monitoring system for smart healthcare. *Journal of Medical Systems, 40*(12), 286.

Zakaria, N. A., Saleh, F. N. B. M., & Razak, M. A. A. (2018). IoT (Internet of Things) based infant body temperature monitoring. In *2018 2nd international conference on biosignal analysis, processing and systems (ICBAPS)* (pp. 148–153). IEEE, July.

Zanjal, S. V., & Talmale, G. R. (2016). Medicine reminder and monitoring system for secure health using IOT. *Procedia Computer Science, 78*, 471–476.

Zhang, Z. K., Cho, M. C. Y., Wang, C. W., Hsu, C. W., Chen, C. K., & Shieh, S. (2014). IoT security: Ongoing challenges and research opportunities. In *2014 IEEE 7th international conference on service-oriented computing and applications* (pp. 230–234). IEEE, November.

Challenges of Handling Data in IoT-Enabled Healthcare

Zeenat Rehena⬤ and **Nandini Mukherjee**⬤

Abstract Internet of Things enables remote healthcare delivery in areas where an adequate number of doctors and healthcare personnel are not available. eHealth sensors are fixed to the patient's body and vital signs are measured and recorded to produce a huge amount of data. The data is mostly unstructured, produced with a high velocity and in a variety of formats. Thus, handling the generated data in real time is challenging and needs to be processed suitably to extract important information from this data. Further, communication and related technologies are crucial for the evolution of future smart healthcare services. In this chapter, these challenges and some solutions to these challenges will be discussed. Primary challenges of integrating e-Health sensors in a remote healthcare framework include heterogeneity of multiple types of sensor devices used for getting the vital signs in real time, communication protocols, and standards. Consequently, this leads to challenges related to data overloading and accuracy. Another challenge related to sensor data is the uncertainty in data that may be caused due to hardware fault, measurement error, and missing data. Various techniques have been applied by the researchers to get rid of uncertainties in data. These include statistical methods, AI techniques, etc., for increasing accuracy and precision in the data. This chapter highlights some of the techniques and presents a case study in this regard.

Keywords e-healthcare · IoT · Challenges · Health data · Uncertainties · Virtual sensors · Statistical methods

Z. Rehena (✉)
Department of Computer Science and Engineering, Aliah University, Kolkata, India
e-mail: zeenatrehena@aliah.ac.in

N. Mukherjee
Department of Computer Science and Engineering, Jadavpur University, Kolkata, India
e-mail: nandini.mukhopadhyay@jadavpuruniversity.in

1 Introduction

Internet of Things (IoT) is a widely used technology in the computing world. It is used in many applications, which impact our daily life and change our business thoughts. IoT interconnects smart objects and devices uniquely within the current internet infrastructure.

Due to the tremendous growth in urbanization and a high number of the elderly population, significant pressure is placed on smart healthcare systems (Baker et al., 2017; Islam et al., 2015; Perrier, 2015). The requirement of resources from hospitals, like beds, ICU, doctors, and caregivers are very high (Perrier, 2015). Therefore, a way out is highly required to decrease this huge demand on the healthcare systems maintaining to offer good quality concern toward critical patients. IoT is identified as a probable solution in the field of eHealth. It has incomparable benefits that give the efficiency of treatment and improve patients' health. This advanced technology reduces hospital costs, reduces hospital stay, and it provides remote, as well as emergency healthcare services, to the patients. IoT is used in health applications, such as medical emergencies like heart attacks, diabetes patients, and remote monitoring. Few IoT applications are focused on providing support to physically challenged and elderly people to live independently in their lives. Applications are also used to take care of patients with chronic diseases avoiding the need for physical check up (Zeadally et al., 2019).

Nowadays, smartphones have become an essential part of daily life. In remote healthcare systems, smartphone devices play an important role. Smartphones are attached with eHealth sensors to monitor the patients. Sometimes wearable devices attached to a patient's body are used to measure the vital signs, like heartbeats, blood sugar level, blood pressure, etc. IoT-based monitoring system obtains various data from hospital wards and medical equipment, sensors attached to a patient's body and processes the data for robust and automatic management of healthcare (Gope & Hwang, 2016; Perrier, 2015) system. The vital signs are measured and recorded from time to time resulting huge amount of data. IoT applications are used to run these healthcare data. Furthermore, the IoT healthcare system improves the quality management of resources for people by providing an efficient monitoring and tracking system (Perrier, 2015). A variety of medical devices, wearable sensors, and other imaging equipment have been viewed as smart devices which form the main component of the IoT. Thus, IoT-based healthcare services seem to cut treatment costs and increase the quality of life.

Remote monitoring in primary healthcare brings great promise for cases involving poor health, weak patients, and old and elderly patients (Larson et al., 2013). It helps to collect vital signs and gives assistance for their illness. It also helps to collect real-time data transmission to healthcare providers (Wasserkrug et al., 2005). Such applications can be developed based on software algorithms, wearable monitoring sensors, and communication technologies.

In this perspective, telemedicine is an amazing mode for supporting patients with long persistent diseases, which guarantees the service of healthcare in distant and interior regions. It improves the assimilation between patients and hospitals. Several research works in this field have revealed that remote health monitoring is reasonable and could offer advantages in different situations. It also helps to keep an eye on less serious patients at home rather than in the hospital, thus dropping the pressure on the hospital's bed, ICU, doctors, etc. Thus, remote medical assistance could be used to support better control of healthcare for the people living in rural or interior areas. It also helps aged people to survive independently at home. Basically, it can get better management of healthcare resources and can give people better control over their own health at all times. However, several issues and challenges come up while implementing telemonitoring systems (Larson et al., 2013). There are a few drawbacks as well to remote health monitoring. The most important drawback include security risk, which arises due to the large amount of sensitive data stored in a single record. In addition, patient data is required to be calibrated regularly to ensure data accuracy and remove uncertainty. Sometimes it may happen that the wearable sensors or other devices engaged to measure vital signs of patients get disconnected from healthcare services when they are out of communication range or run out of battery.

Figure 1 represents an IoT-based healthcare system. The figure shows that real-time big data are generated and collected from various IoT medical devices, body area networks (BAN) attached to remotely located patients. The system uses heterogeneous sources such as body sensors, medical IoT devices, and complaints from patients. Then, advanced data analyses are applied to take the benefits of the IoT cloud to evaluate the complaints of the patients. In healthcare, the huge and versatile eHealth data sets are hard to handle by the traditional systems. It is also hard to process with traditional data managing schemes and methods.

In this chapter, we mainly focus on different challenges related to ehealth data in IoT-based healthcare system. Many services and applications have been noticed in IoT healthcare. These applications undergo several challenges due to their inherent nature. Initially, in this chapter, we discuss various applications and services and then the challenges associated with them.

Fig. 1 Prototype diagram of IoT healthcare system

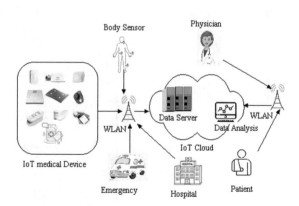

The remainder of this chapter is organized as follows. Section 2 explains various IoT services and applications related to eHealth systems. Section 3 investigates problems of health data generated from multiple health sensors that are used in an IoT healthcare system. Data uncertainty in context of IoT healthcare is discussed in Sect. 4. Types and causes of data uncertainty are also summarized here. Section 5 reviews statistical methods for handling data uncertainty. A case study on blood pressure (BP) vital signs of patients is presented in Sect. 6. Section 7 explains virtual sensors and its infrastructure for IoT-based healthcare system. Section 8 concludes the paper, summarizing the chapter with a future direction of research is required.

2   IoT Healthcare Services and Applications

IoT is projected to facilitate a range of healthcare applications and services. A set of healthcare solutions are generated by each of the services (Islam et al., 2015). There are many scenarios where it is difficult to distinguish between a service and a particular application. This section discusses several services and applications associated with the healthcare domain. Figure 2 shows a list of services and applications.

2.1   Services

Ambient Assisted Living (AAL) is an IoT-based service implemented in conjunction with artificial intelligence that deals with the healthcare of aging and elderly people. The idea of AAL is to widen the self-sufficient living of incapacitated individuals in a suitable and protected way. AAL services offer different solutions that make aged people more secure by ensuring a self-sufficient system and providing them

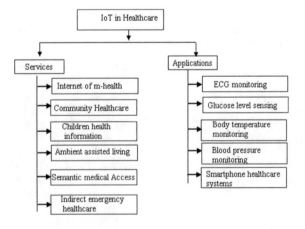

Fig. 2 IoT services and applications in eHealth system

human-caregiver-like support in any emergency situation. There are various IoT-based research works that explained AAL solutions (Istepanian, 2011).

m-IoT is known as Internet of m-health Things. It is a service developed for getting the benefits of ubiquitous computing, wearable body sensors, and communications technologies for healthcare services. The use of m-IoT services has been demonstrated for monitoring the blood sugar level. The design, plan, and implementation scenarios, and challenges of m-IoT are dealt with in Islam et al. (2015); Istepanian et al., 2011).

Community healthcare services appear with the solution of creating a group within the local community (Mondal & Mukherjee, 2016, 2017). For remote healthcare applications, community healthcare plays an important role. With the help of the mobile healthcare delivery system, health assistants diagnose a disease and provide treatment to the patients. One scheme is developed by Das, Mondal, et al., 2018 for assisting the health workers namely ANM (Auxiliary Nurse Midwife) and ASHA (Accredited Social Health Activist), and help them with proper guidelines. In this scheme, the author proposed Mobile-Assisted Remote Healthcare Service (MoRe-Care) for Android mobile device. Further, children's health and the general public health are significant issues in current IoT-based systems. Emotional states of the children, behavioral or mental health problems are also crucial issues. In this regard, children's health information (CHI) services are intended for hospitalized children. It ensures to learn, entertain and empower them. So, this CHI service could be applied to support children to get good nutritional habits.

Semantic medical access is based on IoT to provide medical semantics and ontology. Semantics and ontology use a huge amount of medical information and facts. It has a huge potential to design an IoT-based healthcare system.

Indirect emergency health (IEH) care services include many urgent situations where healthcare issues are seriously engaged. These are bad weather conditions, and transport accidents like air, road, train, etc. IEH suggests a bunch of ways such as data accessibility, alert message, post-accidental cure, and information storing.

2.2 IoT Applications

Like the IoT services, IoT applications also deserve great attention. Health caregivers and patients use IoT applications directly. In this section, some of the important applications are discussed briefly. Blood sugar monitoring finds individual patterns of blood sugar levels and helps patients to schedule their activities and dietary plans. In (Istepanian et al., 2011), the authors proposed an m-IoT-based method for blood sugar monitoring on a real-time basis. For this monitoring, attached sensors collect vital signs from patients and sent them to relevant healthcare providers. They used IPv6 and the IoT devices comprise a blood sugar collector, a smartphone, and a computer. In (Wei et al., 2012), a similar type of work has been done.

Another application is electrocardiogram (ECG) monitoring. The attached sensors are called electrodes and these connect to a monitor. The electrical signals are generated by the heartbeat and recorded. The electrocardiography shows the calculation of the simple heart rate and the pattern of the basic beat (Islam et al., 2015). ECG monitoring has the possibility to furnish the utmost facts and data and can be utilized extensively.

Immunization is one of the main programs to protect children from various life-threatening or infectious diseases. It is a major public health intervention in every country. To alleviate the challenges in the immunization system, MICR (Mobile-Assisted Immunization of Child in Remote Healthcare), a mobile-based child immunization system has been implemented and discussed in Mondal and Mukherjee (2020). It is an android based mobile app which sends alert messages to the registered mobile numbers of new mothers or caregivers as a reminder of vaccination for each child within a given time schedule.

3 Challenges of Health Data

In the previous sections, we have discussed several applications and their benefits in IoT-based eHealth care system. However, several challenges are there which need to be addressed. In this section, some of the current challenges of eHealth care (Firouzi et al., 2018) have been discussed.

3.1 Inter-Domain Authentication and Interoperability

In IoT-based systems, different systems work in different domains. Thus, inter-domain authentication is necessary for systems working in different domains. Healthcare is a very crucial and sensitive domain. Thus, while executing eHealth transaction, it is important to create confidence in the data. There are various eHealth systems that do not have proper accomplishments due to the lack of services to host separate entities. This may be within a country or may be across all the same types of eHealth organizations. The lack of expertise in IT and essential financial support, especially in developing countries, delays the ready approval of the systems.

The other important feature is that there is no policy for universal collaboration among countries for a swap of sensitive medical data. For telemedicine and remote health care, such data exchange is necessary. Further, there is also a lack of interoperability between eHealth ICT infrastructures of various countries. The lack of interoperability among the various devices and platforms makes inter-domain authentication more vulnerable and direct to loss of data isolation.

3.2 Security and Privacy

IoT devices are very much critical with respect to patients' security and privacy. Unlawful right of control to IoT gadgets and sensors might make a severe threat to patients' health as well as to their confidential data (Zeadally et al., 2016). Attached wearable devices collect the critical data from the patient's body. Aggregated and processed data are transferred to the cloud. There are many types of attacks occurred during this process. Devices are vulnerable to security attacks.

Denial of service (DoS) attacks may influence healthcare systems and change patients' personal data. It concerns about patient safety. Using multiple devices, DoS can be easily solvable. However, in the healthcare environment, multiple resources or doubling of resources may not be always feasible as the devices are connected with life-saving systems. In addition, due to the advancement in technology, with the help of powerful search engines, it is possible to locate wearable devices. Also, the lack of security principles of these devices makes them susceptible to different types of security attacks (Das et al., 2018).

Nowadays, many wireless networking technologies, namely: Wi-Fi, BLE, and ZigBee have been deployed in the healthcare environment to give connectivity to various types of medical gadgets and sensors in BAN (Zeadally & Bello, 2019). Security shield of these wireless devices against security attacks like eavesdropping, and sinkhole attacks must compulsory. Personal data, past narration of family, e-medical testimonies, and gene-related data must also be saved from unauthorized access and suspicious software and it imposes safety and isolation (Nambiar et al., 2017). Again, confidentiality and privacy are equally important for doctors. Further, patients do not wish to distribute their sensitive medical information, for example, cancer, TB, or HIV.

3.3 Device Communication

Due to the heterogeneity of the devices used in eHealth infrastructure, each of the devices often communicates with the server with their own languages and communication stack. Therefore, it is difficult for the devices to interact with each other. This gap hinders the main idea behind IoT health care services (Dimitrov, 2016).

Moreover, in some cases Wireless Personal Area Network (WPAN)-allowed devices are worked arbitrarily (Shahamabadi et al., 2013). Hence, the free movement can make in a clash when multiple WPANs work in a parallel frequency domain. This clash in WPANs has some negative impacts because it lessens the performance. It may result in unsuccessful situations, especially when healthcare delivery is concerned. Therefore, it is a crucial concern that IoT gadgets for healthcare operate properly when connected using various types of wireless communication technologies (Gawanmeh, 2016).

Interoperability is essential between health caregivers and service providers within particular IoT fields. It makes big disputes since various IoT devices are operated by a varied group of controlling companies (Firouzi et al., 2018).

In an interoperable connected health system, data floods with one-to-one and one-to-many connections. It may also lead to the switching of data within several interfaces which need systems to help each other.

3.4 Management of Data

The eHealth data generates either from wearable sensors or from medical diagnostic devices that are attached or embedded inside the human body or in the life critical systems. Since the condition of the human body is continuously varying, therefore, a huge amount of data is produced. Also, the data are generated from various medical gadgets. Therefore, these sensed data are heterogeneous in nature. For example, ECG records are frequently obtained in binary or XML format, and data received from camera-based IoT gadgets are generally stored as a different variety of image standards.

Due to the nature (volume and velocity) of the data generated in healthcare systems, several challenges exist. The absence of standardized data collection formats makes it more complex. Integrity is another crucial aspect of big data. Erroneous data may lead to false decisions and consequently to future planning. Since healthcare data frequently comes from heterogeneous devices, therefore, a robust authentication system is needed to make sure that healthcare data are collected from genuine authentic health centers, hospitals, and medical organizations (Tse et al., 2018).

4 Uncertainties in Data

Uncertainty is one of the common characteristics of data. It originates due to various reasons like incomplete data or deficient context of sensor data. It can also be defined as a limitation of data.

Recently, the demand for IoT has increased in various types of applications in healthcare. It provides different supports like remote patient observation, and a smart home system for diabetic and aged patients.

Nowadays, uncertainty gains a lot of attention in healthcare due to several limitations of knowledge. In healthcare, it is difficult to express many problems for the layman, patients, caregivers, technicians, doctors, and health policymaker. Uncertainty has several theoretical definitions, which are not much notable (Han et al., 2011). In the following section, types and sources of uncertainty in healthcare are discussed briefly.

4.1 Types of Uncertainty in Healthcare

According to Hayes (2011), uncertainty is broadly divided into four classes such as: (i) epistemic, (ii) linguistic, (iii) ambiguity, and (iv) variability.

While considering the literature on a patient's illness, Mishel has classified uncertainty as "the inability to determine the meaning of illness-related events" (Mishel, 1988).

In case of ambiguity, the patient's perception of illness is fuzzy and imprecise. Epistemic uncertainty occurs due to limited data (Swiler, 2009). It is also known as subjective uncertainty and reducible uncertainty. Further, variability means people's trust in a range of possibilities. For linguistic uncertainty, the linguistic data "John has a fever" results some uncertainty regarding John's illness, but it cannot be clear about the particular disease. This type of uncertainty is known as linguistic uncertainty.

4.2 Sources of Uncertainty in IoT System

Many reasons could direct the amount of ambiguity in IoT system. Heterogeneity of devices or Interoperability is one of the main reasons that influence the uncertainty in IoT devices. Interoperability shows a vital contribution to smart healthcare. It provides links between multiple devices using diverse internetworking technologies. IoT gadgets that are used for healthcare comprise of a collection of sensors. These sensors are tiny in size and battery-operated. Therefore, an uninterrupted source of energy is required to run these gadgets. This makes a severe challenge in terms of cost and battery life. On the other hand, their computational and storage capabilities are also limited and do not supports complex operations.

On the other hand, a smart healthcare network comprises of billions of devices. Hence, data transmission is another crucial issue. Data transferred from the sensor to another sensor and the control device may affect the quality of the original data due to the outside noise. The better architecture will help to transmit the data without disturbing its originality during transmission.

In the next section, several methods for dealing with these uncertainties have been discussed.

5 Statistical Methods

Various techniques or methods have been in the literature for examining uncertainty. Some of the uncertainty analysis techniques are discussed in this section. Widely varied techniques are probabilistic analysis and fuzzy analysis of data. Several other techniques are also briefly summarized here.

A.   Probabilistic Analysis

Probability analysis is used for finding out uncertain events or outcomes. Probability analysis makes both qualitative and quantitative calculations of uncertainties. While finding likelihood sharing, the individual outcomes are already defined. Here, the associated probabilities with every event have been used to measure the uncertainties. The frequency of the occurrences of the event controls the probability of that event. In (Bilcke et al., 2011), the authors propose a probabilistic method for extracting high-level events from RFID data. In another work (Wasserkrug et al., 2008), the authors propose a framework for comprehension illustration and interpretation enabling the event interface. According to the probabilistic approach, the demonstration of the linked uncertainty value is defined. Additionally, they have defined the likelihood space, and they have explained the formulation of relevant probabilities.

B.   Fuzzy Analysis

Fuzzy analysis is another statistical method. It gives a very helpful way of understanding, quantifying, and handling unclear, ambiguous, and uncertain data. To manage and examine the uncertainty of data, environmental data fuzzy sets are extensively used. While fuzzy logic is used to handle incorrect reasoning in knowledge-based models. It helps to justify ambiguity and doubt of data in the human understanding, and permits to describe in linguistic expressions.

C.   Bayesian Analysis

Bayesian network analysis is another important tool in the family of probabilistic Graphical Models. In literature, the Bayesian network is known as belief networks or Bayes nets. These models are used to characterize facts about a tentative realm.

   Bayes networks are comprised of nodes and edges. Each node in the graph signifies a random variable and the edges correspond to the conditional relationship or dependencies among the variables. The variables may be continuous or discrete. The relationships are estimated using statistical and computational methods. Bayes network always forms a directed acyclic graph and it provides a visible, mathematical expression to state one's certainty in a conceptual model. Bayesian networks work as a risk estimation mechanism and it has been used as a practical and technical method having a system with "high uncertainty".

   Bayesian Networks have the property to contain a large number of contacting devices, and therefore, it is used as an efficient uncertainty modeling technique. However, for a large data set or domain, Bayes Net is not suitable.

D.   Soft Computing Technique

Fuzzy logic, neural networks, and probabilistic analysis are part of soft computing techniques. The primary objective of soft computing is to deal with precision making, and decrease cost by exploiting the tolerance for uncertainty. Fuzzy system is more efficient in extracting facts since its representation of it allows rescheduling the knowledge extracted from the system reverse into linguistic terms. Hence, fuzzy systems have a high possibility of finding out knowledge.

E.   Rule-Based Classification Technique

To classify uncertain data, rule-based classification and prediction algorithms are used. For pruning data, creating new rule-based classification, and improving rules, several new features are introduced in the algorithms. Uncertain data interval and probability distribution function are used to compute these new measures. The sequential covering method is used to extract features from the data.

6   Case Studies

In this section, a case study on blood pressure (BP) vital signs of patients is presented. The experiments have been carried out by the authors (Wasserkrug et al., 2005), where they have conducted a real-time BP measurement using manual analog sphygmomanometer and another digital cooking Hacks eHealth biometric sensor. The goal of this study has been to understand the nature of the error by considering two cases.

Case1: BP of multiple persons has been collected in a kiosk using a Mercury Sphygmomanometer and the Cooking Hacks eHealth sensor. Data of every person has been taken once and randomly. The total number of sample data was 116.

Case2: BP of specific individuals was collected over varied time periods with data of every person being taken multiple times in a day. The table below shows the sample data.

Table 1 represents the sample data of individual persons for Case 2.

In this study, the authors focused on understanding the accuracy and precision-related errors in digital BP sensors, considering the manual ones as accurate. They first find out the accuracy-related error and then determined the precision error, if any, generated by the digital sensor. For accuracy-related error, they analyzed the relationship between digital and analog sensors. In the second case, model or pattern of BP of each individual has been determined, and once understood how the blood pressure varies precision error has been calculated.

Table 1 Sample data of individual persons over varied time periods (Gupta & Mukherjee, 2017)

No. of sample	No. of days data collected	Sample sizes
Person 1	9	34
Person 2	7	13
Person 3	4	10
Person 4	6	13
Person 5	6	8
Person 6	9	14
Person 7	5	10
Person 8	3	10
Person 9	9	16
Person 10	3	4

The steps are as follows:

Step 1: Accuracy-Related Error Reduction:

This is done by finding a relationship between analog and digital sensors dynamically using regression and neural network.

Step 2: Precision-Related Error Reduction:

During the entire experiment, blood pressure has been measured using both the manual, as well as digital BP sensors for the same person multiple times. The corresponding mean and standard deviation are calculated to analyze the preciseness of the sensor data. Based on the analysis of the collected data, a pattern for each individual has been generated. For example, if the general tendency of the systolic and the diastolic pressure for a person is above normal, then it is obvious that future readings will follow the hypertension reads as well for the same person. Otherwise, if suddenly the BP shows low readings from the mentioned range, then it is likely to be an instrumental error or some sudden sickness of the concerned person and further readings are to be taken for checking.

Step 3: Combining both to find the Correct Pressure:

To find out the correct final digital BP, it is required to find the relationship between analog systolic and analog diastolic BP. Therefore, there is a need to merge these two datasets. They have done this merging using a fuzzy mapping model.

6.1   Accuracy-Related Error Prediction

In the first part of the experiment, the author (Gupta & Mukherjee, 2017) focused on understanding the nature of errors by plotting the deviation of the digital sensor data from the analog sensor data. The histograms generated through this process are shown in Fig. 3.

Next, a model was developed; so that future prediction can be done based on the model and any error associated with the digital sensor data can be removed based on this model. With the sample data size of 278, 80% of data have been used for deriving or constructing the model, and the remaining 20% of data have been used to validate the prediction process. After analyzing the data, the corresponding error is predicted.

6.2   Results for Precision Error Reduction

In this section, the precision error calculation has been depicted for the previously mentioned data. Table 2 shows the standard BP range variants as suggested by

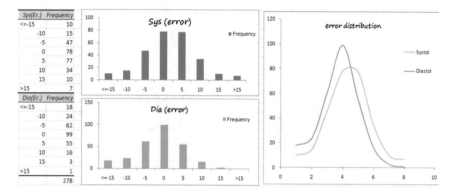

Fig. 3 Histograms corresponding to the systolic-diastolic error distributions

Table 2 Standard BP range variants

Bp range variants	Systolic (mmHg)	Diastolic (mmHg)
Normal	<120 and	<80
Pre-hypertension	120–139 or	80–89
Stage1 hypertension	140–159 or	90–99
Stage 2 hypertension	>160 or	>100
Hypertensive crisis	>180 or	>110
Hypotension	<=90 or	<=60

the American Heart Association (Nag, 2018) which the authors have used while categorization of behavioral patterns of an individual.

As mentioned in Case 2, the BP readings are sampled over varied time periods with data of every person being taken multiple times. Figure 4 shows the corresponding systolic and diastolic readings for person 1 using both the analog and digital devices. In this chapter, we have included only one graph from Gupta and Mukherjee, (2017).

From the graph, the normal tendency of the blood pressure of a person can be determined, which can be classified in Table 2. Any deviation from the normal range while measuring the BP may be due to an error in the instrument or may be due to a sudden change in the health condition of the patient. Thus, advanced techniques, such as neural network or fuzzy logic may be implemented to decide the actual reason for the deviation. Here also a model may be derived and used to predict any kind of precision-related error.

7 Virtual Sensor-Based Infrastructure

A Virtual sensor is a software sensor, which provides the abstraction of one or more physical sensors in the cloud and can be enabled as per the requirement (Wasserkrug

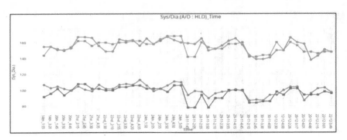

1. Time(1:30 pm to 4:30pm) Person 1 (total 4 samples /hour.),collected for 11 days.

2. Analog range : (Sys) [139 – 167] (Dia) [87 -113] , Digital range : (Sys) [139 –
167]   (Dia) [87 -113]

3. As most number of readings fall in the 140-160/90-100 zone for the entire 11 days
experiment. Therefore, person is indicative of ' hypertension Stage 1'.

4. errors: Sys = 167 Dia = 113 may be due to erroneous sensor read/ sickness

Fig. 4 Systolic and Diastolic measurements using both analog and digital devices of person 1

et al., 2005). The advantage of such abstraction has primarily been to hide heterogeneity. Each physical sensor is set with its purpose beforehand, while the virtual
sensor is designed to act as per application demand. Thus, virtual sensors offer indirect measurements of the environmental states by uniting sensed data from a group
of various sensors.

A virtual sensor network (VSN) consists of multiple subsets of sensor networks
(Mukherjee et al., 2016) and each subset is dedicated to a certain task or an application. Thus, VSN consists of various diverse sensor networks from different sensor
infrastructure provider (SIP). VSN is a promising skill that separates the real sensor
deployment from the applications running on it. It supports several services and applications for the end users. VSN provides manifold logical networks over a single real
network infrastructure (Circulation, 2010).

For recent development in technology, it is likely to segregate the services from the
infrastructure to provide multiple services on top of WSN. Using the virtualization
technique, physical resources can be presented logically over a physical WSN for
sharing and efficient use. Thus, virtualization of WSN can be considered to split the
roles of traditional WSN service providers into two parts, namely: sensor infrastructure provider (SIP) and sensor virtualization network service provider (SVNSP). SIP
manages the physical sensor infrastructure and SVNSP provides multiple services
(Circulation, 2010).

Therefore, a virtual sensor layer contains logical occurrences of sensors that set
up multiple applications or services. For example, if VSN permits p number of
applications, then it should have at least p number of virtual sensor layers, each layer
dedicated to a particular task.

The above logical representation of physical resources based on virtualization
technologies enables the end users to share the resources and request services on
"as and when required basis". It also enables the infrastructure providers to place

the sensing resources in a shared resource pool and make them available in an open market place anytime anywhere (Das et al., 2014).

Furthermore, in eHealth applications, sensor data needs to be analyzed in real time, thus requiring sufficient computational power. However, physical sensing devices are resource-constrained and may not be able to analyze the data efficiently if sufficient computational power is not available. Uncertainty reduction, as discussed in the previous section, also involves computations which need to be performed in real time. Virtual sensors created in the edge devices or in the cloud can be engaged to carry out these tasks.

Figure 5 represents the virtual sensor infrastructure for eHealth system. In this scenario, multiple real sensors are placed on the patient's body and virtual sensors are deployed in the middle layer. The cloud gateway is used to connect the user layer and middle layer. The virtual sensor receives data from the real sensors. Then the interleaving process has done and sends the merged data for exploitation by an application or a service (Bose et al., 2015).

Fig. 5 Layered structure of IoT sensor-cloud in ehealth system

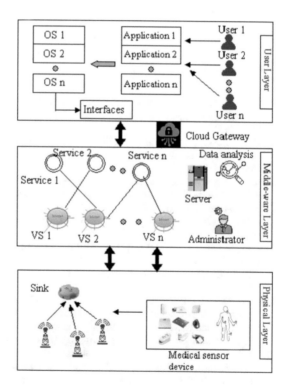

8 Conclusion

In the field of eHealth, IoT has been extensively recognized as potential solution. This advanced technology provides remote as well as emergency healthcare services to the patients. It is also used as eHealth application with different features such as early detection of vital signs, emergency warning and computer-assisted therapy. It focuses on helping physically challenged and elderly people to live independently in their lives. It also takes care of patients with chronic diseases since there is no need for physical check up. In spite of these facilities, IoT-based healthcare system poses various challenges in it. The challenges like privacy and security, inter-domain authentication and interoperability of devices, device communication, and data management are discussed. Data uncertainty is another challenge which is also explained here. Statistical methods for removing erroneous and vague readings from the data have been discussed. Finally, case studies regarding BP measurements of multiple persons have been illustrated. In this study, error patterns regarding the uncertainty of measured data have been demonstrated.

References

Baker, S. B., Xiang, W., & Atkinson, I. (2017). Internet of things for smart healthcare: Technologies, challenges, and opportunities. *IEEE Access, 5*, 26521–26544. https://doi.org/10.1109/ACCESS. 2017.2775180

Bilcke, J., Beutels, P., Brisson, M., & Jit, M. (2011). Accounting for methodological, structural, and parameter uncertainty in decision-analytic models: A practical guide. *Medical Decision Making, 31*(4), 675–692.

Bose, S., Gupta, A., Adhikary, S., & Mukherjee, N. (2015). Towards a sensor-cloud infrastructure with sensor virtualization. In: *Proceedings of the Second Workshop on Mobile Sensing, Computing and Communication* (pp. 25–30).

Circulation. (2010). 122, pp. S640–S656. https://doi.org/10.1161/CIRCULATIONAHA.110. 970889.

Das, R., Mondal, S., & Mukherjee, N. (2018a). MoRe-care: Mobile-assisted remote healthcare service delivery. In: *10th International Conference on Communication Systems & Networks (COMSNETS)* (pp. 677–681). Bengaluru: India. https://doi.org/10.1109/COMSNETS.2018a.832 8294.

Das, H., Naik, B., Pati, B., & Panigrahi, C. R. (2014). A Survey on Virtual Sensor Networks Framework. *International Journal of Grid and Distributed Computing, 7*, 121–130.

Das, A. K., Zeadally, S., & He, D. (2018). Taxonomy and analysis of security protocols for internet of things. *Future Generation Computer Systems, 89*, 110–125.

Dimitrov, D. V. (2016). Medical internet of things and big data in healthcare. *Healthcare Informatics Research, 22*(3), 156–163. www.ncbi.nlm.nih.gov/pmc/articles/PMC4981575/.

Firouzi, F., Farahani, B., Ibrahim, M., & Chakrabarty, K. (2018). From EDA to IoT eHealth: Promise, challenges, and solutions. *IEEE Transactions on Computer-Aided Design of Integrated Circuits and Systems, 37*(12), 2965–2978.

Gawanmeh, A. (2016). Open issues in reliability, safety, and efficiency of connected health. In: *First IEEE Conference on Connected Health: Applications, Systems and Engineering Technologies.* Washington, DC.

Gope, P., & Hwang, T. (2016). BSN-care: A secure IoTBased modern healthcare system using body sensor network. *IEEE Sensors Journal, 16*(5), 1368–1376.

Gupta, A., & Mukherjee, N. (2017). Can the challenges of IOT be overcome by virtual sensors. In: *2017 IEEE International Conference on Internet of Things (iThings) and IEEE Green Computing and Communications (GreenCom) and IEEE Cyber, Physical and Social Computing (CPSCom) and IEEE Smart Data (SmartData), Exeter* (pp. 584–590). https://doi.org/10.1109/iThings-GreenCom-CPSCom-SmartData.2017.92.

Han, P. K., Klein, W. M., & Arora, N. K. (2011). Varieties of uncertainty in health care: a conceptual taxonomy. *Medical Decision Making, 31*(6), 828–838. https://doi.org/10.1177/0272989x11393976. PMID: 22067431; PMCID: PMC3146626.

Hayes, K. R. (2011). Uncertainty and uncertainty analysis methods.

Istepanian, R. S. H. (2011). The potential of Internet of Things (IoT) for assisted living applications. In: *Proceeding IET Seminar Assistance Living* (pp. 1–40).

Istepanian, R. S. H., Hu, S., Philip, N. Y., & Sungoor, A. (2011). The potential of Internet of m-health Things 'm-IoT' for non-invasive glucose level sensing. In: *Proceeding IEEE Annual International Conferences Enggineering Medical Biological Society (EMBC)* (pp. 5264–5266).

Islam, S. M. R., Kwak, D., Kabir, M. H., Hossain, M., & Kwak, K. (2015). The internet of things for health care: A comprehensive survey. *IEEE Access, 3*, 678–708. https://doi.org/10.1109/ACCESS.2015.2437951

Larson, E. C., Goel, M., Redeld, M., Boriello, G., Rosenfeld, M., & Patel, S. N. (2013). Tracking lung function on any phone. In: *Proceedings of ACM Symposium Computer Development*, Art. ID 29.

Mondal, S., & Mukherjee, N. (2016). Mobile-assisted remote healthcare delivery. In: *2016 Fourth International Conference on Parallel, Distributed and Grid Computing (PDGC)* (pp. 630–635). Waknaghat. https://doi.org/10.1109/PDGC.2016.7913199.

Mondal, S., & Mukherjee, N. (2017). A framework for ICT-based primary healthcare delivery for children. In: *2017 9th International Conference on Communication Systems and Networks (COMSNETS)* (pp. 525–529). Bangalore. https://doi.org/10.1109/COMSNETS.2017.7945447.

Mondal, S., & Nandini, M. (2020). MICR: mobile-assisted immunization of child in remote healthcare. In: *4th International Conference on Intelligent Computing and Communication (ICICC–2020)*.

Mishel, M. H. (1988). Uncertainty in illness. *Image: The Journal of Nursing Scholarship Winter, 20*(4), 225–232. [PubMed: 3203947]

Mukherjee, N., Bhunia, S. S., & Bose, S. (2016). Virtual sensors in remote healthcare delivery: Some case studies. HEALTHINF 484–489.

Nag, A. (2018) A study on measurement errors in e-health sensors. M. Tech Thesis, Department of Computer Science and Engineering, Jadavpur University, India.

Nambiar, A. R., Reddy, N., & Dutta, D. (2017). Connected health: Opportunities and challenges. In: *IEEE International Conference on Big Data* (pp. 1658–1662). IEEE: Boston, MA.

Perrier, E. (2015). Positive disruption: Healthcare, ageing & participation in the age of technology. Australia: The McKell Institute.

Shahamabadi, M. S., Ali, B. B. M., Varahram, P., & Jara, A. J. (2013). A network mobility solution based on 6LoWPAN hospital wireless sensor network (NEMO-HWSN). In: *Proceedings 7th International Conferences Innovation Mobile Internet Services Ubiquitous Comput. (IMIS)* (pp. 433–438).

Swiler, L. P., Paez, T. L., & Mayes, R. L. (2009). Uncertainty Analysis. In: *Proceeding of IMAC*.

Tse, D., Chow, C. K., Ly, T. P., Tong, C. Y. & Tam, K. W. (2018). The challenges of big data governance in healthcare. In: *17th IEEE International Conference on Trust, Security and Privacy in Computing and Communications*. New York.

Wasserkrug, S., Gal, A., & Etzion, O. (2005). A model for reasoning with uncertain rules in event composition systems. In: *Proceedings of 21st Conferences Uncertainty in Artificial Intelligence (UAI '05)* (pp. 599–606).

Wasserkrug, S., Gal, A., Etzion, O., & Turchin, Y. (2008). Complex event processing over uncertain data. In: *Proceeding of Second International Conferences Distributed Event-Based Systems (DEBS '08)* (pp. 253–264).

Wei, L., Heng, Y., & Lin, W. Y. (2012). Things based wireless data transmission of blood glucose measuring instruments. Chinese Patent 202 154 684 U, Mar. 7.

Zeadally, S., Isaac, J. T., & Baig, Z. (2016). Security attacks and solutions in electronic health (E-health) systems. *Journal of Medical Systems, 40*(12), 263.

Zeadally, S., & Bello, O. (2019). Harnessing the power of internet of things based connectivity to improve healthcare. *Internet of Things* 100074. https://doi.org/10.1016/j.iot.2019.100074.

Zeadally, S., Siddiqui, F., Baig, Z., & Ibrahim, A. (2019). Smart healthcare: Challenges and potential solutions using internet of things (IoT) and big data analytics. *PSU Research Review, 4*(2), 149–168.

Context and Body Vitals Monitoring Systems

Human Activity Recognition Systems Based on Sensor Data Using Machine Learning

Seemanti Saha and **Rajarshi Bhattacharya**

Abstract An increase in life expectancy is leading to an aging society, where gradual degradation in physical/cognitive health could result in fall injuries, cardiovascular, neurological/psychological problems, or a sedentary lifestyle. Sensor-based human activity recognition (HAR) is found to be a potential assistive technology in this context to improve the quality of life of an aging society. This chapter presents the state of the art and future trends of Internet of Things (IoT)-enabled sensor data-based Human Activity Recognition (HAR) systems, where machine learning (ML)/deep learning (DL) is used to classify human actions in the context of healthcare applications. In particular, the impact of IoT on the healthcare industry is so immense that a dedicated specialization, termed as Internet of Healthcare Things (IoHT), has emerged. Smart healthcare systems are equipped with different categories of sensors (wearable, wireless, and ambient). The huge amount of sensor data acquired by IoHT sensors allows for performing accurate HAR. The HAR involves detection/classification problems, e.g. fall detection and seizer detection, where ML is used extensively, at its heart. A lot of ML/DL techniques are being used in HAR including support vector machine (SVM), artificial neural network (ANN), recurrent neural network (RNN), convolutional neural network (CNN), deep neural network (DNN), long short-term memory (LSTM), etc. However, there are a few special aspects of HAR sensor data that make it difficult to handle. Involved research is still being pursued across the globe to solve these problems.

Keywords IoT · IoHT · Health care · HAR · Sensor · Machine learning (ML) · Deep learning (DL)

S. Saha (✉) · R. Bhattacharya
Department of Electronics and Communication Engineering, National Institute of Technology, Patna, India
e-mail: seemanti@nitp.ac.in

R. Bhattacharya
e-mail: r.b.1980@ieee.org

1   Introduction

This chapter aims to provide a comprehensive discussion on the state of the art and future of Internet of Things (IoT)-enabled sensor data-based Human Activity Recognition (HAR) systems in the context of smart health care. The chapter focuses on machine learning (ML) (Bhoi et al., 2020; Bishop, 2006) /deep learning (DL) (Goodfellow et al., 2016) -based HAR for healthcare applications. Along with rapid advancement in fog/edge computing, cloud computing, etc., and unprecedented growth of ML/DL-based techniques, IoT has become a disruptive technology in the context of big data, smart homes, smart hospitals, smart cities, etc. (Cui et al., 2018). In recent years, the proliferation of IoT is seen almost in all sectors: From health care to industry, from consumer services to infrastructure management, and from governance to military applications. With this explosion in the placement of IoT devices, IoT is playing a pivotal role in the healthcare industry and healthcare management to make them more personalized, operational, practical, proactive, and of course cost-effective. Hence, a new paradigm termed as Internet of Healthcare Things (IoHT) or Internet of Medical Things (IoMT) has been coined (Habibzadeh et al., 2020). A representative diagram of an IoHT is shown below in Fig. 1.

The key features of IoT take into account energy-efficient IoT devices embedded with sensors connected over a network that helps in sensing followed by data acquisition. The definition of "IoT," given by IEEE, is *"a network of items each of which*

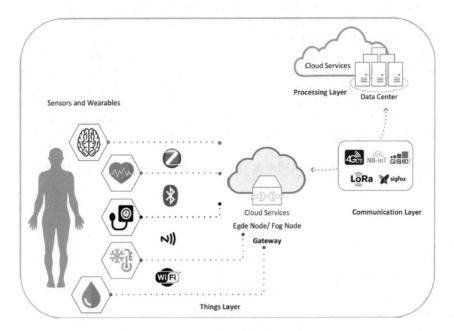

Fig. 1 A representative diagram of an IoHT. The enabling communication technologies along with Fog/Edge and Cloud computing at different layers are depicted (Qadri et al., 2020)

is embedded with sensors and these sensors are connected to the Internet" (Qadri et al., 2020). Smart healthcare systems are equipped with *different categories of IoT sensors*, viz.,

(i)   Wearable sensors, which are classically used in wireless body area networks (WBAN);
(ii)   Ambient sensors, e.g. surveillance cameras and passive infrared sensors;
(iii)   Smartphones, smartwatches, smart clothes, etc.;
(iv)   Wi-Fi hub, RFID, Frequency-Modulated Continuous Wave (FMCW) radar, etc.

The huge amount of sensor data, gathered by different IoHT devices, allows us to perform accurate human activity recognition (HAR). HAR plays an important role in a wide-ranging application in the context of IoHT-enabled smart health care (Dinarević et al., 2019). Acquired sensor data is evaluated and analyzed with an aim to recognize activities leading to a healthy lifestyle that includes physical activities on a daily basis. Lack of daily physical activities results in cardiovascular disorders, diabetes, a higher risk of stress, and musculoskeletal disorders (Dinarević et al., 2019). In health care, the detection and prevention of numerous chronic diseases could be done by HAR (Li et al., 2018). In patients with Parkinson's, dementia, and other psychological disorders, HAR-based monitoring can help in recognizing the abnormalities in regular lifestyle, which, in turn, prevents undesirable consequences (Lara & Labrador, 2013). Also, HAR can effectively be used in psychological health-care applications as it can recognize sedentary behaviors. Most importantly, in elderly health care, non-intrusive activity sensing can play a pivotal role in long-term monitoring, fall/seizure detection, etc. and/or providing remote medical help (Chen et al., 2018). In HAR, we try to solve involved detection/classification problems, e.g. fall detection and seizer detection, which are depicted in Fig. 2.

1.1   Classification of HAR According to Sensor Deployment

HAR systems are classified into three modalities in terms of the *sensor deployment in the IoHT* environment (Wang et al., 2019):

(i)   HAR based on Ambient Sensor (AS-HAR);
(ii)   HAR based on Wearable Sensor (WS-HAR);
(iii)   HAR based on Hybrid Sensor (HS-HAR).

AS-HAR systems recognize human activities from the data acquired from ambient sensors that are installed in surroundings like doors, walls, floors, kettles, furniture, etc. The ambient sensors include a read switch sensor, light sensor, passive infrared (PIR), radio frequency identification (RFID), pressure sensor, flow sensor, temperature (Debes et al., 2016; Wang et al., 2019), etc. AS-HAR sensor is less intrusive as there is no on-body deployment. But it is less flexible and demands more complex sensor placement at home. Further, AS-HAR operates in a restricted area, in which

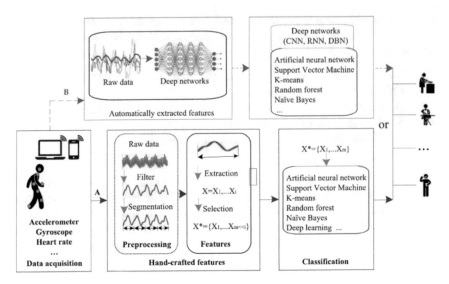

Fig. 2 Human activity recognition from sensing data; the basic enabling technologies include the enabling ML/DL algorithms that perform the HAR (Wang et al., 2019)

the sensors are installed. Further, ambient sensors become non-functional when the consumer does not communicate with the objects containing those sensors or does not move in the operational area of an ambient sensor.

Alternatively, WS-HAR gathers the data from wearable sensors and performs HAR by mining the data using ML algorithms. The functioning area of WS-HAR is relatively large compared to the AS-HAR area when the person is on the move. Of late, smartphones, smart clothes, smartwatches, and other specially designed devices with embedded sensors are used as wearable devices in HAR (Bianchi et al., 2019; Lara & Labrador, 2013; Qi et al., 2019a; Wang et al., 2019; Zhou et al., 2020). Generally, the performance and robustness of WS-HAR are enhanced by placing more sensors on different body parts (e.g. wrists, feet, head, legs, and waist) (Wang et al., 2019). However, complex sensor deployment with more number of sensors on the body results in higher costs, difficulties in deployment, and intrusions for aging people with an independent lifestyle.

AS-HAR and WS-HAR both have their own merits and demerits. It is evident that recognition accuracy could be enhanced by combining different sensor modalities (Muaaz et al., 2020). In (Bianchi et al., 2019), the authors proposed WiWeHAR— which combines Wi-Fi and wearable sensing modalities to sense human activities. More accurate information about human actions could be obtained from the blend of different sensor modalities, which, in turn, improves the HAR performance. Nonetheless, HS-HAR would increase both the complexity and cost of HAR in comparison to a single sensor-based HAR. Moreover, data fusion along with sensing synchronization from multiple sensor modalities are required in HS-HAR.

Among all three sensor modalities, WS-HAR is a more attractive solution due to its flexibility in daily use, low cost, and acceptable performance (Wang et al., 2019). Hence, WS-HAR has found extensive usage in assisted living, such as rehabilitation (Hermanis et al., 2016), gait analysis (Anwary et al., 2018), fall detection (Jung et al., 2015), sports assessment (Qi et al., 2019b), and daily activity analysis (Wang et al., 2018).

1.2   General Components of HAR System

The HAR in IoHT is a complex process, and could be accomplished in the following steps:

(i)   *Selection* and *deployment* of appropriate sensors on the human body or in the surroundings to acquire the user's health data for a long duration.

(ii) *Data acquisition* from the deployed IoHT sensors, *Data Communication,* and *Data preprocessing* of gathered data at *edge/fog/cloud.*

(i)   Selection and deployment of appropriate sensors to acquire health data

A generic data acquisition architecture is depicted in Fig. 3 (Lara & Labrador, 2013). Sensor data is collected in integration devices, viz., smartphones, PDA, laptops, or in a customized embedded system. Preprocessed data from integration devices are communicated through Wi-Fi or cellular networks to edge/cloud servers for real-time monitoring, visualizing, and/or analyzing. Previously, researchers have done a lot of work on HAR in IoHT with wearable sensors typically used in WBAN (Lara & Labrador, 2013), wireless sensing using Wi-Fi hub and FMCW radar (Liu et al., 2020), contactless sensing (Dinarević et al., 2019), and smartphones () with tri-axial gyroscope, tri-axial accelerometer, magnetometer, proximity sensor, GPS, etc. A detailed discussion on wearable sensors for HAR in health care is presented in Wang et al., 2019. Contactless sensing incorporates different ambient sensors

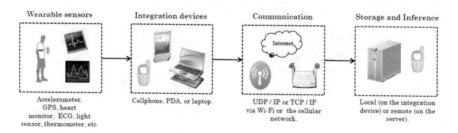

Fig. 3 Data acquisition and communication architecture for HAR (Lara & Labrador, 2013)

Table 1 Smartphone sensors used for health monitoring

Monitored health issues	Typically used smartphone sensors
Cardiovascular activity, e.g. heart rate (HR) and HR variability (HRV)	Image sensor (camera), microphone
Eye health	Image sensor (camera)
Respiratory and lung health	Image sensor (camera), microphone
Skin health	Image sensor (camera)
Daily activity and fall	Motion sensors (accelerometer, gyroscope, proximity sensor), Global Positioning System (GPS)
Ear health	Microphone
Cognitive function and mental health	Motion sensors (accelerometer, gyroscope), camera, light sensor, GPS

(MacHot et al., 2018), like temperature sensors, motion sensors, a door/burner sensor, hot/cold water sensors, image and video sensors (Acharya & Gantayat, 2015), etc. Table 1 presents the monitored health issues using different embedded sensors of the smartphone (Majumder & Deen, 2019). The data acquired by the sensors could be analyzed/displayed on the phone through some mobile App and/or transmitted to a remote healthcare facility or healthcare provider through various wireless communication platforms.

Wireless sensing using Wi-Fi signals and radar signals is depicted in Fig. 4. Since the performance level in activity recognition depends on sets of activities (Liu et al., 2020), different authors used various sets of possible activities in their research. They also can use the public datasets available for HAR to evaluate their proposed methods or compare their methods with other studies on the same datasets (Wang et al., 2019), e.g. *PAMAP2, SBHAR, mHealth, WISDM, REALDISP, MobiAct, and OPPORTUNITY*. Besides, discussion on all kinds of IoHT sensors, not limited to HAR and the commercially available IoHT sensors, is detailed in Ray et al. (2020). However, the scope of this chapter is limited to sensor data-based HAR in IoHT.

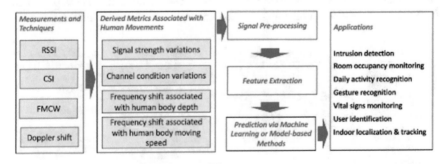

Fig. 4 A typical workflow of human activity recognition using wireless sensing (Liu et al., 2020)

(ii)   **Data acquisition from the deployed IoHT sensors, Data communication, and Data preprocessing of gathered data at edge/fog/cloud**

These sensors should communicate with an integration device (ID), which can be a smartphone, a PDA, a laptop, or a customized embedded system. The main purpose of the ID is to preprocess the data received from the sensors and, in some cases, send them to an application server for real-time monitoring, visualization, and/or analysis (Qadri et al., 2020). The communication protocol might be UDP/IP or TCP/IP, according to the desired level of reliability. Most of the connectivity from an IoHT perspective is provided by Wireless Personal Area network technologies, viz., Bluetooth, ZigBee, and/or Wi-Fi technologies to send the acquired data to nearby access points or at the edge devices for edge computing. To send the healthcare data to a remote server, WiMax and cellular networks play a key role. An interconnected network of WiMax, the IP protocol network, and access service networks stream the healthcare data for remote patient monitoring (Dhanvijay & Patil, 2019).

The processing unit for extracting the useful features from the collected data can be implemented either on a local processing unit or at a remote cloud server (Qadri et al., 2020). A cloud-based solution is more practical as the amount of gathered healthcare data is huge. However, the delay induced by transporting the data from the sensor to the cloud is more significant than the delay incurred by processing the data at a local processing unit known as an *edge node*. Furthermore, an additional layer of distributed computing resources is included in the structure. This layer is known as the *fog layer*. The advantages of the fog layer include reduced latency, improved data processing, enhanced security, and being increasingly interoperable.

1.3   *Few Challenges of HAR in IoHT with Their Solution*

There are lot many challenges that motivate the research in HAR to enhance its accuracy under a more realistic scenario as follows:

(1)   One of the major challenges in the design and optimization of HARs is to envisage a clear picture of the activities under consideration and understand their characteristics (Bulling et al., 2014). With this goal, a few indexing tools like the *Activities of Daily Living* (ADLs) index have been developed in elderly care.

(2)   There are also experimental challenges accompanying data acquisition and the validation of HAR systems under realistic conditions. Data acquisition poses wide-ranging requirements, viz., high data quality, long-term recordings, large numbers of sensors, and so on. A closer look reveals that the analog-to-digital converter (ADC) and battery are two critical components in this respect. It is well known that a huge amount of research is going on the battery to reduce the cost, weight, size, form factor, etc. and increase the charge storage capacity, battery life, etc. Research is also going on designing low power, low cost, high

sampling-rate ADC (Petrie et al., 2020; Jotschke et al., 2020, Verma et al., 2020).

(3) Many of the health-monitoring sensors are classically intrusive in nature and it creates a true hazard in IoHT, especially in the context of assisted daily living of elderly people. Throughout the world, research is being carried out to invent low-cost noninvasive sensors of small form-factor and superior accuracy. Presently, low-cost non-invasive sensors are available for monitoring blood pressure and heart rate (Queyam et al., 2018; Wang et al., 2018), hemoglobin (Acharya et al., 2020; Hasan et al., 2019), plasma glucose (Choi et al., 2015; Kim et al., 2018), blood oxygen level (Bui et al., 2017), core body temperature (Mazgaoker et al., 2017), etc.

(4) Furthermore, HAR system design and implementation also face tough challenges regarding a trade-off between system latency, processing power, and accuracy. 5G communication reduces the latency to less than 1 ms. The required processing power has been achieved through the onset of fog/edge/cloud computing. Apart from the choice of the proper algorithms, the accuracy of HAR largely depends upon successful data collection as well. With the advent of big data technology, the problem of data collection is likely to be alleviated.

(5) Another challenge in HAR is handling weakly labeled data. Handling of weakly labeled data is dealt with in Sect. 3 (Qi, Yang, et al., 2019).

2 Activity Recognition Method: A Machine Learning (ML) Approach

ML-based classification algorithms are extensively being used in HAR to solve various involved detection/classification problems, e.g. fall detection and seizer detection, which have serious consequences in elderly and/or in ill patients. Therefore, in this section, we begin our discussion with the necessity of ML in HAR problems followed by a discussion on the basic steps of ML-based HAR.

2.1 Why ML is to Be Used in HAR

Classification of different human activities is a involved problem in the sense the human activities are ambiguous themselves and are often weekly labeled. Furthermore, the effect of such human activities on different sensor data is not always logically interpretable in a straightforward manner. Hence, a sensitive task like HAR, where misdetection and false alarm could be heavily consequential, is accomplished using advanced statistical tools of machine learning. On the other hand, massive growth in the IoHT sector owes to providing a huge amount of training and testing data to solve different types of HAR problems in connection with healthcare services. This has sparked the opportunity of using the demanding deep learning algorithms utilizing the edge computing facility of modern wireless network architecture, and a huge amount of research is initiated throughout the globe in ML/DL-based HAR (Cui et al., 2018; Ravi et al., 2017).

2.2 Data Preprocessing:

Raw data preprocessing is a very important step in any pattern recognition system and HAR is also no exception to that. In simple language, preprocessing is a sort of "cleaning" of the data/signal and making it ready for further operations like feature classification, prediction, etc. The very first step for data preprocessing, especially in the case of ML, is normalization. The subsequent steps of preprocessing HAR sensor data are as follows:

(i)   *Denoising* through low-pass filtering or by using Discrete Wavelet Transform (DWT), etc.
(ii) *Conversion of time-domain signal or data log to image like* $2D$ *matrix* to facilitate the usage of the plethora of deep learning techniques, developed mainly in connection with image processing. However, this step is not mandatory.
(iii) *Segmentation* using different algorithms as per the origin of the signal.
(iv) *Feature Extraction.*
(v)   *Feature Selection and Dimensionality Reduction.*

First, we will introduce the typical HAR signals, as depicted in Figs. 5, 6, 7, 8 and Fig. 9, before discussing the data preprocessing techniques.

(i)   Denoising

The typical raw sensor data shown above are evidently highly noisy in nature. Therefore, the very first step in HAR is denoising. Generally, Butterworth (Wang et al., 2020; Yan et al., 2020), Chebyshev, or Elliptic filter (Qi et al., 2020; Qi et al., 2019b) is used depending upon the requirement (Lutovac et al., 2001). Two examples of such filtering are shown below in Figs. 10 and 11.

However, care is taken so that vital information is not lost during denoising. This is especially applicable in the cases, where the edge information of the signal is used for the detection of human activity as shown in Fig. 12.

In these cases, discrete wavelet transform (DWT) is used and the approximation coefficient, which automatically removes the fast-changing component of the signal, is used (Bhat et al., 2019; Kumar et al., 2018).

(ii) Conversion of time-domain signal or data log to image like 2—D matrix:

This step is not mandatory. In many cases, the 1—D time-domain signal is directly used in ML. Two such cases are elaborated in Sect. 4.3 (Abdel-Basset et al., 2020; Qi et al., 2019a). However, in many cases the measured time-domain signal is converted

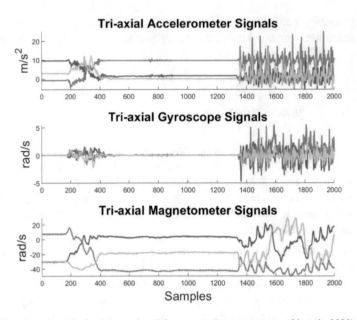

Fig. 5 Signal produced by body-worn inertial sensor and magnetometer (Qi et al., 2020)

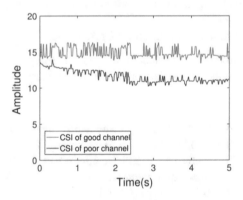

Fig. 6 Comparison of CSI values of two radio channels of different quality (Wang et al., 2020)

into a 2—D matrix so that the modern ML/DL techniques, which were mostly developed in connection with image processing, could be applied. Obtaining a spectrogram of a time-varying signal is very useful for this purpose. A spectrogram of an inertial signal $x[\xi]$ is a representation of the same as a function of frequency-index ϖ and time-index ξ. Generally, a spectrogram is generated using short-time Fourier transform (STFT). A brief outline of the technique is given below.

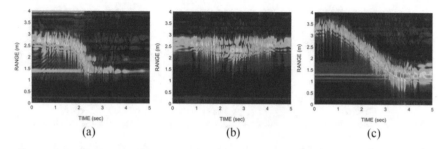

Fig. 7 CSI of a radio channel, which could easily be extracted from Wi-Fi nodes using freely available dedicated tool (Chowdhury, 2018; Wang et al., 2020)

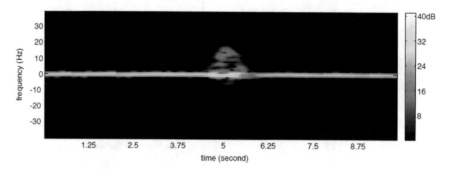

Fig. 8 Frequency-time Doppler profile obtained from pulse-Doppler radar of an example gesture (Pu et al., 2013). The user moves her hand toward the receiver

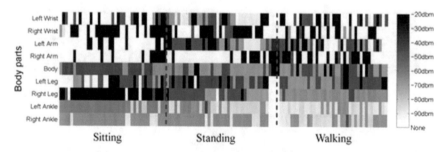

Fig. 9 Average RSS with different activities over time (Wang et al., 2017a) obtained from wearable RFID tag

$$STFT\{x[\xi]\} = X(\zeta, \varpi) = \sum_{\xi=-\infty}^{\infty} x[n]\Xi[\xi - \zeta]e^{-j\varpi\xi} \tag{1}$$

Here, $x[\xi]$ is the signal to be represented in the time–frequency domain and $\Xi[\xi - m]$ is the window function, shifted by ζ points. The spectrogram is given by

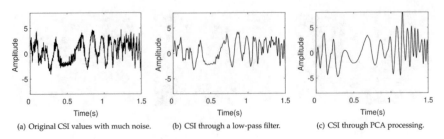

(a) Original CSI values with much noise.   (b) CSI through a low-pass filter.   (c) CSI through PCA processing.

Fig. 10 Denoising of noisy CSI signal using Butterworth filter and/or PCA (Wang et al., 2020)

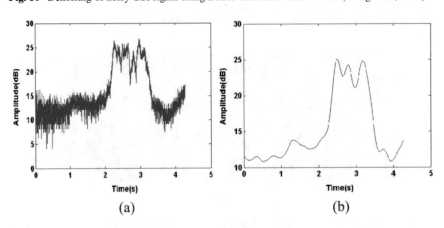

(a)   (b)

Fig. 11 Raw CSI and its denoising results for kicking action: **a** The raw CSI; **b** Butterworth low-pass filtered signal (Yan et al., 2020)

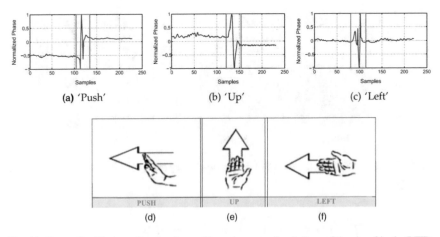

(a) 'Push'   (b) 'Up'   (c) 'Left'

(d)   (e)   (f)

Fig. 12 Example of fast varying signal: **a–c** Show the normalized phase of the signal in the RFID-based HAR system, corresponding to various gestures, shown in **d–f** (Zou et al., 2017)

the magnitude squared of the STFT:

$$spectrogrm\{x(\xi)\}(\zeta, \varpi) = |X(\zeta, \varpi)|^2 \tag{2}$$

At present days, dedicated block/command is available for spectrogram in NI LabVIEW and MATLAB (Kehtarnavaz, 2011; Klapper, 2010). In Fig. 13, we show examples of the spectrograms of signals of 3-axis inertial sensors for different activities.

DWT-based spectrum spectrogram is also used for superior time–frequency resolution (Wang et al., 2020). Figure 14 represents the DWT spectrograms of CSI during three typical activities. Spectrogram of walking shows a persistent high-frequency component. The spectrogram of falling depicts an initial high-frequency disturbance in CSI followed by a quiet episode. Figure 14c shows a periodic onset of high-frequency signal due to the waving of the hand. It is needless to mention that such spectrograms assist in activity recognition.

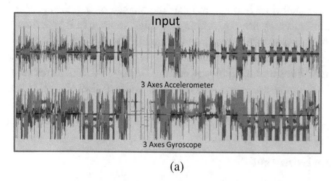

(a)

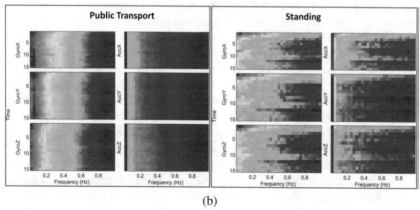

(b)

Fig. 13 Spectrogram of the signals of inertial sensors during different human activity (Acharya et al., 2020)

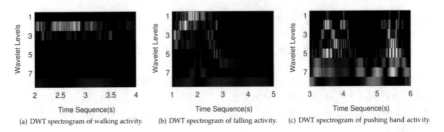

(a) DWT spectrogram of walking activity.   (b) DWT spectrogram of falling activity.   (c) DWT spectrogram of pushing hand activity.

Fig. 14 Extracted DWT spectrograms of CSI during three typical HAR activities (Wang et al., 2020)

(iii) Segmentation

Segmentation is done to remove the "inactive portion" of the sensor data (Yan et al., 2020). Classification of only those portions of the sensor data that contain the activity-related information not only enhances the performance of the HAR system in terms of the computational time but also reduces the chance of overfitting. Furthermore, when different activities are performed one after another in a practical scenario, segmentation of sensor data is required to "isolate" one period of activity from the following one (Gu et al., 2011; Wang et al., 2017b). A very standard technique of segmentation is thresholding (Cuevas et al., 2012). However, different dedicated algorithms for the same are introduced in several works (Gu et al., 2011; Wang et al., 2017c; Yan et al., 2020). Figure 15 clearly indicates that their proposed Adaptive Activity Cutting Algorithm (AACA) outperforms the standard thresholding-based segmentation algorithm (Fig. 16).

(iv) Feature Extraction

After segmenting the sensor data, feature extraction is adopted to extract useful features from each time window. In general, two approaches have been applied for FE: statistical and structural (Dhanvijay & Patil, 2019). Statistical methods (FT, DFT, DCT, STFT, DWT, etc.) use quantitative characteristics of the data to extract features, whereas structural approaches consider the interrelationship among data (Lara & Labrador, 2013). In existing works, researchers have used extracted time-domain and frequency-domain hand-crafted features based on domain knowledge (Wang et al., 2019). Conversely, state-of-the-art research focuses on deep learning approaches in HAR to automatically learn features for HAR (Bulling et al., 2014). The key advantage of using hand-crafted features is that the features are computationally lightweight, whereas the strengths of the automatically learned features by the deep networks are that the learning can be very deep, and the learning process does not rely on domain knowledge (Wang et al., 2019b). Some well-applied time-domain features are mean, median, variance, Kurtosis, skewness, zero-crossing rate, autoregressive coefficient (AR), peak-to-peak, and so on (Dinarević et al., 2019). Frequency-domain features indicate the periodicity of signals. To produce frequency-domain features, a segment of the sensor data should first be applied to a transformation function, such as Fast Fourier Transform (FFT), Discrete Wavelet Transform (DWT), or Discrete

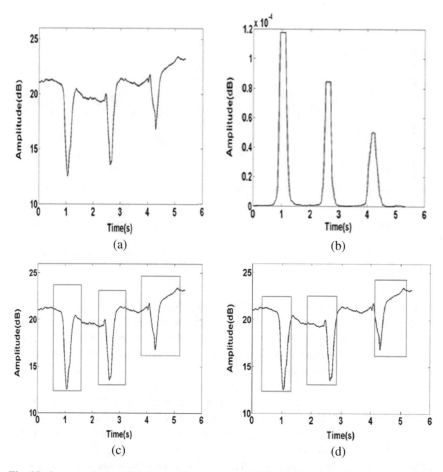

Fig. 15 Segmentation on CSI data: **a** The preprocessed CSI data for push action; **b** The signal of Fig. 15 **a**, processed through AACA algorithm; **c** Signal, segmented using the standard thresholding technique; **d** Signal, segmented using AACA technique with improved performance (Yan et al., 2020)

Cosine Transform (DCT). Frequency-domain features based on FFT include spectral energy, entropy, dominant frequency, etc. In (Petrie et al., 2020), the authors employ wavelet packet decomposition (WPD), DWT, and empirical mode decomposition (EMD) as feature extractors for automated seizure detection and prediction based on EEG measurements. Recently, deep features using deep networks like convolutional neural network (CNN), long short-term memory (LSTM) network, recurrent neural network (RNN), deep neural network (DNN), etc. are effectively used in HAR (Bulling et al., 2014; Jotschke et al., 2020, 2020; Wang et al., 2018) especially in IoHT applications.

A quite exhaustive list of standard features, used in HAR, is tabulated in Villar et al. (2015). Among many such important features, here we will touch upon a few of

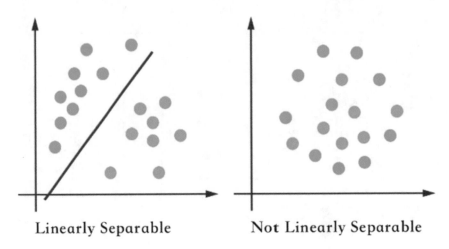

Fig. 16 Linearly and non-linearly separable feature vectors in a representative 2D feature space (Duda et al., 2006; Yen et al., 2020)

them just to give a flavor of the subject. *Time warping* that finds "similarity" between two time sequences, which are misaligned in phase, is used for feature extraction in HAR (Salvador & Chan, 2007; Zou et al., 2017). *Pearson correlation*, which could easily be evaluated for scattered data without finding out the ensemble mean of the feature vectors, finds extensive usage in HAR systems (Janidarmian et al., 2017; Liu et al., 2020; Ud Din et al., 2019). *Combined features* are also used many a time and a considerable amount of research has been carried out on feature selection as well (Villar et al., 2015). The presence of unnecessary features not only increases the computational complexity by increasing the dimensionality of the feature space, but the presence of misleading features is observed to hamper the performance of ML techniques (Pal & Saha, 2008; Wang et al., 2019). A substantial amount of discussion on dimensionality reduction of feature space and feature selection is available in Wang et al., 2019. However, it is worth mentioning that feature extraction and feature selection for detection using CNN-like deep learning networks are supposed to be done automatically and that is one of the lucrative features of CNN.

(v)   **Feature Selection and Dimensionality Reduction**

By the procedure of feature selection, we eliminate the redundant/irrelevant features that negatively affect the accuracy in HAR, and we construct a new feature vector. These methods can be classified into three categories, i.e. wrapper-based, filter-based, and correlation-based approaches (Wang et al., 2019). Moreover, Principal Component Analysis (PCA), Autoencoder, Sparse filtering, etc. are also used to reduce the dimensionality of a feature vector to facilitate more accurate and faster learning and improve generalization and interpretability (Lara & Labrador, 2013).

Among these, PCA is very commonly used on HAR signals to reduce its dimensionality. An apt introduction to PCA is available in Shlens (2014). A thorough treatment of PCA is available in Jollife and Cadima (2016). Loosely speaking, PCA does away with the undesired components of the signal and thereby pronounces the features to be used during classification. This is accomplished by keeping only a few significant eigenvectors, i.e. eigenvectors with lower eigenvalues. For example, PCA has been used for noise elimination in Wang et al. (2020); Yan et al., 2020; Zhang et al., 2020. This effect is depicted in Fig. 10c. The misleading effect of orientation on HAR is nullified in Chen et al. (2017) using PCA.

2.3   Learning and Inference

After the feature extraction phase, classification is performed to identify/recognize human activities. Classifiers interpret the extracted input features and predict the activity, e.g. fall detection and seizure detection. In connection to HAR, the classification problems could be broadly categorized into two types: *i)* Classification of *linearly separable classes* and *ii)* Classification of *classes, not linearly separable*. A typical representative diagram of both the genre is given below.

Unfortunately, the classes of HAR are non-separable in nature as shown in Fig. 17. Therefore, ML models and their training algorithms are required to be applied to HAR

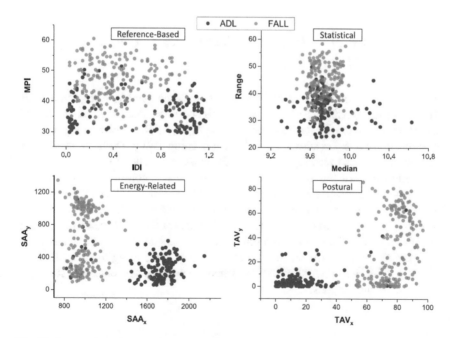

Fig. 17 Scatter plots of some of the extracted features from accelerometer signals using waist location dataset in order to compare the activities of daily leaving (ADL) and fall events. (Shahzad & Kim, 2019)

problems. The first step of working with such ML algorithms is the training of the models and the next step is testing of the model's accuracy (Goodfellow et al., 2016).

The state-of-the-art classification algorithms can be classified into the following two categories: conventional methods and deep learning algorithms. Conventional algorithms involve probabilistic models, viz., dynamic Bayesian network (DBN) and hidden Markov model (HMM) and some supervised classifiers that map inputs (features) to outputs (recognized activity) like Artificial Neural Network (ANN), Support Vector Machines (SVMs), Decision trees (DT), Naïve Bayes (NB), k-Nearest Neighbors (kNN), Multilayer Perceptron (MLP), Random Forest (RF), etc. In unsupervised learning, the sensor data are utilized to automatically identify data clusters that indicate specific human activity. A few unsupervised learning algorithms including k-Means, Gaussian mixture models (GMM), etc. and Fuzzy and deep fuzzy-based classifiers are also being used in HAR. In (Duda et al., 2006), an inclusive discussion on conventional classifiers is presented in detail. In recent years, deep networks that include CNN, RNN, Restricted Boltzmann machine (RBM), etc. are popularly used in HAR. Deep networks are capable of learning deep features from input data and performing classification in a simultaneous fashion as shown in Fig. 2. The state-of-the-art ML/DL-based classification algorithms are discussed in Sect. 3. However, prior to discussing that we further investigate the very need for modern ML techniques and DL in HAR in the following sub-section.

2.4   Why to Prefer Modern ML Techniques and Deep Learning

There exists a lot of classical ML technique-based pattern recognition tools, viz., Bayesian classifier, SVM, k-Nearest neighborhood, decision tree, and HMM. However, the modern ML techniques involving ANN, RNN, etc. give an edge over the classical techniques because of their efficient learning ability. The prominent advantage of ANN-based techniques owes to the massive parallel connection of ANN, inspired by the structure of the human brain, the inherent non-linearity of ANN that let it work as a non-linear discriminant, and above all the well-developed training algorithms for neural (Duda et al., 2006). On the other hand, the DL techniques involving CNN-like structures allow convenient use of the spectrogram data, which contain important features of both time and frequency domains as shown above in the example of typical HAR sensor data. The reason for using modern ML techniques and DL will be further clarified when we will discuss some case studies in the forthcoming sections.

3   Different State-Of-The-Art ML/DL Techniques

At present, extensive research is going on HAR, and everywhere the classification of human activity is accomplished using ML/DL techniques almost without any exception. A good review of modern machine learning techniques, widely used in HAR, is available in Wang et al., 2019. In (Suto & Oniga, 2019), the efficacy of the deep neural models over the shallow ones is depicted in a systematic way.

However, in terms of feature selection, modern research is showing that augmentation of the so-called shallow features, which are mostly statistical features of the data itself and its first-order difference, in the DL paradigm improves the performance of human activity classifier (Wang et al., 2019). Some typical shallow features, used in HAR, are tabulated below in Table 2.

A technique of augmenting shallow features with the deep ones, obtained from CNN, is graphically presented in Ravi et al. (2017). First, the deep and shallow features are computed and merged together into a unique combined feature vector. Next, the combined feature vector is classified through a fully connected layer and a soft-max layer as shown in Fig. 18.

Table 2 Typical shallow features used in HAR

Features		
Interquartile range	**Amplitude**	**Kurtosis**
Root mean square	Variance	Mean
Standard deviation	Skewness	Min
Mean-cross	Median	Max

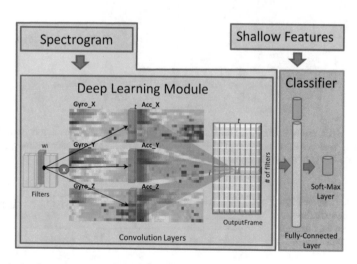

Fig. 18 A simple way to augment the deep and shallow features in a HAR classifier (Ravi et al., 2017)

Similar work on concatenating hand-crafted features with the deep features obtained from CNN is reported in Huynh-The et al. (2020). Figure 19 shows the generic block schematic diagram of the model. In this work, first, data acquired from a multi-sensor system are converted to activity image, to be used in deep learning. Afterwards, deep CNN is used to simultaneously extract the signal-level and sensor-level correlation from the activity image. This deep CNN is designed employing several stacks of the residual convolutional blocks, where each block consists of multiple convolutional layers defined using different kernels. The deep visual features are extracted at the global average pooling layer of the deep CNN. Finally, the deep features, thus extracted, are concatenated with the hand-crafted shallow features, and the combined featured vector is classified using SVM. In this work, the result presented in Table 3 clearly indicates that augmentation of deep and hand-crafted features improves the HAR accuracy up to 96% for different datasets.

Here, we present a tentative list of neural network structures, used in current works:

(1) **DNN:** Feedforward MLP with deep layers (Qadri et al., 2020; Qi et al., 2019);
(2) **CNN:** Convolutional neural network (Qi et al., 2019; Ravi et al., 2017; Seyfioğlu et al., 2018; Zhang et al., 2020);
(3) **LSTM:** A gated recurrent ANN (RNN), i.e. ANN with feedback; typically used in deep learning (Abdel-Basset et al., 2020; Zhang et al., 2020; Zhou et al., 2020);

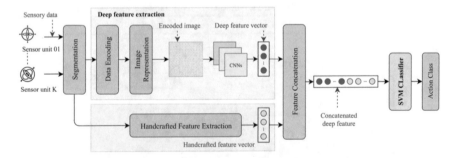

Fig. 19 A HAR example, based on wearable sensor data, where both the deep features and the hand-crafted features are concatenated to successfully train an SVM classifier ensuring improved performance (Huynh-The et al., 2020)

3 Variation in percentage accuracy due to feature augmentation for different datasets (Huynh-The et al., 2020)	Features\ Dataset	Sport	DaLiAc	RealWorld
	Hand-crafted	88.2	89.4	82.7
	Deep	93.2	96.2	91.1
	Hybrid: Deep + Hand-crafted	96.1	97.2	96.2

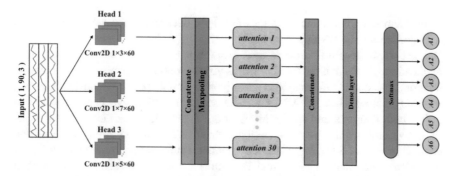

Fig. 20 A HAR example, where both the CNN and Attention models are used to ensure improved classification performance (Zhang et al., 2020). It is a six-class recognition problem, where A1–A6 are the class labels

(4)   **AM:** Attention model assigns a score value to each feature allowing the deep network to focus on the important part of the data (Chen et al., 2019, 2020; Zhang et al., 2020);

(5)   **DBN:** Deep belief network that uses Bayesian statistics (Hassan et al., 2018);

(6)   **SAE:** Stacked autoencoder; a feedforward neural network that learns through decoding–encoding (Seyfioğlu et al., 2018; Zhou et al., 2020);

(7)   **Hybrid Combination** of different DL models (Qi, Yang, et al., 2019) (Abdel-Basset et al., 2020; Huynh-The et al., 2020; Qi & Aliverti, 2020; Zhang et al., 2020; Zhou, Liang, et al., 2020).

In the following three examples of HAR, as depicted in Figs. 20–22, we show the block diagrams of a few relevant *hybrid DL models* to shed some light on this concept:

Case–I: A hybrid HAR technique, where *both CNN and attention mechanism (AM)* are used, is presented in Zhang et al., 2020. The proposed hybrid ML model is depicted in Fig. 20. A "3-head CNN" is used for feature extraction. The *jth* feature map at the *ith* layer of *cth* head of the multi-head CNN and the value at the *xth* row is denoted as $v_{i,j}^{x,c}$, and it is given by

$$v_{i,j}^{x,c} = f_{ReLU}\left(f_{Conv2D}\left(v_{i-1}^{x+p}\right)\right), \forall c = 1, 2, 3 \tag{3}$$

where f_{ReLU} is the activation function and f_{Conv2D} is the convolution function (Zhang et al., 2020). AM is used after feature extraction to emphasize the relatively more relevant features to improve the classifier performance:

$$Attention(Q, K, V) = softmax\left(\frac{QK^T}{\sqrt{d_k}}\right)V, \tag{4}$$

where Q is the query matrix, and V is the matrix of keys and K is the matrix of keys values. Experimentations are conducted on public domain WISDM data. The results demonstrate a higher accuracy of the hybrid learning approach in comparison with conventional CNN as shown in Table 4.

Case–II: Exhaustive literature survey on DL-based HAR in many IoHT-relevant applications shows that most of the works give suboptimal performance as both the temporal and spatial information is not exploited simultaneously. A novel DL model for HAR, called ST-deepHAR (Abdel-Basset et al., 2020), has been proposed to utilize both temporal and spatial information. A generic block diagram of the ST-deepHAR comprising two computational channels is depicted in Fig. 21. The first channel includes LSTM for efficient sequential feature extraction, trailed by Attention Mechanism that enhances and fine-tunes the temporal features. The second channel is designed using $1D$ convolutional residual network (ResNet) that effectively extracts spatial features. An adaptive squeeze and excite (SE) operation is adopted to enhance the spatial feature extraction. The *temporal* features obtained from *LSTM + AM* and *spatial* features obtained from *ResNet + SE* are concatenated to classify various activities finally. In the second channel, each layer extracts spatial features using the following mechanisms that use F convolutional filters for extraction of internal features and an F feature map is constructed. Raw sensor data were convolved ($*$) with a filter of width w and depth d along the time axis. Here, d indicates the channel size of the former layer. ReLU operation is adopted for the activation of the convolution layer owing to its capability to handle vanishing gradient issues. Two public HAR datasets are used to validate the performance of the proposed algorithm. The contribution of each building block of the hybrid DL model and their comparison with the proposed hybrid model on UCI-HAR data are summarized in Table 5.

Case–III: A two-layer HAR framework is proposed in Qi, Yang, et al., 2019 for classifying different gym physical activities (GPA). In layer one, a one-class SVM is applied to coarsely classify the free weight and non-free weight activities, whereas in the second layer, an ANN is used for recognition of aerobic and sedentary activities.

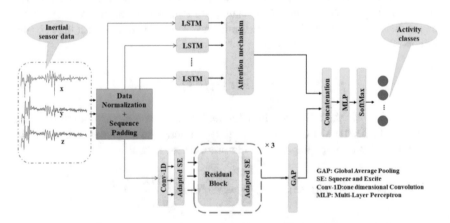

Fig. 21 A HAR example, where both the LSTM and MLP classifier are used to ensure improved performance (Abdel-Basset et al., 2020)

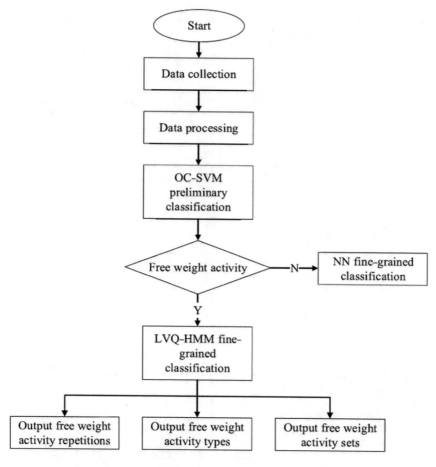

Fig. 22 Flow diagram of hybrid hierarchical gym physical activity recognition and measurement framework (Qi et al., 2019)

Apart from these, an HMM is incorporated to classify free weight activities. The proposed framework is found to perform better than other approaches in recognizing and measuring GPAs as depicted in Table 3 and 4 of Qi et al., (2019a).

It is well known that one of the central problems of HAR is its weakly labeled sensor data. In recent work, this problem is alleviated by introducing a deep Q-network (DQN)-based auto-labeling mechanism (Zhou, Liang, et al., 2020). The corresponding HAR scheme is shown in Fig. 23. The attention-based CNN model is also proposed to combat such a situation of detecting ambiguous human activities (Wang et al., 2019).

Table 4 Test accuracy comparison of different CNN-based methods for a shorter segment (48 data points) and longer segment (64 data points)

K	Class	1D-CNN	2D-CNN	Multi-head 2D-CNN	Multi-head Convolutional Attention
48	A1	92.0	74.0	96.1	96.0
	A2	94.2	96.0	91.2	93.0
	A3	90.0	89.0	96.7	98.0
	A4	92.0	97.0	89.0	98.0
	A5	88.6	90.0	97.8	97.0
	A6	86.0	91.0	87.4	93.0
	Overall	90.5	89.5	93.0	**95.8**
64	A1	93.5	70.0	96.1	96.0
	A2	91.0	98.0	91.2	94.0
	A3	94.0	89.0	97.0	97.0
	A4	93.5	98.0	89.0	98.0
	A5	89.5	90.0	98.0	99.0
	A6	86.0	93.0	87.8	92.0
	Overall	91.3	89.7	93.2	**96.0**

Table 5 Performance comparison considering each building block of the hybrid DL model (Abdel-Basset et al., 2020) (AM = Attention Model, ResNet = Residual block, SE = squeeze)

Methods	Accuracy
Basic LSTM	92.5%
Basic LSTM + AM	93.7%
Basic LSTM + ResNet	94.82%
Basic LSTM + AM + ResNet	95.65%
Basic LSTM + AM + ResNet + SE	96.54%
ST-deepHAR (Abdel-Basset et al., 2020)	**97.70%**

4 Future Direction of Research

With the advent of HAR-based supportive technologies in IoHT, users' quality of life is continuously being improved, especially for the aging society and also for the physically or mentally challenged. Nonetheless, HAR systems still have lot many challenges regarding their accuracy, robustness, cost, unobtrusiveness, security, user compliance, etc. A few open research problems are summarized as follows:

(i)   Design and implementation of a HAR system to cater to the needs of aged people who are not that much conversant with information technology and who desire to live independently in home comfort is an open research problem to tackle with the present technology.

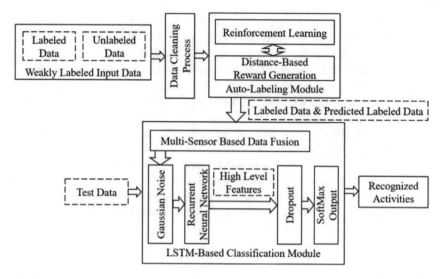

Fig. 23 A HAR system for handling weakly labeled sensor data (Zhou, Liang, et al., 2020)

(ii)　In the case of wrist-worn sensors like smartwatches for HAR, the sensor data suffer high intra-class variance due to the similar activities done by wrist movements, which, in turn, decreases the recognition accuracy due to being easily misclassified like brushing of teeth and eating/feeding, etc. This problem of misclassification of similar activities by wrist-worn devices could be overcome by adding additional sensors that provide enough information to perform more robust and accurate HAR from multiple sensor modalities.

(iii)　Under-utilization of sensing data, obtained from multiple sensors, for feature extraction is an open problem to date.

(iv)　More practical and effective data fusion mechanisms are required to combine the information obtained from multiple modality sensors.

(v)　What kind of FE should we use for accurate HAR is an open research problem: Hand-crafted features or automatically learned deep features or a combination of both? This is still an open issue to be investigated by the researchers.

(vi)　For wireless sensing in HAR, RSSI- and CSI-based sensing need to generate a training profile, which could be easily changed by surrounding changes (e.g. furniture movements, opening/closing of a (window/door), and leading to inconsistency). A huge additional effort has to be given to retraining the profiles, which results in a hike in labor cost and system downtime.

(vii)　Besides, the users' orientation and location influence the performance of HAR by wireless signal-based sensing. The change in users' orientation and location could induce different variation patterns of RSSI/CSI measurements. Thus, for the existing HAR systems, user has to keep the same location and orientation during the training and testing phases. Overcoming this limitation in RSSI- and CSI-based sensing is an open research problem.

(viii) The safety and security of user-health data are of utter importance and the research scope is there to provide security in different layers for the protection of user data.

(ix) CrowdHAR: Most of the HAR systems predict a single user. Information gathered from social networks or from a target sample population could be effectively used to recognize activity levels of sedentariness, exercise habits, and health conditions. Such data received from thousands/millions of users may be utilized to train classifiers thereby improving the overall recognition accuracy. CrowdHAR is still open for doing involved research.

References

Abdel-Basset, M., Hawash, H., Chakrabortty, R. K., Ryan, M., Elhoseny, M., & Song, H. (2020). ST-DeepHAR: Deep Learning Model for Human Activity Recognition in IoHT Applications. *IEEE Internet of Things Journal, 4662*, 1–1. https://doi.org/10.1109/jiot.2020.3033430.

Acharya, S., Swaminathan, D., Das, S., Kansara, K., Chakraborty, S., Kumar R, D., Francis, T., Aatre, K.R.: Non-Invasive Estimation of Hemoglobin Using a Multi-Model Stacking Regressor. IEEE J. Biomed. Heal. Informatics. 24, 1717–1726 (2020). https://doi.org/10.1109/JBHI.2019. 2954553.

Anwary, A. R., Yu, H., & Vassallo, M. (2018). Optimal Foot Location for Placing Wearable IMU Sensors and Automatic Feature Extraction for Gait Analysis. *IEEE Sensors Journal, 18*, 2555–2567. https://doi.org/10.1109/JSEN.2017.2786587.

Bhat, G., Tuncel, Y., An, S., Lee, H.G., Ogras, U.Y.: An ultra-low energy human activity recognition accelerator for wearable health applications. In: ACM Transactions on Embedded Computing Systems. pp. 1–22. Association for Computing Machinery (2019). https://doi.org/10.1145/335 8175.

Bhoi, A. K., Mallick, P. K., Liu, C.-M., Balas, V. E. (2020). Bio-inspired Neurocomputing.

Bianchi, V., Bassoli, M., Lombardo, G., Fornacciari, P., Mordonini, M., & De Munari, I. (2019). IoT Wearable Sensor and Deep Learning: An Integrated Approach for Personalized Human Activity Recognition in a Smart Home Environment. *IEEE Internet of Things Journal, 6*, 8553–8562. https://doi.org/10.1109/JIOT.2019.2920283.

Bishop, C.M. (2006). Pattern recognition and machine learning. springer.

Bui, N., Truong, H., Nguyen, A., Ashok, A., Nguyen, P., Dinh, T., Deterding, R., Vu, T. (2017). PhO2: Smartphone based blood oxygen level measurement systems using near-IR and RED wave-guided light. In: SenSys 2017 - Proceedings of the 15th ACM Conference on Embedded Networked Sensor Systems. pp. 1–14. , Delft, Netherlands (2017). https://doi.org/10.1145/313 1672.3131696.

Bulling, A., Blanke, U., & Schiele, B. (2014). A tutorial on human activity recognition using body-worn inertial sensors. *ACM Computing Surveys, 46*, 1–33. https://doi.org/10.1145/2499621.

Chen, Z., Zhu, Q., Soh, Y. C., & Zhang, L. (2017). Robust human activity recognition using smartphone sensors via CT-PCA and online SVM. *IEEE Trans. Ind. Informatics., 13*, 3070–3080. https://doi.org/10.1109/TII.2017.2712746.

Chen, Y., Yu, L., Ota, K., & Dong, M. (2018). Robust activity recognition for aging society. *IEEE J. Biomed. Heal. Informatics., 22*, 1754–1764. https://doi.org/10.1109/JBHI.2018.2819182.

Chen, K., Yao, L., Zhang, D., Wang, X., Chang, X., & Nie, F. (2020). A Semisupervised Recurrent Convolutional Attention Model for Human Activity Recognition. *IEEE Trans. Neural Networks Learn. Syst., 31*, 1747–1756. https://doi.org/10.1109/TNNLS.2019.2927224.

Chen, Z., Zhang, L., Jiang, C., Cao, Z., & Cui, W. (2019). WiFi CSI based passive human activity recognition using attention based BLSTM. *IEEE Transactions on Mobile Computing, 18*, 2714–2724. https://doi.org/10.1109/TMC.2018.2878233.

Choi, H., Naylon, J., Luzio, S., Beutler, J., Birchall, J., Martin, C., & Porch, A. (2015). Design and in Vitro Interference Test of Microwave Noninvasive Blood Glucose Monitoring Sensor. *IEEE Transactions on Microwave Theory and Techniques, 63*, 3016–3025. https://doi.org/10.1109/TMTT.2015.2472019.

Chowdhury, T.Z.: Using Wi-Fi channel state information (CSI) for human activity recognition and fall detection, (2018).

Cuevas, E., Sención, F., Zaldivar, D., Pérez-Cisneros, M., & Sossa, H. (2012). A multi-threshold segmentation approach based on artificial bee colony optimization. *Applied Intelligence, 37*, 321–336. https://doi.org/10.1007/s10489-011-0330-z.

Cui, L., Yang, S., Chen, F., Ming, Z., Lu, N., Qin, J.: A survey on application of machine learning for Internet of Things. Int. J. Mach. Learn. Cybern. Springer-Verlag GmbH Ger. part Springer Nat. 9, 1399–1417 (2018). https://doi.org/10.1007/s13042-018-0834-5.

Debes, C., Merentitis, A., Sukhanov, S., Niessen, M., Frangiadakis, N., & Bauer, A. (2016). Monitoring activities of daily living in smart homes: Understanding human behavior. *IEEE Signal Processing Magazine, 33*, 81–94. https://doi.org/10.1109/MSP.2015.2503881.

Dhanvijay, M. M., & Patil, S. C. (2019). Internet of Things : A survey of enabling technologies in healthcare and its applications. *Comput. Networks., 153*, 113–131. https://doi.org/10.1016/j.comnet.2019.03.006.

Dinarević, E.C., Husić, J.B., Baraković, S. (2019). Issues of Human Activity Recognition in Healthcare. 2019 18th Int. Symp. INFOTEH-JAHORINA, INFOTEH 2019 - Proc. 20–22 (2019). https://doi.org/10.1109/INFOTEH.2019.8717749.

Duda, R. O., Hart, P. E., & Stork, D. G. (2006). *Pattern classification.* Wiley.

Goodfellow, I., Bengio, Y., Courville, A., Bengio, Y. (2016). Deep learning. MIT press Cambridge.

Gu, T., Wang, L., Member, S., & Wu, Z. (2011). A Pattern Mining Approach to Sensor-Based Human Activity Recognition. *IEEE Transactions on Knowledge and Data Engineering, 23*, 1359–1372. https://doi.org/10.1109/TKDE.2010.184.

Habibzadeh, H., Dinesh, K., Rajabi Shishvan, O., Boggio-Dandry, A., Sharma, G., & Soyata, T. (2020). A Survey of Healthcare Internet of Things (HIoT): A Clinical Perspective. *IEEE Internet of Things Journal, 7*, 53–71. https://doi.org/10.1109/JIOT.2019.2946359.

Hasan, M. K., Aziz, M. H., Zarif, M. I. I., Hasan, M., Hashem, M. M. A., Guha, S., Love, R., & Ahamed, S. (2019). HeLP ME: Recommendations for non-invasive hemoglobin level prediction in mobile-phone environment (preprint). *JMIR mHealth and uHealth.* https://doi.org/10.2196/16806.

Hassan, M. M., Uddin, M. Z., Mohamed, A., & Almogren, A. (2018). A robust human activity recognition system using smartphone sensors and deep learning. *Future Generation Computer Systems, 81*, 307–313. https://doi.org/10.1016/j.future.2017.11.029.

Hermanis, A., Cacurs, R., Nesenbergs, K., Greitans, M., Syundyukov, E., Selavo, L. (2016). Demo: Wearable Sensor System for Human Biomechanics Monitoring, 247–248.

Huynh-The, T., Hua, C.-H., Tu, N. A., & Kim, D.-S. (2020). Physical Activity Recognition with Statistical-Deep Fusion Model using Multiple Sensory Data for Smart Health. *IEEE Internet of Things Journal, 4662*, 1–1. https://doi.org/10.1109/jiot.2020.3013272.

Janidarmian, M., Fekr, A. R., Radecka, K., Zilic, Z. (2017). A comprehensive analysis on wearable acceleration sensors in human activity recognition. Sensors (Switzerland), 17. https://doi.org/10.3390/s17030529.

Jollife, I. T., Cadima, J. (2016). Principal component analysis: A review and recent developments. Philos. Trans. R. Soc. A Math. Phys. Eng. Sci. 374. https://doi.org/10.1098/rsta.2015.0202.

Jotschke, M., Carvajal Ossa, W., Reich, T., Mayr, C. (2020). A 10.5μW programmable SAR ADC frontend with SC reamplifier for low-power IoT sensor nodes. IEEE World Forum Internet Things, WF-IoT 2020—Symp. Proc. 1–6. https://doi.org/10.1109/WF-IoT48130.2020.9221058.

Jung, S., Hong, S., Kim, J., Lee, S., Hyeon, T., Lee, M., & Kim, D. H. (2015). Wearable Fall Detector using Integrated Sensors and Energy Devices. *Science and Reports, 5,* 1–9. https://doi.org/10.1038/srep17081.

Kehtarnavaz, N.: Digital Signal Processing System Design: LabVIEW-Based Hybrid Programming. (2011).

Kim, J., Campbell, A. S., & Wang, J. (2018). Wearable non-invasive epidermal glucose sensors: A review. *Talanta, 177,* 163–170. https://doi.org/10.1016/j.talanta.2017.08.077.

Klapper, J. (2010). *Discrete Fourier Analysis and Wavelets.* https://doi.org/10.1080/02664760902919762.

Kumar, A., Saha, S., & Bhattacharya, R. (2018). Wavelet transform based novel edge detection algorithms for wideband spectrum sensing in CRNs. *AEU - Int. J. Electron. Commun., 84,* 100–110. https://doi.org/10.1016/j.aeue.2017.11.024.

Lara, Ó. D., & Labrador, M. A. (2013). A survey on human activity recognition using wearable sensors. *IEEE Commun. Surv. Tutorials., 15,* 1192–1209. https://doi.org/10.1109/SURV.2012.110112.00192.

Li, W., Tan, B., & Piechocki, R. (2018). Passive Radar for opportunistic monitoring in e-health applications. *IEEE J. Transl. Eng. Heal. Med., 6,* 1–10. https://doi.org/10.1109/JTEHM.2018.2791609.

Liu, J., Liu, H., Chen, Y., Wang, Y., & Wang, C. (2020). Wireless sensing for human activity: A survey. *IEEE Commun. Surv. Tutorials., 22,* 1629–1645. https://doi.org/10.1109/COMST.2019.2934489.

Liu, Y., Mu, Y., Chen, K., Li, Y., & Guo, J. (2020). Daily activity feature selection in smart homes based on Pearson correlation coefficient. *Neural Processing Letters, 51,* 1771–1787. https://doi.org/10.1007/s11063-019-10185-8.

Lutovac, M. D., Tošić, D. V., Evans, B. L. (2001). Filter design for signal processing using MATLAB and mathematica.

MacHot, F. Al, Mosa, A. H., Ali, M., Kyamakya, K. (2018). Activity recognition in sensor data streams for active and assisted living environments. *IEEE Trans. Circuits Syst. Video Technol.* 28, 2933–2945. https://doi.org/10.1109/TCSVT.2017.2764868.

Majumder, S., & Deen, M. J. (2019). Smartphone sensors for health monitoring and diagnosis. *Sensors (Switzerland)., 19,* 1–45. https://doi.org/10.3390/s19092164.

Mazgaoker, S., Ketko, I., Yanovich, R., Heled, Y., & Epstein, Y. (2017). Measuring core body temperature with a non-invasive sensor. *Journal of Thermal Biology, 66,* 17–20. https://doi.org/10.1016/j.jtherbio.2017.03.007.

Muaaz, M., Chelli, A., Abdelgawwad, A. A., Mallofre, A. C., & Patzold, M. (2020). WiWeHAR: Multimodal Human Activity Recognition Using Wi-Fi and Wearable Sensing Modalities. *IEEE Access., 8,* 164453–164470. https://doi.org/10.1109/access.2020.3022287.

Pal, N.R., Saha, S. (2008). Simultaneous structure identification and fuzzy rule generation for Takagi-Sugeno models. IEEE Trans. Syst. Man, Cybern. Part B Cybern. 38, 1626–1638. https://doi.org/10.1109/TSMCB.2008.2006367.

Petrie, A., Kinnison, W., Song, Y., Chiang, S.H.W., Layton, K. (2020). A 0.2-V 10-bit 5-kHz SAR ADC with Dynamic Bulk Biasing and Ultra-Low-Supply-Voltage Comparator. *Proc. Cust. Integr. Circuits Conf.* 2020-March, 31–34. https://doi.org/10.1109/CICC48029.2020.9075917.

Pu, Q., Jiang, S., & Gollakota, S. (2013). Whole-home gesture recognition using wireless signals. *Comput. Commun. Rev., 43,* 485–486. https://doi.org/10.1145/2534169.2491687.

Qadri, Y. A., Nauman, A., Zikria, Y. Bin, Vasilakos, A. V., Kim, S.W. (2020). The Future of Healthcare Internet of Things: A Survey of Emerging Technologies. IEEE Commun. Surv. Tutorials. 22, 1121–1167. https://doi.org/10.1109/COMST.2020.2973314.

Qi, W., & Aliverti, A. (2020). A multimodal wearable system for continuous and real-time breathing pattern monitoring during daily activity. *IEEE J. Biomed. Heal. Informatics., 24,* 2199–2207. https://doi.org/10.1109/JBHI.2019.2963048.

Qi, W., Su, H., & Aliverti, A. (2020). A smartphone-based adaptive recognition and real-time monitoring system for human activities. *IEEE Trans. Human-Machine Syst., 50,* 414–423. https://doi.org/10.1109/THMS.2020.2984181.

Qi, J., Yang, P., Hanneghan, M., Tang, S., & Zhou, B. (2019a). A hybrid hierarchical framework for gym physical activity recognition and measurement using wearable sensors. *IEEE Internet of Things Journal, 6,* 1384–1393. https://doi.org/10.1109/JIOT.2018.2846359.

Qi, W., Su, H., Yang, C., Ferrigno, G., De Momi, E., Aliverti, A. (2019b). A fast and robust deep convolutional neural networks for complex human activity recognition using smartphone. Sensors (Switzerland). 19, 3731. https://doi.org/10.3390/s19173731.

Queyam, A. Bin, Pahuja, S.K., Singh, D. (2018). Doppler ultrasound based non-invasive heart rate telemonitoring system for wellbeing assessment. *Int. J. Intell. Syst. Appl.* 10, 69–79 (2018). https://doi.org/10.5815/ijisa.2018.12.07.

Ranjan Acharya, B., Kumar Gantayat, P. (2015). Recognition of human unusual activity in surveillance videos surveillance view project environment view project recognition of human unusual activity in surveillance videos.

Ravi, D., Wong, C., Lo, B., & Yang, G. Z. (2017). A deep learning approach to on-node sensor data analytics for mobile or wearable devices. *IEEE J. Biomed. Heal. Informatics., 21,* 56–64. https://doi.org/10.1109/JBHI.2016.2633287.

Ray, P. P., Dash, D., & Kumar, N. (2020). Sensors for internet of medical things: State-of-the-art, security and privacy issues, challenges and future directions. *Computer Communications, 160,* 111–131. https://doi.org/10.1016/j.comcom.2020.05.029.

Saha, J., Chowdhury, C., Chowdhury, I.R., Biswas, S., Aslam, N. (2018a). An ensemble of condition based classifiers for device independent detailed human activity recognition using smartphones. Inf. 9. https://doi.org/10.3390/info9040094.

Saha, J., Chowdhury, C., & Biswas, S. (2018b). Two phase ensemble classifier for smartphone based human activity recognition independent of hardware configuration and usage behaviour. *Microsystem Technologies, 24,* 2737–2752. https://doi.org/10.1007/s00542-018-3802-9.

Salvador, S., & Chan, P. (2007). Toward accurate dynamic time warping in linear time and space. *Intell. Data Anal., 11,* 561–580.

Seyfioğlu, M. S., Özbayoğlu, A. M., & Gürbüz, S. Z. (2018). Deep convolutional autoencoder for radar-based classification of similar aided and unaided human activities. *IEEE Transactions on Aerospace and Electronic Systems, 54,* 1709–1723. https://doi.org/10.1109/TAES.2018.2799758.

Shahzad, A., & Kim, K. (2019). FallDroid: An automated smart-phone-based fall detection system using multiple kernel learning. *IEEE Trans. Ind. Informatics., 15,* 35–44. https://doi.org/10.1109/TII.2018.2839749.

Shlens, J. (2014). A Tutorial on Principal Component Analysis.

Suto, J., & Oniga, S. (2019). Efficiency investigation from shallow to deep neural network techniques in human activity recognition. *Cognitive Systems Research, 54,* 37–49. https://doi.org/10.1016/j.cogsys.2018.11.009.

Ud Din, I., Almogren, A., Guizani, M., & Zuair, M. (2019). A Decade of Internet of Things: Analysis in the Light of Healthcare Applications. *IEEE Access., 7,* 89967–89979. https://doi.org/10.1109/ACCESS.2019.2927082.

Verma, D., Shehzad, K., Khan, D., Ain, Q.U., Kim, S.J., Lee, D., Pu, Y., Lee, M., Hwang, K.C., Yang, Y., Lee, K.Y. (2020). A Design of 8 fJ/Conversion-Step 10-bit 8MS/s Low Power Asynchronous SAR ADC for IEEE 802.15.1 IoT Sensor Based Applications. IEEE Access. 8, 85869–85879. https://doi.org/10.1109/ACCESS.2020.2992750.

Villar, J. R., González, S., Sedano, J., Chira, C., Trejo-Gabriel-Galan, J.M. (2015). Improving human activity recognition and its application in early stroke diagnosis. Int. J. Neural Syst. 25. https://doi.org/10.1142/S0129065714500361.

Wang, L., Gu, T., & Member, S. (2017a). Toward a wearable RFID system for real-time activity recognition using radio patterns. *IEEE Transactions on Mobile Computing, 16*, 228–242. https://doi.org/10.1109/TMC.2016.2538230.

Wang, H., Member, S., & Zhang, D. (2017b). RT-Fall : A real-time and contactless fall detection system with commodity WiFi devices. *IEEE Transactions on Mobile Computing, 16*, 511–526.

Wang, G., Atef, M., & Lian, Y. (2018a). Towards a Continuous Non-Invasive Cuffless Blood Pressure Monitoring System Using PPG: Systems and Circuits Review. *IEEE Circuits and Systems Magazine, 18*, 6–26. https://doi.org/10.1109/MCAS.2018.2849261.

Wang, Y., Cang, S., & Yu, H. (2018a). A Data Fusion-Based Hybrid Sensory System for Older People's Daily Activity and Daily Routine Recognition. *IEEE Sensors Journal, 18*, 6874–6888. https://doi.org/10.1109/JSEN.2018.2833745.

Wang, Y., Cang, S., & Yu, H. (2019a). A survey on wearable sensor modality centred human activity recognition in health care. *Expert Systems with Applications, 137*, 167–190. https://doi.org/10.1016/j.eswa.2019.04.057.

Wang, J., Chen, Y., Hao, S., Peng, X., & Hu, L. (2019b). Deep learning for sensor-based activity recognition: A survey. *Pattern Recognit. Lett., 119*, 3–11. https://doi.org/10.1016/j.patrec.2018.02.010.

Wang, F., Gong, W., Liu, J., & Wu, K. (2020). Channel selective activity recognition with WiFi: A deep learning approach exploring wideband information. *IEEE Trans. Netw. Sci. Eng., 7*, 181–192. https://doi.org/10.1109/TNSE.2018.2825144.

Wang, K., He, J., Zhang, L. (2019c). Attention-based convolutional neural network for weakly labeled human activities recognition with wearable sensors.

Yan, H., Zhang, Y., Wang, Y., & Xu, K. (2020). WiAct: A passive WiFi-based human activity recognition system. *IEEE Sensors Journal, 20*, 296–305. https://doi.org/10.1109/JSEN.2019.2938245.

Yen, N. Y., Chang, J. W., Liao, J. Y., & Yong, Y. M. (2020). Analysis of interpolation algorithms for the missing values in IoT time series: A case of air quality in Taiwan. *The Journal of Supercomputing, 76*, 6475–6500. https://doi.org/10.1007/s11227-019-02991-7.

Zhang, H., Xiao, Z., Wang, J., Li, F., & Szczerbicki, E. (2020). A Novel IoT-Perceptive Human Activity Recognition (HAR) Approach Using Multihead Convolutional Attention. *IEEE Internet of Things Journal, 7*, 1072–1080. https://doi.org/10.1109/JIOT.2019.2949715.

Zhang, J., Wu, F., Wei, B., Zhang, Q., Huang, H., Shah, S.W., Cheng, J. (2020a). Data Augmentation and Dense-LSTM for Human Activity Recognition using WiFi Signal. *IEEE Internet Things J. XX*, 1–1 (2020a). https://doi.org/10.1109/jiot.2020a.3026732.

Zhou, X., Liang, W., Wang, K. I. K., Wang, H., Yang, L. T., & Jin, Q. (2020a). Deep-Learning-Enhanced Human Activity Recognition for Internet of Healthcare Things. *IEEE Internet of Things Journal, 7*, 6429–6438. https://doi.org/10.1109/JIOT.2020.2985082.

Zhou, Z., Yu, H., & Shi, H. (2020b). Human Activity Recognition Based on Improved Bayesian Convolution Network to Analyze Health Care Data Using Wearable IoT Device. *IEEE Access., 8*, 86411–86418. https://doi.org/10.1109/ACCESS.2020.2992584.

Zou, Y., Member, S., Xiao, J., & Han, J. (2017). GRfid : A Device-Free RFID-Based Gesture Recognition System. *IEEE Transactions on Mobile Computing, 16*, 381–393. https://doi.org/10.1109/TMC.2016.2549518.

Human Activity Recognition Systems Based on Audio-Video Data Using Machine Learning and Deep Learning

Dipanwita Thakur, Suparna Biswas, and Arindam Pal

Abstract Human Activity Recognition (HAR) has attracted great attention from the researchers in pervasive computing for smart healthcare. Patients with cardiac disease, obesity, diabetes have to perform some routine physical exercises as a treatment of their disease. Some of the mental disorder patients have to monitor their daily physical activities to prevent undesirable conditions. Therefore, identification and monitoring of physical human activities are helpful to provide the health assessment to the health person regarding patients behaviour. So, it is necessary to make HAR system available to the end users for the safety measures of their health. However, it is important to design the HAR system with proper experimental data set. Various research communities evolved and came up with various datasets for HAR. Audio-Video data are very much useful to create an appropriate HAR system along with smartphone based sensory data. Different types of data have their own advantages and disadvantages. This chapter discusses the implications of various types of data in HAR. Moreover, the primary objective is to enhance the performance of the identification of the human physical activities to make the HAR system reliable. So far, various "Machine Learning" (ML) and "Deep Learning" (DL) approaches are applied to enhance the recognition accuracy of various human physical activities. Analysis of the performance of various HAR systems on audio-video and sensory data using various ML and DL algorithms is discussed. Moreover, detailed case study on the application HAR is also discussed in this chapter.

D. Thakur (✉)
Banasthali Vidyapith, Vanasthali, Rajasthan, India
e-mail: dipanwitathakur@ieee.org

S. Biswas
Maulana Abul Kalam Azad University of Technology, Kolkata, West Bengal, India

A. Pal
Data61, Commonwealth Scientific and Industrial Research Organization (CSIRO) and Cyber Security Cooperative Research Centre (CSCRC), Sydney, NSW, Australia

© The Author(s), under exclusive license to Springer Nature Singapore Pte Ltd. 2022   151
S. Biswas et al. (eds.), *Internet of Things Based Smart Healthcare*, Smart Computing and Intelligence, https://doi.org/10.1007/978-981-19-1408-9_7

1   Introduction

Societies in developed and developing nations are aging rapidly. Worldwide, almost 500 million individuals were 65 years old or higher in 2006. It is appraised that the total number of aged people will rise to 1 billion by 2030. Developing countries are seeing the highest rise in aging populations, which will see a 140% leap by 2030 ((NIA), 2007). In addition, by 2050, the world population is projected to hit 9.3 billion, and people over 60 years of age will make up 28% of the world population (Department of Economic and Social Affairs and Population Division, 2004). It would take immense financial resources to cope with this situation in order to sustain the ever growing cost of living, where human longevity is projected to exceed 81 years by 2100 (Department of Economic and Social Affairs and Population Division, 2004).

The necessity of smart health assistance programs grows every year as elderly people may have body function problems or undergo any age-related illnesses. Actual perception is a typical strategy for following geriatric patients, which is costly, requires a ton of human personnel, and is progressively impossible taking into account the enormous maturing of the populace, in the forthcoming years. Many "Ambient Assisted Living" (AAL) devices need human activity identification, such as "care-providing robots", "video monitoring systems", and "assistive human-computer interaction technologies". Of course, although the main users of AAL systems are the aged people. This principle of AAL systems useful for people with mentally and physical disabilities, individuals suffering from diabetes, nerve related disease and obesity, people, who need medical assistance at home and also for the people, who are interested in personal health monitoring (Chahuara et al., 2016).

Figures 1, 2 and 3, shows the framework of AAL system for remote patient monitoring, weable computing for health monitoring system and mobile health monitoring system respectively.

In light of exponential growth of recent technology of sensor data and our extremely busy lifestyle, the need for real-time HAR solutions has increased substantially due to its application in health care. There are several applications of HAR in health care such as cardiac rehabilitation (Bidargaddi et al., 2007), physical rehabilitation (Katoch, 2017), remote health monitoring (Thakur and Biswas, 2020), smart home, nursing and athletics (Li et al., 2019; Morales and Akopian, 2017).

2   HAR

In the literature, the definition of HAR is indifferent according to the level of granularity under consideration. In most of the research work, different human movements. Essentially "jogging", "standing", "running" or "walking" are treated as human physical activities (Khan et al., 2010). The activities can be static ("sitting", "standing"

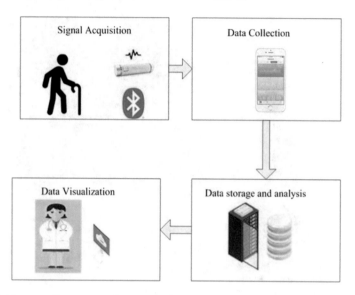

Fig. 1 AAL system for remote patient monitoring

Fig. 2 Wearable computing
for health monitoring system

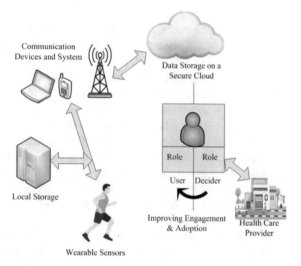

or "laying") and also can be dynamic ("jogging", "walking" or "cycling"). These activities are identified using wearable sensors or smartphone sensors on the basis of different body movements. These activities are categorized as indoor or outdoor activities and the interpretation of these activities can be used in medical assessment to provide health assistance. Apart from these activities some other complex activities are also there such as making tea, coffee, peeling fruits or preparing meals (Okeyo et al., 2014). Recognition of such activities need several sensors as each activity is

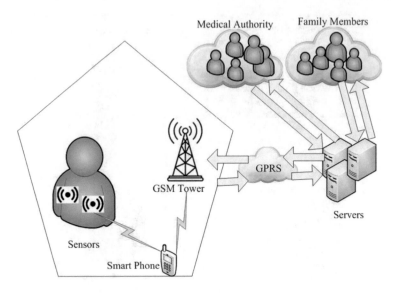

Fig. 3 Mobile health monitoring system

a special task of a casual task and also the collection of several subtasks. Some of the subtasks can only be recognized using a specific sensor. In certain utilizations of observation out in the open spots, activities are judged as communications among individuals. For example, video recognition systems are very fruitful to distinguish several complex activities, such as "fighting" and "stealing" (Artikis et al., 2010; Chahuara et al., 2016; Lin et al., 2008; Rota and Thonnat, 2000). Apart from the granularity level of the activity, there are several ways towards the solution of HAR such as online and offline. The offline HAR solutions are based on a static dataset (Bao and Intille, 2004). For instance, while evaluating the wellbeing condition of a patient in an emergency clinic, the sensor information of a past period of time is utilized to perceive the relating activities and also to distinguish a difference in behaviour. The benefit of aforesaid investigation is that all transient relations can be misused permitting better exactness since for each example previous and future occasions are accessible (Chahuara et al., 2016). However, in case of on-line recognition (Htike et al., 2010; Krishnan and Cook, 2014), the examination is conducted from an information flow while the subject is playing out the movement. For this situation the point is to recognize as fast as conceivable the current movement at a specific moment depending just on previous and present data. Table 1, demonstrates several characteristics of HAR systems.

Approaches for activity framework can be isolated generally into two characterizations: "knowledge-driven" and "data-driven" (Chahuara et al., 2016). In the previous class, a rationale based methodology offers an ideal system to show unequivocal information which can be given by a domain specialist. Ontologies have been broadly utilized for activity recognition (Chen et al., 2012) since they give intelligibility and

Table 1 Characteristics of HAR systems. *Source* (Bulling et al., 2014; Spinsante et al., 2016)

Type	Characteristics	Description
Generalization	User Independent	This HAR models are optimized in such a way that can be used by large number of users
	User Specific	These HAR systems are used by an individual user. Normally, the performance of this system is more than the user independent but it can not be generalize for others
	Temporal	The scheme should be stable in order to cope with temporal fluctuations caused by external situations such as sensor displacement, drifting sensor response such as barometer and gyroscope
Execution	Offline	The sensor data is proposed first. Then the recognition is performed. This is useful in health monitoring which is used for non-interactive applications
	Online	In real time, the collection and analysis of data is carried out. It is used in interactive application and activity-based computing such as human-computer interaction
Recognition	Continuous	The machine "spots" the presence of events automaticallyOr movements in the data of the streaming sensor
	Isolated	In case of complex activities, the collected data used to identify the human activity in a segmented way
Activities	Periodic	It express periodic activities such as walking, running etc. Generally, frequency domain features and sliding window segmentation are used for classification
	Static	The system deals with detecting static postures or posturesGestures of static pointing
	Sporadic	Sporadic activities scattered with other activities. Segmentation can be used to separate the subset of data containing the activity
System Model	Stateless	Activities are identified by spotting any particular sensor signals
	Stateful	The HAR system influenced by the environment. Here, context-aware activities are mapped with the location of the object. In case of identifying complex activities, it is suitable

formal definitions while the surmising can be performed by an ontology reasoner as an issue of satisfiability (Chahuara et al., 2016). Additionally, within a model, the logic rules encourage the execution of specialized knowledge under a description-based approach (Storf et al., 2009). For example, in (Augusto and Nugent, 2004), the recognition of activities was performed using logical models to establish the temporal relations among events. Artikis et al. (Artikis et al., 2010), used event calculus for activity recognition. Event calculus is capable of modeling complex activity and temporal relations. In (Chen et al., 2008), a framework to assist a person in a smart environment has been proposed. In this proposed framework, using event calculus was used for behaviour reasoning. Despite the fact that logical methods are highly articulate, they don't deal with vulnerability while smart home input data is incredibly noisy. Data-driven methodologies may be either supervised or unsupervised. Unsupervised identification of activity is relevant when it isn't needed to perceive explicit activities; for example, a change in the inhabitant's everyday pattern. Some related studies (Clarkson, 2003; Minnen, 2008) have considered techniques to find repetitive patterns, or themes, from a flood of sensory data; the segmentation is considered by other approaches and data clustering in order to construct models capable of marking a segment within one of the clusters (Chahuara et al., 2016; Flanagan et al., 2002; Rsnen, 2012).

Table 2, depicts several HAR solutions using Audio-video and wearable sensor and smartphone sensory data using various ML & DL methods. From this table, we can conclude that most of the audio based HAR systems are implemented for various indoor activities. Smartphone based HAR systems are popularly used to identify outdoor activities. HAR solutions are based on two different categories. One is vision based and another one is sensor based. In vision based HAR solutions, audio, video or image data are used. In sensor based HAR solutions, various wearable sensors and smartphone based sensors are used. Recently, fusion strategies are used to identify several complex activities in an efficient manner. Generally, "data fusion", "feature fusion" and "decision fusion" strategies are popularly used in HAR literature. Therefore, multi sensor data fusion is another popular approach in HAR solution to enhance the recognition accuracy.

3 Sensory Data, Audio and Video Data for HAR

Data obtained from the deployed heterogeneous sensors in intelligent environments or from body-attached sensors(wearables) in datasets are processed. Thusly, various modalities of information assortment have been proposed: compact wearable sensors, accelerometers, gyroscopes are deployed on the body (Rashidi and Mihailidis, 2013; Yen et al., 2020), smartphone in-built sensors (Anguita et al., 2013), binary sensors (van Kasteren et al., 2011; Singla et al., 2010), audio (Oliver et al., 2002; Stork et al., 2012) and video (Ajmal et al., 2019; Popoola and Wang, 2012; Zhang and Parker, 2016). After the data collection, the dataset is used to train various ML strategies to predict the actions of individuals for various purposes, such as sending early alerts to medical practitioners or any caregivers and mitigating the risks associated with the individuals whose health is deteriorating. There are several standard datasets available publicly for HAR. Therefore, it is a very complicated task to choose the appropriate dataset to evaluate the HAR system. Several datasets have their own advantages and disadvantages.

Table 2 Some HAR solutions using several sensory data

Reference	Data source	Description
Stork et al. (2012)	Audio	Robustly apprehend 22 different kind sounds that correspond to some of human sports in a toilet and kitchen context. NEV method is used to classify activities using audio stram
Galván-Tejada et al. (2016)	Audio	Use audio features to identify several indoor activities
Jung and Chi (2020)	Audio	Develop a sound recognition based human activity model. Several indoor activities are considered in this work
Ntalampiras and Potamitis (2018)	Audio	Audio-based HAR system using HMM is developed to identify indoor activities
Ajmal et al. (2019)	Video	A video-based HAR system using SVM to identify complex activities
Popoola and Wang (2012)	Video	A video-based abnormal activity recognition system
Zhang and Parker (2016)	Video	A video-based HAR system
Jiang and Yin (2015)	Wearable Sensor	A wearable sensor based HAR system for outdoor activities
Zubair et al. (2016)	Wearable Sensor	A wearable accelerometer based HAR system usin DT and RF classifier
Attal et al. (2015)	Wearable Sensor	Three inertial sensor based HAR system using K-NN, SVM, GMM, RF, k-means and HMM classifiers
Wang et al. (2020)	Wearable Sensor	Wearable sensor based HAR system using in combination of CNN and LSTM
Katoch (2017)	Wearable Sensor	Wearable sensor fusion based HAR system using CNN
Yen et al. (2020)	Wearable Sensor	Wearable Inertial Sensors based HAR system using DL methods
Natarajasivan and Govindarajan (2016)	Smartphone	Smartphone-based sensor fusion using ML methods
Chen and Xue (2015)	Smartphone	A smartphone-based HAR system using CNN
Tran and Phan (2016)	Smartphone	A smartphone-based HAR system using SVM
Wang et al. (2016)	Smartphone	A smartphone-based HAR system using KNN
Ronao and Cho (2016)	Smartphone	A smartphone-based HAR system using deep CNN
Tian and Chen (2016)	Smartphone	A smartphone-based HAR system using SVM
Song-Mi et al. (2017)	Smartphone	Smartphone-based HAR system using CNN and Co-training based ME

(continued)

Table 2 (continued)

Reference	Data source	Description
Mejia-Ricart et al. (2017)	Smartphone	A smartphone-based HAR system using unsupervised learning
Nurhanim et al. (2017)	Smartphone	Smartphone-based HAR system using multiclass SVM and MC-SVM-Polynomial
Ravi et al. (2017)	Smartphone	Smartphone-based HAR system using DL methodology
Li et al. (2017)	Smartphone	Smartphone-based HAR system using adaboost-stump
Cvetkovic et al. (2017)	Smartphone	Smartphone-based HAR system using DT, SVR, multi-layer perceptron - neural network, linear regression, RF and Reptree-DT
Bulbul et al. (2018)	Smartphone	Smartphone-based HAR system using DT, SVM, k-NN and ensemble classification methods (boosting, bagging, stacking)
Yu and Qin (2018)	Smartphone	A Smartphone-based HAR system using RNN
Jain and Kanhangad (2018)	Smartphone	Smartphone-based HAR system using SVM and KNN
Chen et al. (2019)	Smartphone	A Smartphone-based HAR system using ELM
Barua et al. (2019)	Smartphone	A Smartphone-based HAR system using K-NN, RF, SVM and deep CNN
Voicu et al. (2019)	Smartphone	A Smartphone-based HAR system using Multi-layer Perceptron

3.1 Sensory Data

Wearable sensor datasets are highly popular to evaluate a HAR system. In order to infer descriptions of human behaviors and transport modes, sensor data is obtained using smartphone or wearable sensors positioned at various locations of the body. In human movement investigation, action following and identification, the utility of tactile information given by cell phones and other wearable sensor gadgets has affected the exploration scene because of their conspicuous focal points over other sensor modalities. Normally, smartphones and wearable sensor based physical HAR systems sensors are motivated by their ubiquity, discretion, inexpensive installation procedures and ease of use (Nweke et al., 2018). The proliferation of the age of smartphones with multiple in-built sensors enable researchers to gather human physiological signals to track daily living activity has made human physical activity analysis an intrinsic part of our everyday lives. Smartphones have an extensive range of sensors with access to "accelerometer", "gyroscope", "proximity", "magnetometer", "Bluetooth", "Wi-Fi", "microphones" and "light sensor" and "cellular radio" sensors that can be utilized to deduce various human physical activities (Nweke et al., 2018). In coarse grain and context-aware HAR, user location and social interaction between users can be monitored using an accelerometer, gyroscope, heart rate and GPS sensors (Nweke et al., 2018). "Accelerometer", "gyroscope" and "magnetometer motion" sensors are used to identify and monitor various human physical activities. Other in-built smartphone sensors such as proximity and light sensors are used to identify the light intensity of the users' position such as light or dark place (Incel, 2015).Similarly, barometers, air humidity, pedometers and thermometers are used for ambient assisted living and to maintain the healthy information of elderly people (Gong et al., 2012).

Advantages:

- Smartphones have become part of our daily life and can be found in each home and conveyed wherever we go. Cell phones and wearable sensors are regular elective strategies for construing action data in this unique circumstance. (Nweke et al., 2018).
- Smartphone sensors take advantage of statistical and frequency based features to identify human physical activities (Nweke et al., 2018). Statistical features take less time and complexity for computation (Figo et al., 2010).
- Cell phones and wearable gadgets are area free, savvy, simple to convey and don't represent any radiation-initiated wellbeing peril (Alsheikh et al., 2015).

Given the conspicuous advantages of the execution of human movement dependent on smartphone and wearable sensors, a scope of studies have been proposed by utilizing the information delivered utilizing these gadgets (Morales and Akopian, 2017).

Disadvantages:

- Wearing a sensor for a long duration is problematic.
- Battery life is less.
- Data collected using smartphone sensors are noisy.
- Continuous use of smartphone in-built sensor can cause battery discharge.

3.2   Audio Data

Audio data based HAR has been addressed in the wearable computing community (Clarkson and Pentland, 1998), for auditory surveillance systems (Eronen et al., 2006), multimedia systems (Zhang and Kuo, 2001). In HAR, audio datasets are not alone sufficient to recognize various static or dynamic activities such as sitting or walking. Audio datasets can be helpful to identify some indoor activities such as brushing the teeth. Since sound is relatively easy to reflect and refract, physical barriers in indoor space are less influenced by the propagation of sound. In addition, as sound can be assessed remotely, movement data from people who do not wear sensing devices can be obtained (Jung and Chi, 2020).There are various advantages and disadvantages of audio data.

Advantages:

- Easy to collect.
- No wearable sensors are needed to collect audio information.
- No need to install any other hardware device. Using a smartphone one can capture the audio information.

Disadvantages:

- Audio datasets are noisy.
- Sometimes it may be difficult to differentiate between two audio information.
- Only audio data is not sufficient to recognize some basic activities.

HAR using audio data has a significant difference compared to any other HAR techniques (Jung and Chi, 2020). First, the approach based on sound recognition does not need the identification phase of the individual who is conducting the activity. A video-based approach, for example, typically begins by locating an object (e.g., an individual) performing various physical activities and distinguishing its various parts of the body and their association, which differentiates between various patterns of the activities, and eventually finds the operation performed by the object (Ji et al., 2013; Jung and Chi, 2020; Du et al., 2015). However, an audio based HAR system simplifies data processing process and modeling as it is relied upon on sound activity generated information. Moreover, an audio based HAR system eliminates the effect of multiple errors that can arise in the recognition of artifacts (e.g. sensing error, detecting error, classification error) (Jung and Chi, 2020).

Moreover, the sound recognition-based approach classifies categories of operation by not only considering the sounds produced by individuals who are doing tasks, but also those of people-related artifacts (Jung and Chi, 2020).

3.3 Video Data

Video data is easily collected after installing a camera. Using the collected video frames or images one can identify various human activities. Video datasets are more useful to identify various complex activities such as cooking food, peeling orange etc. as complex activities are the combination of different basic activities. While cooking food standing and movement of hand both are two different activities. Moreover, using video data one can take location as a feature to identify the activities more accurately. To capture the location in video data, we don't need any other sensors. There are several advantages and disadvantages of video dataset.

Advantages:

- To collect the video data only the camera is sufficient.
- Easy to install.
- One video frame or an image gives the total information regarding the object, the location and the activity performed by the object.

- Well established feature selection methods are available to extract several features from video data.

Disadvantages:

- It can be problematic to collect the video data from a populated location or from the location where many physical obstacles exist or from the places where brightness is low (Wang et al., 2015).
- To collect the indoor data using a camera, privacy can be another issue.
- Feature extraction can be complex while recognizing the complex activities.

4 ML and DL in HAR

HAR is a multi-class classification problem. Several ML and DL algorithms are used in HAR solutions so far.

4.1 ML in HAR

The popular ML algorithms such as "Decision Tree" (DT), "Random Forest" (RF), "Naive Bayes" (NB), "Support Vector Machine" (SVM), "K-nearest Neighbour" (KNN), "Neural Networks" (NN), "Hidden Markov Model"(HMM), "Gaussian Mixture Model" (GMM) and "Extreme Learning Machine" (ELM) (Thakur and Biswas, 2020). The performance of any of the machine learning classifiers primarily depends on the dataset. Raw sensor data or vision based data both are noisy. So, data preprocessing is essential to process the data. The aforementioned classification algorithms are supervised algorithms. The input in these algorithms is the labelled data. That means, each feature vector or instance of a dataset is mapped with a class label. Therefore, feature extraction and selection both are very important phases in ML. Using various feature extraction and selection techniques depend on the dataset, the relevant and important features are fed to the ML classifiers to get the result.

4.2 Challenges of ML in HAR

In HAR, several ML techniques have been employed. This sector still faces many technological challenges. However, some of the issues are correlated with other fields of recognition such as computer vision and processing of natural language, while others are unique to recognizing sensor-based behavior and involve dedicated methods for real-life applications (Chen et al., 2021). Here are a few categorizations of issues that should be discussed by the activity recognition group.

- Data collection is the first and foremost challenge to implement a HAR system. As there are several types of data (sensory, audio and video) that can be used to implement a HAR model, so deciding the type of data is a crucial task. Recently, researchers used fusion of sensors to enhance the recognition accuracy of HAR models. In case of data collection, it is difficult to manage the adequate number of volunteers to perform several physical activities.
- Data preprocessing is another critical challenge in this domain. There are several data preprocessing techniques in ML literature. The data preprocessing techniques are very much dependent on the source of the data. The preprocessing technique which is fruitful in audio data may not be useful in sensory data. Imbalance dataset is another problem to apply ML strategies. In case of imbalance in the dataset the performance of the classifier degrades. Hence, in the data preprocessing phase, it is necessary to take care of several problems that can be associated with the collected dataset.
- Feature extraction is a big challenge in the domain of HAR. The human physical activities are inter-activity related. Therefore, it is very difficult to identify the relevant and important features for better performance of the ML classifier. Moreover, the relevancy of the features totally depend on the type of the datasets. The features which are relevant in case of sensor data the features may not work well in case of audio or video data.
- Dimensionality reduction is another important challenge. In case of huge numbers of extracted features, it may be possible that some features are correlated. That means redundant features are there. As a result, time complexity has increased. Thus, computation cost will be higher. Several dimensionality reduction techniques are there to reduce the dimension of the feature set. However, it may cause data loss. Therefore, selection of the appropriate features is a challenging issue.
- Recognition of human behavior requires three factors: users, time, and dataset (Chen et al., 2021). First, patterns of activity are person-dependent. Different users can have various types of operation. Second, over time, activity pattern definitions differ. It is impractical to presume that users retain their pattern of activities unchanged over a long period of time. In addition, when in use, innovative activities are likely to occur. Thirdly, the source of the collected datasets are different. In case of sensor data, the configuration of the different sensors varies. In case of audio-video data, there are several challenges such as the impacts of illumination condition and privacy concerns.
- Overfitting is a crucial challenge in ML. In case of ML, sometimes it may happen that the training accuracy of any ML based model is much higher but in case of new data, the testing accuracy is very poor. It may happen, when the information and noise in the training data is learned by a model to the degree that it negatively affects the model's output on new data.

4.3 DL in HAR

DL techniques such as "Convolution Neural Networks" (CNN), "Long-Short Term Memory" (LSTM), "Recurrent Neural Network" (RNN) are popularly used for HAR. DL methods are capable of learning the features automatically. Therefore, there is no need for feature engineering in DL methods. But DL methods are data hungry and the computational complexity of DL methods are higher than ML. Figure 4, depicts recent DL methods that are used in HAR (Nweke et al., 2018).

4.4 Challenges of DL in HAR

- DL methods are data hungry. To get good performance using DL methods, the dimension of the dataset should be large.
- The computational complexity of the DL methods are high. Instead of CPU-based systems, GPU-based systems are much more fruitful to get the result in some permissible time.

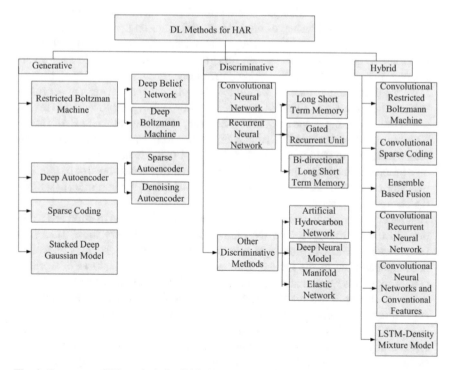

Fig. 4 Taxonomy of DL methods for HAR (Nweke et al., 2018)

- DL algorithms are capable of learning the features automatically. Therefore, some-times DL methods do not properly recognize the similar human physical activities.
- Several learning parameters such as drop-out rate, number of epochs etc. are used in DL methods. Deciding the values of the hyperparameters is a very challenging task. There are several hyperparameter optimization techniques. Choosing a suitable hyperparameter optimization technique is also very challenging.

5 Implementation of HAR

Efficiency of the HAR model is a big challenge. Healthcare is a sensitive issue. So, researchers are continuously trying to enhance the effectiveness of the HAR model. There are several directions to enhance the effectiveness of the HAR model. The HAR model can be efficient regarding accuracy, response time, simplicity, security etc. The main concern is accuracy. To enhance the accuracy of the HAR solutions, several approaches are used. ML and/or DL approaches consist of various phases. All the phases have some role to enhance the efficiency of the HAR model. Figure 5, shows the steps of HAR system implementation.

- Data Collection Phase: This phase is a critical and time-consuming phase. Ulti-mately, the overall efficiency of the HAR model relies on the data set. Relevancy of the collected data is a major concern. The sensors used to collect the data are an important issue because different sensors give us the data set in different formats. For example, the data collected using smartphone sensors are very noisy data.
- Data Pre-processing Phase: As mentioned, the collected data set has a major role to enhance the efficiency of the HAR model, the raw data is pre-processed in several ways. Preprocessing of the raw data is necessary to build an efficient HAR model. Noise removal, removing of missing data, outliers removal, data normalization are major concerns in data preprocessing. Different datasets need different types of data preprocessing techniques. For instance, the audio datasets need to be digitized using the concept of sampling. In case of video based data, it is important to subtract the background information.
- Feature engineering: Feature engineering consists of feature extraction and selec-tion. In the healthcare sector, the dimensions of data is very high. Therefore, feature engineering is required to enhance the classification accuracy as well as the response time of the model. The selection of relevant features is a crucial task. There are several statistical approaches proposed in HAR literature for the selection of the relevant features. Using the proper feature extraction and selection approach, one can increase the efficiency of the HAR model. Handcrafted features work well in HAR. Extraction of handcrafted features need expert domain knowl-edge. Many kinds of low-level characteristics are widely used in literature, such as "zero-crossing rate", "band-energy ratio", "spectral roll-off", "spectral flux", "spectral centroid", "spectral comparison", "mel-frequency cepstral coefficients" (MFCCs) and "gammatone frequency cepstral coefficients" (Cruciani et al., 2020).

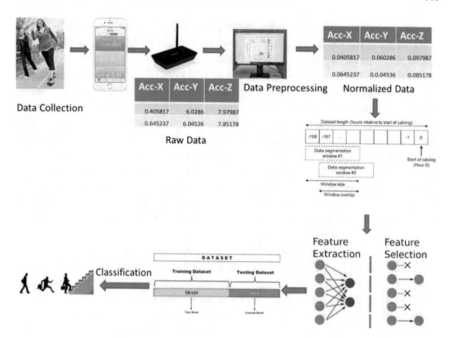

Fig. 5 Different Phases of HAR system (Thakur and Biswas, 2020)

Many of the above features function well with particular datasets, but others can fail. DL methods can learn the features automatically.

- Classification: There are several classification approaches in machine learning and deep learning. These classification algorithms are used to classify different human activities. To enhance the accuracy of the HAR model, some researchers use various ensemble ML and/or DL algorithms or hybrid ML and/or DL algorithms.

ML and/or DL methods give the opportunity to increase the efficiency of the HAR model in each and every phase. Implementation of HAR model using several ML and/or DL methods open a new horizon in the domain of smart healthcare.

5.1 Experimental Environment

Experimental setup to address all the aforementioned challenges is an issue for the new researchers. There are several tools such as the MATLAB machine learning toolbox, deep learning toolbox, WEKA tool can be used in all the experiments to create a HAR model using ML and/or DL. MATLAB is one of the very popular tools to perform the experiment related to HAR in ML and/or DL. Though, to use the ML and DL toolbox of MATLAB, someone has to purchase the licence from MathWorks. MathWorks is the provider of MATLAB. WEKA tool is freely available and very simple to use. One can easily download the WEKA tool from the web and can use it for medical data classification. Another very common ML tool is R. This can also be used to build ML and/or DL HAR models. Now-a-days, python is getting popularity due to its rich library which is related to ML and/or DL. In this chapter, the step-by-step procedure is shown to develop a HAR model. Starting from the installation and the hardware and software specifications the step-by-step procedure will be helpful for a new researcher in this domain. Starting from the data collection pictorial representation of each and every step will be helpful for the users. Data can be collected using various sensors. It depends on the type of the experiment. For example, if someone wants to collect the data for fall detection, smartphone inbuilt sensors can be used to collect the data. There are several mobile applications such as SenSee, which are available to run the "accelerometer" and "gyroscope" sensors of smartphones to gather the data while performing several activities. As smartphones are available to almost every person so its the easiest way to collect the data using a smartphone. After collection of data, the data will be transferred to the laptop or PC for further computation. The data transfer can be done using data cable or Bluetooth or wirelessly. Now the raw data will be pre-processed using several ML techniques. Here, the data preprocessing is done using python libraries. If someone wants to go for supervised learning then the data should be labelled manually. Again, feature extraction and selection can be done in python. Then we have to use machine learning algorithms for prediction. Several performance measures are used to check the prediction accuracy of the implemented HAR model.

6   Evaluation of HAR Systems

6.1   *Evaluation Methodologies*

Evaluation of any ML or DL method needs the disjoint set of training and testing. The target to evaluate any ML or DL methods is to check its effectiveness for unseen data. One instinctive strategy is known as random splitting. In a random split, the total dataset is splitted into training and testing dataset. Generally, two third of the total dataset is used for training purposes and the remaining one third of the dataset is used for testing purposes. Random split is the simplest method to split the data in training and testing. However, a random split method can be biased to a particular feature set. In that case, the model learns some of the specific features. As a result, the actual performance of the classifier is hampered. Therefore, another approach came into picture, known as k-cross validation. In this approach, the dataset is divided in k numbers of equally size folds. In k-fold cross validation, k number of iterations are there. In the first iteration, the first fold data is used for testing and k-1 folds are used for training. Similarly, in the next iteration 2 folds data are used for training and remaining k-2 folds are used for testing and so on. Finally, the evaluation metrics are calculated based on the average performance of all the iterations. In practical terms, the tenfold cross validation method is widely used. However, if the aim is to compare to different classifiers to select the most accurate one, a 5X2-fold cross validation with a pair t-test is endorsed. Actually, this is the 5 repetitions of twofold cross validation with different dataset combinations, which is generated using a random number generator using different seed values. In case of comparison of two different classifiers using 5X2- fold cross validation, five different accuracies are available for both the classifiers. If there is significant statistical difference among the accuracies of both the classifiers then statistical paired t-test is used to identify the most accurate classifier. Here, the null hypothesis is the similar accuracy or error rate of both the classifiers. The $\tilde{t}$ statistics is defined as follows:

$$\tilde{t} = \frac{p_i^{(j)}}{\sqrt{\frac{1}{5}\sum_{i=1}^{5} s_i^2}} \tag{1}$$

where p_i^{j} are the accuracies of the two classifiers, $1 \leq i \leq 5$ and $1 \leq j \leq 2$ in 5X2-fold cross validation. In Eq. 1, $s_i^2 = (p_i^{(1)} - \bar{p})^2 + (p_i^{(2)} - \bar{p})^2$ where $\bar{p}$ is the average of $p_i^{(1)}$ and $p_i^{(2)}$. $\tilde{t}$ follows the Students t distribution with five degrees of freedom under the null hypothesis. The 5X2-fold cross validation with the paired t-test has been found to be more successful than the non-parametric McNemar's test and gives a better estimate of the differences due to the choice of the training range (Dietterich, 1998).

6.2 Evaluation Metrics

In general, only observational evidence has confirmed the selection of a classification algorithm for HAR. Cross validation with statistical tests is used by the vast majority of research to compare the performance of classifiers with a given dataset. For a classification problem of c groups, the classification results for a specific approach may be ordered in a confusion matrix M_{cxc}. The confusion matrix shows the element M_{ij} is the number of instances from class i that were classified as class j (scar et al., 2012). From the confusion matrix various performance measures of the classifiers such as "precision", "recall", "F-Measure" and "accuracy" are calculated using "Ture Positive (TP)", "True Negative (TN)", "False Positive (FP)" and "False Negative (FN)". The equations of the performance measures are as follows:

- Accuracy: It is the most remarkable presentation measure to sum up the general characterization execution of the relative multitude of classes. The following equation is used to calculate the accuracy of the model:

$$Accuracy = \frac{TP + TN}{TP + TN + FP + FN} \tag{2}$$

- Precision: It gives the level of positive occasions appropriately grouped to the general number of positive cases ordered. Precision is defined using the following equation:

$$Precision = \frac{TP}{TP + FP} \tag{3}$$

- Recall: It gives the proportion of positive occurrences effectively ordered to the complete number of positive occasions. Recall is defined using the following equation:

$$Recall = \frac{TP}{TP + FN} \tag{4}$$

- F-Measure: It is the harmonic mean of precision and recall.

$$F - Measure = \frac{Precision.Recall}{Precision + Recall} \tag{5}$$

where

- TP: The sum of accurately categorized instances that are correctly classified.
- TN: The number of wrongly-identified cases that are incorrectly classified.
- FP: The number of incorrect instances which are properly identified.
- FN: The number of right instances that are wrongly listed.

Finally, the "False Positive Rate" (FPR) and "False Negative Rate" (FNR) Are calculated as follows:

$$FPR = \frac{FP}{TN + FP} \tag{6}$$

$$FNR = \frac{FN}{TP + FN} \tag{7}$$

7   Case Studies

Studies of different human activity patterns are helpful to identify various lifestyle diseases such as obesity, diabetes. Moreover, it can also be used for rehabilitation purposes such as cardiac rehabilitation or any neurological rehabilitation.Therefore, the research community is always trying to enhance the HAR systems using various ML or DL methods based on sensory or audio-video data.In this section some case study has been discussed. Recently, in (Wang et al., 2021), the authors proposed a "SpatioTemporal Human Activity Model (STHAM), for simulating SARS-CoV-2 transmission dynamics". The movement of the people and their interaction with individuals in the society is the primary cause of the flow of "SARS-COV-2" (Wang et al., 2021). Social determinants of wellbeing, for example, levels of training, family size, populace thickness, work environment school-family unit area designs, age-construction, and zone level neediness, joined with propensities, for example, cigarette smoking that debilitate wellbeing, will influence prompt and long haul pandemic impacts straightforwardly and by implication. The only realistic scientific approach to designing successful modelling is simulation that will minimize the adverse side effects and explain the treatments' efficacy (Gates, 2015, 2018). With the essential driver of the spread of "SARS-CoV-2" being the development and contact of individuals inside a gathering, displaying ought to be guided by patterns of human conduct as different individuals would dependent on their temperament, interact with tainted people exercises each day (Shereen et al., 2020). Therefore, there is a need for a HAR model. In this work, the human activity patterns which are recorded by "American Time Use Survey" (ATUS) (Statistics usdolbotl, 2015) is classified and used to simulate human activity in the context of estimating personal exposure to PM 2.5 (Albert et al., 2020; Lund et al., 2020; Wang et al., 2021). Hence, the authors develop STHAM, based the grouping of human exercises to deliver and order development directions and movement designs (Bellemans et al., 2010; Bhat et al., 2004; Bradley et al., 2010) and to combine spatial distributions of exposure agents to approximate overall geographical distributions in wide populations, human exposure. Therefore, the authors illustrated that the by and large noticed examples of "SARS-CoV-2" transmission inside the number of inhabitants here can be rehashed by a disease model dependent on the STHAM framework to reenact human development in the Wasatch Front of the State of Utah, United States of America[US] (Lund et al., 2020). Moreover, the authors uncover that disease rates are unequivocally reliant on the movement examples of the thought about specialists.

Stork *et al.* proposed an audio based HAR system using "Non-Markovian Ensemble Voting" (NEV) (Stork et al., 2012). In this work, 22 unique sounds identified with various sorts of human exercises in the restroom and kitchen are recognized. Sound stream is partitioned into different brief span casings to handle further to distinguish the human activities. Identification of these activities are helpful to monitor the health activities for elderly people or a person living alone.

Galvn-Tejada *et al.* proposed an audio based HAR system to identify different kitchen activities using neural networks, genetic algorithms and random forests (Galván-Tejada et al., 2016). The authors also analyse the various audio features to develop an efficient HAR solution.

Jung and Chi proposed an HAR system to identify some indoor activities using sound (Jung and Chi, 2020). In this work, Using the Log Mel-filter bank energy system, the sound data characteristics were extracted and a residual neural network model with 34 convolutional layers was trained using the data.

A HAR model based on recurrent neural networks for health and social care services was proposed in (Park et al., 2016). In this work, the authors have used joint angles from many time-changing body joints that are represented as a spatiotemporal function matrix (i.e., multiple body joint angles in time). With these derived characteristics, the authors train and test the recurrent neural network for HAR.

Therefore, from the aforementioned case studies we are able to understand that the various ML and DL approaches have significant impact in HAR based on sensory or audio-video data.

8   Conclusion

This chapter discusses the audio-video based HAR models using various ML and DL approaches. Addressing various issues and challenges of the different phases of the implementation of HAR system. There are several applications of HAR systems in modern healthcare, which motivate the researchers to investigate the HAR solutions using various datasets such as sensory data and audio-video data. The several case studies, which are discussed in this chapter demonstrate that HAR models are gaining popularity in several healthcare domains including the recent global pandemic.

References

Ajmal, M., Ahmad, F., Naseer, M., & Jamjoom, M. (2019). Recognizing human activities from video using weakly supervised contextual features. *IEEE Access, 7,* 98420–98435. https://doi.org/10.1109/ACCESS.2019.2929262.

Albert, L., Ramkiran, G., & Julio, C. (2020). Generation and classification of activity sequences for spatiotemporal modeling of human populations. *Online Journal of Public Health Informatics,* **12**(1). https://doi.org/10.5210/ojphi.v12i1.10588

Alsheikh, M. A., Selim, A., Niyato, D., Doyle, L., Lin, S., & Tan, H. P. (2015). Deep activity recognition models with triaxial accelerometers. CoRR abs/1511.04664. http://arxiv.org/abs/1511.04664

American Time Use Survey (ATUS). (2015). Statistics USdolbotl, United States (2016)

Anguita, D., Ghio, A., Oneto, L., Parra, X., & Reyes-Ortiz, J. L. (2013). A public domain dataset for human activity recognition using smartphones. In *European Symposium on Artificial Neural Networks, Computational Intelligence and Machine Learning.*

Artikis, A., Skarlatidis, A., & Paliouras, G. (2010). Behaviour recognition from video content: A logic programming approach. *International Journal on Artificial Intelligence Tools, 19*(2), 193–209. https://doi.org/10.1142/S021821301000011X.

Attal, F., Mohammed, S., Dedabrishvili, M., Chamroukhi, F., Oukhellou, L., & Amirat, Y. (2015). Physical human activity recognition using wearable sensors. *Sensors, 15*(12), 31314–31338.

Augusto, J. C., & Nugent, C. D. (2004). The use of temporal reasoning and management of complex events in smart homes. In *Proceedings of the 16th European Conference on Artificial Intelligence, ECAI'04* (pp. 778–782).

Bao, L., Intille, S. S. (2004). Activity recognition from user-annotated acceleration data. In *Pervasive Computing 2004.* Lecture Notes in Computer Science, Vol. 3001. https://doi.org/10.1007/978-3-540-24646-6-1

Barua, A., Masum, A. K. M., Hossain, M. E., Bahadur, E. H., & Alam, M. S. (2019). A study on human activity recognition using gyroscope, accelerometer, temperature and humidity data. In *2019 International Conference on Electrical, Computer and Communication Engineering (ECCE)* (pp. 1–6).

Bellemans, T., Kochan, B., Janssens, D., Wets, G., Arentze, T., & Timmermans, H. (2010). Implementation framework and development trajectory of feathers activity-based simulation platform. *Transportation Research Record, 2175*(1), 111–9. https://doi.org/10.3141/2175-13.

Bhat, C., Guo, J., Srinivasan, S., & Sivakumardoi, A. (2004). Comprehensive econometric microsimulator for daily activity-travel patterns. *Transportation Research Record, 1894*(1), 57–66. https://doi.org/10.3141/1894-07.

Bidargaddi, N., Sarela, A., Klingbeil, L., & Karunanithi, M. (2007). Detecting walking activity in cardiac rehabilitation by using accelerometer. In *2007 3rd International Conference on Intelligent*

Sensors, Sensor Networks and Information (pp. 555–560). https://doi.org/10.1109/ISSNIP.2007. 4496903

Bradley, M., Bowman, J., & Griesenbeck, B. (2010). Sacsim: An applied activity-based model system with fine-level spatial and temporal resolution. *Journal of Choice Modelling,33*(1), 5–31. https://doi.org/10.1016/S1755-5345(13)70027-7

Bulbul, E., Cetin, A., & Dogru, I. A. (2018). Human activity recognition using smartphones. In *2018 2nd International Symposium on Multidisciplinary Studies and Innovative Technologies (ISMSIT)* (pp. 1–6).

Bulling, A., Blanke, U., & Schiele, B. (2014). A tutorial on human activity recognition using body-worn inertial sensors. *ACM Computing Surveys (CSUR)46*(3) (2014). https://doi.org/10.1145/ 2499621

Chahuara, P., Fleury, A., Portet, F., & Vacher, M. (2016). On-line Human Activity Recognition from Audio and Home Automation Sensors: comparison of sequential and non-sequential models in realistic Smart Homes. *JAISE-Journal of Ambient Intelligence and Smart Environments, 8*(4), 399–422.

Chen, Y., & Xue, Y. (2015). A deep learning approach to human activity recognition based on single accelerometer. In *2015 IEEE International Conference on Systems, Man, and Cybernetics* (pp. 1488–1492)

Chen, K., Zhang, D., Yao, L., Guo, B., Yu, Z., & Liu, Y. (2021). Deep learning for sensor-based human activity recognition: Overview, challenges and opportunities

Chen, L., Nugent, C., Mulvenna, M., Finlay, D., Hong, X., & Poland, M. (2008). A logical framework for behaviour reasoning and assistance in a smart home. *International Journal of Assistive Robotics and Mechatronics, 9*(4), 20–34.

Chen, L., Nugent, C. D., & Wang, H. (2012). A knowledge-driven approach to activity recognition in smart homes. *IEEE Transactions on Knowledge and Data Engineering, 24*(6), 961–974. https:// doi.org/10.1109/TKDE.2011.51.

Chen, Z., Jiang, C., & Xie, L. (2019). A novel ensemble elm for human activity recognition using smartphone sensors. *IEEE Transactions on Industrial Informatics, 15*(5), 2691–2699.

Clarkson, B. (2003). *Life patterns : Structure from wearable sensors*. Ph.D. thesis, Massachusetts Institute of Technology, USA

Clarkson, B., & Pentland, A. (1998). Extracting context from environmental audio. In *Second International Symposium on Wearable Computers (Cat. No.98EX215), (Digest of Papers)* (pp. 154–155). https://doi.org/10.1109/ISWC.1998.729542

Cruciani, F., Magnani, A., & Maio, D. (2020). Feature learning for human activity recognition using convolutional neural networks. *CCF Transactions on Pervasive Computing and Interaction, 21,* 18–32.

Cvetkovic, B., Szeklicki, R., Janko, V., Lutomski, P., & Lustrek, M. (2017). Real-time activity monitoring with a wristband and a smartphone. *Information Fusion*

Department of Economic and Social Affairs and Population Division. (2004). *World population to 2300.* United Nations, New York, NY, USA: Department of Economic and Social Affairs and Population Division.

Dietterich, T. G. (1998). Approximate statistical tests for comparing supervised classification learning algorithms. *Neural Computation, 10,* 1895–1923.

Du, Y., Wang, W., & Wang, L. (2015). Hierarchical recurrent neural network for skeleton based action recognition. In *2015 IEEE Conference on Computer Vision and Pattern Recognition (CVPR)* (pp. 1110–1118). https://doi.org/10.1109/CVPR.2015.7298714

Eronen, A. J., Peltonen, V. T., Tuomi, J. T., Klapuri, A. P., Fagerlund, S., Sorsa, T., et al. (2006). Audio-based context recognition. *IEEE Transactions on Audio, Speech, and Language Processing, 14*(1), 321–329. https://doi.org/10.1109/TSA.2005.854103.

Figo, D., Diniz, P., Ferreira, D., & Cardoso, J. (2010). Preprocessing techniques for context recognition from accelerometer data. *Personal and Ubiquitous Computing, 14,* 645–662. https://doi. org/10.1007/s00779-010-0293-9.

Flanagan, J. A., Mantyjarvi, J., & Himberg, J. (2002). Unsupervised clustering of symbol strings and context recognition. In *2002 IEEE International Conference on Data Mining* (pp. 171–178). https://doi.org/10.1109/ICDM.2002.1183900

Galván-Tejada, C. E., Galván-Tejada, J. I., Celaya-Padilla, J. M., Delgado-Contreras, J. R., Magallanes-Quintanar, R., Martinez-Fierro, M. L., Garza-Veloz, I., López-Hernández, Y., Gamboa-Rosales, H. (2016). An analysis of audio features to develop a human activity recognition model using genetic algorithms, random forests, and neural networks. *Mobile Information Systems, 2016*, 1784,101. https://doi.org/10.1155/2016/1784101

Gates, B. (2015). The next epidemic-lessons from Ebola. *New England Journal of Medicine, 372*(15), 1381–4. https://doi.org/10.1056/NEJMp1502918.

Gates, B. (2018). Innovation for pandemics. *New England Journal of Medicine, 378*(22), 2057–2060. https://doi.org/10.1056/NEJMp1806283.

Gong, J., Cui, L., Xiao, K., & Wang, R. (2012). MPD-Model: A distributed multipreference-driven data fusion model and its application in a WSNs-based health- care monitoring system. *International Journal of Distributed Sensor Networks, 8*(12)

Htike, Z. Z., Egerton, S., Chow, K. Y. (2010). Real-time human activity recognition using external and internal spatial features. In *2010 Sixth International Conference on Intelligent Environments* (pp. 52–57). https://doi.org/10.1109/IE.2010.17

Incel, D. O. (2015). Analysis of movement, orientation and rotation-based sensing for phone placement recognition. *Sensors, 15*(10), 25474–25506.

Jain, A., & Kanhangad, V. (2018). Human activity classification in smartphones using accelerometer and gyroscope sensors. *IEEE Sensors Journal, 18*(3), 1169–1177.

Ji, S., Xu, W., Yang, M., & Yu, K. (2013). 3d convolutional neural networks for human action recognition. *IEEE Transactions on Pattern Analysis and Machine Intelligence, 35*(1), 221–231. https://doi.org/10.1109/TPAMI.2012.59.

Jiang, W., & Yin, Z. (2015). Human activity recognition using wearable sensors by deep convolutional neural networks. In *Proceedings of the 23rd ACM International Conference on Multimedia* (pp. 1307–1310). Association for Computing Machinery

Jung, M., & Chi, S. (2020). Human activity classification based on sound recognition and residual convolutional neural network. *Automation in Construction, 114*, 103,177. https://doi.org/10.1016/j.autcon.2020.103177

Katoch, E. (2017). Human activity recognition for physical rehabilitation using wearable sensors fusion and artificial neural networks. In *2017 Computing in Cardiology (CinC)* (pp. 1–4). https://doi.org/10.22489/CinC.2017.296-332

Khan, A. M., Lee, Y., Lee, S. Y., & Kim, T. (2010). A triaxial accelerometer-based physical-activity recognition via augmented-signal features and a hierarchical recognizer. *IEEE Transactions on Information Technology in Biomedicine, 14*(5), 1166–1172. https://doi.org/10.1109/TITB.2010.2051955.

Krishnan, N. C., & Cook, D. J. (2014). Activity recognition on streaming sensor data. *Pervasive and Mobile Computing, 10*, 138–154. https://doi.org/10.1016/j.pmcj.2012.07.003.

Lara, O. D., Preza, A. J., Labradora, M. A., & Posada, J. D. (2012). Centinela: A human activity recognition system based on acceleration and vital sign data. *Pervasive and Mobile Computing, 8*, 717–729

Lee, S. M., Yoon, S. M., Cho, H. (2017). Human activity recognition from accelerometer data using convolutional neural network. In *2017 IEEE International Conference on Big Data and Smart Computing (BigComp)* (pp. 131–134)

Li, P., Wang, Y., Tian, Y., Zhou, T., & Li, J. (2017). An automatic user-adapted physical activity classification method using smartphones. *IEEE Transactions on Biomedical Engineering, 64*(3), 706–714.

Li, J., Tian, L., Wang, H., An, Y., Wang, K., & Yu, L. (2019). Segmentation and recognition of basic and transitional activities for continuous physical human activity. *IEEE Access, 7*, 42565–42576. https://doi.org/10.1109/ACCESS.2019.2905575.

Lin, W., Sun, M., Poovendran, R., & Zhang, Z. (2008). Activity recognition using a combination of category components and local models for video surveillance. *IEEE Transactions on Circuits and Systems for Video Technology, 18*(8), 1128–1139. https://doi.org/10.1109/TCSVT.2008.927111.

Lund, A., Gouripeddi, R., & Facelli, J. (2020). Stham: an agent based model for simulating human exposure across high resolution spatiotemporal domains. *Journal of Exposure Science & Environmental Epidemiology*. https://doi.org/10.1038/s41370-020-0216-4.

Mejia-Ricart, L. F., Helling, P., & Olmsted, A. (2017). Evaluate action primitives for human activity recognition using unsupervised learning approach. In *2017 12th International Conference for Internet Technology and Secured Transactions (ICITST)* (pp. 186–188)

Minnen, D. (2008). *Unsupervised discovery of activity primitives from multivariate sensor data.* Ph.D. thesis, Georgia Institute of Technology, USA

Morales, J., & Akopian, D. (2017). Physical activity recognition by smartphones, a survey. *Biocybernetics and Biomedical Engineering, 37*(3), 388–400. https://doi.org/10.1016/j.bbe.2017.04.004.

Natarajasivan, D., & Govindarajan, M. (2016). Filter based sensor fusion for activity recognition using smartphone. *International Journal of Computer Science and Telecommunications, 7*(5), 26–31.

Ntalampiras, S., & Potamitis, I. (2018). Transfer learning for improved audio-based human activity recognition. *Biosensors, 8*(3)

Nurhanim, K., Elamvazuthi, I., Izhar, L. I., & Ganesan, T. (2017). Classification of human activity based on smartphone inertial sensor using support vector machine. In *2017 IEEE 3rd International Symposium in Robotics and Manufacturing Automation (ROMA)* (pp. 1–5)

Nweke, H. F., Teh, Y. W., Al-garadi, M. A., & Alo, U. R. (2018). Deep learning algorithms for human activity recognition using mobile and wearable sensor networks: State of the art and research challenges. *Expert Systems with Applications, 105,* 233–261. https://doi.org/10.1016/j.eswa.2018.03.056.

Okeyo, G., Chen, L., Wang, H., & Sterritt, R. (2014). Dynamic sensor data segmentation for real-time knowledge-driven activity recognition. *Pervasive and Mobile Computing, 10,* 155–172. https://doi.org/10.1016/j.pmcj.2012.11.004.

Oliver, N., Horvitz, E., & Garg, A. (2002). Layered representations for human activity recognition. In *Proceedings of the 4th IEEE International Conference on Multimodal Interfaces, ICMI '02* (p. 3). IEEE Computer Society. https://doi.org/10.1109/ICMI.2002.1166960

Park, S., Park, J., Al-masni, M., Al-antari, M., Uddin, M., & Kim, T. S. (2016). A depth camera-based human activity recognition via deep learning recurrent neural network for health and social care services. *Procedia Computer Science, 100,* 78–84. https://doi.org/10.1016/j.procs.2016.09.126 (International Conference on ENTERprise Information Systems/International Conference on Project MANagement/International Conference on Health and Social Care Information Systems and Technologies, CENTERIS/ProjMAN/HCist 2016)

Popoola, O. P., & Wang, K. (2012). Video-based abnormal human behavior recognition-a review. *IEEE Transactions on Systems, Man, and Cybernetics, Part C (Applications and Reviews), 42*(6), 865–878. https://doi.org/10.1109/TSMCC.2011.2178594

Rashidi, P., & Mihailidis, A. (2013). A survey on ambient-assisted living tools for older adults. *IEEE Journal of Biomedical and Health Informatics, 17*(3), 579–590. https://doi.org/10.1109/JBHI.2012.2234129.

Ravi, D., Wong, C., Lo, B., & Yang, G. (2017). A deep learning approach to on-node sensor data analytics for mobile or wearable devices. *IEEE Journal of Biomedical and Health Informatics, 21*(1), 56–64.

Ronao, C. A., & Cho, S. B. (2016). Human activity recognition with smartphone sensors using deep learning neural networks. *Expert Systems with Applications, 59,* 235–244.

Rota, N. A., & Thonnat, M. (2000). Activity recognition from video sequences using declarative models. In *Proceedings of the 14th European Conference on Artificial Intelligence, ECAI'00* (pp. 673–677). IOS Press, NLD

Rsnen, O. (2012). Hierarchical unsupervised discovery of user context from multivariate sensory data. In *2012 IEEE International Conference on Acoustics, Speech and Signal Processing (ICASSP)* (pp. 2105–2108). https://doi.org/10.1109/ICASSP.2012.6288326

Shereen, M. A., Khan, S., Kazmi, A., Bashir, N., & Siddique, R. (2020). Covid-19 infection: Origin, transmission, and characteristics of human coronaviruses. *Journal of Advanced Research, 24,* 91–98. https://doi.org/10.1016/j.jare.2020.03.005.

Singla, G., Cook, D. J., & Schmitter-Edgecombe, M. (2010). Recognizing independent and joint activities among multiple residents in smart environments. *Journal of Ambient Intelligence and Humanized Computing, 1*(1), 57–63. https://doi.org/10.1007/s12652-009-0007-1.

Spinsante, S., Angelici, A., Lundström, J., Espinilla, M., Cleland, I., & Nugent, C. (2016). A mobile application for easy design and testing of algorithms to monitor physical activity in the workplace. *Mobile Information Systems, 2016,* 5126,816

U.S. State Department and National Institute on Aging (NIA). (2007). Why population aging matters: A global perspective. U. S. State Department and National Institute on Aging (NIA)

Storf, H., Becker, M., & Riedl, M. (2009). Rule-based activity recognition framework: Challenges, technique and learning. In *2009 3rd International Conference on Pervasive Computing Technologies for Healthcare* (pp. 1–7). https://doi.org/10.4108/ICST.PERVASIVEHEALTH2009.6108

Stork, J. A., Spinello, L., Silva, J., & Arras, K. O. (2012). Audio-based human activity recognition using non-markovian ensemble voting. In *2012 IEEE RO-MAN: The 21st IEEE International Symposium on Robot and Human Interactive Communication*, pp. 509–514. https://doi.org/10.1109/ROMAN.2012.6343802

Thakur, D., & Biswas, S.: A novel human activity recognition strategy using extreme learning machine algorithm for smart health. In *2nd International Conference on Emerging Technologies in Data Mining and Information Security(IEMIS2020)*. Kolkata

Thakur, D., & Biswas, S. (2020). Smartphone based human activity monitoring and recognition using ml and dl: A comprehensive survey. *Journal of Ambient Intelligence and Humanized Computing, 11*(11), 5433–5444.

Tian, Y., & Chen, W. (2016). Mems-based human activity recognition using smartphone. In *2016 35th Chinese Control Conference (CCC)* (pp. 3984–3989).

Tran, D. N., & Phan, D. D. (2016). Human activities recognition in android smartphone using support vector machine. In *2016 7th International Conference on Intelligent Systems, Modelling and Simulation (ISMS)* (pp. 64–68).

van Kasteren, T. L. M., Englebienne, G., & Krse, B. J. A. (2011). Human activity recognition from wireless sensor network data: benchmark and software. In *Activity recognition in pervasive intelligent environments* Vol. 4, pp. 165–186. Atlantis Press

Voicu, R. A., Dobre, C., Bajenaru, L., & Ciobanu, R. I. (2019). Human physical activity recognition using smartphone sensors. *Sensors, 19*(3)

Wang, Y., Li, B., Gouripeddi, R., & Facelli, J. C. (2021). Human activity pattern implications for modeling sars-cov-2 transmission. *Computer Methods and Programs in Biomedicine, 199,* 105,896. https://doi.org/10.1016/j.cmpb.2020.105896

Wang, Y., Jiang, X., Cao, R., & Wang, X. (2015). Robust indoor human activity recognition using wireless signals. *Sensors, 15*(7), 17195–17208. https://doi.org/10.3390/s150717195.

Wang, A., Chen, G., Yang, J., Zhao, S., & Chang, C. (2016). A comparative study on human activity recognition using inertial sensors in a smartphone. *IEEE Sensors Journal, 16*(11), 4566–4578.

Wang, H., Zhao, J., Li, J., Tian, L., Tu, P., Cao, T., et al. (2020). Wearable sensor-based human activity recognition using hybrid deep learning techniques. *Security and Communication Networks, 2020,* 12.

Yen, C. T., Liao, J. X., & Huang, Y. K. (2020). Human daily activity recognition performed using wearable inertial sensors combined with deep learning algorithms. *IEEE Access, 8,* 174,105–174,114. https://doi.org/10.1109/ACCESS.2020.3025938

Yu, S., & Qin, L. (2018). Human activity recognition with smartphone inertial sensors using bidir-lstm networks. In *2018 3rd International Conference on Mechanical, Control and Computer Engineering (ICMCCE)* (pp. 219–224).

Zhang, T., & Kuo, C. J. (2001). Audio content analysis for online audiovisual data segmentation and classification. *IEEE Transactions on Speech and Audio Processing, 9*(4), 441–457. https://doi.org/10.1109/89.917689.

Zhang, H., & Parker, L. E. (2016). Code4d: Color-depth local spatio-temporal features for human activity recognition from rgb-d videos. *IEEE Transactions on Circuits and Systems for Video Technology, 26*(3), 541–555. https://doi.org/10.1109/TCSVT.2014.2376139.

Zubair, M., Song, K., & Yoon, C. (2016). Human activity recognition using wearable accelerometer sensors. In *2016 IEEE International Conference on Consumer Electronics-Asia (ICCE-Asia)* (pp. 1–5). https://doi.org/10.1109/ICCE-Asia.2016.7804737

On Body Vitals Monitoring for Disease Prediction: A Systematic Survey

Tanuja Das, Partha Pratim Kalita, Ramesh Saha, and Nizara Das

Abstract With the increase in the number of people influenced by chronic ailments such as diabetes, hypertension, obesity and many more, promoting a healthy mind and body for a liberated way of life is the need of the hour. A possible way to achieve this to be aware of the vital body signs and monitor them continuously, so as to detect any anomalies in the body of an individual. The traditional way of monitoring the vital body signs becomes insufficient as the frequency of monitoring is not enough to reveal the underlying degradation of the patient health (Mei and Gül, 2019). Internet of things (IOT) in healthcare have come forward as a promising field for remote monitoring of the vital body signs, thereby emerging as a necessary component of the medical systems in the course of time (Wu et al., 2019). These remote monitoring systems have the potential to uncover the latent causes responsible for a particular disease and is an active research area grabbing the interest of the academia and the industries as well. For people having serious health concerns, these systems can be particularly life-saving. Also, these systems can diminish the load on the existing healthcare framework by decreasing the number of repetitive visits to the hospital. Due to the accelerated advancement in technology, the purview of the remote health-care systems has improved to a considerable extent (Tokognon et al., 2017). These systems are essentially established on the grounds of advanced wireless networks and wearable sensor technologies. The paradigm shift of the current healthcare systems from clinic-centric to patient-centric has been possible due to the assimilation of mobile communication approaches with wearable sensor technology (Bonato, 2003). Wearable health monitoring system has the capability of providing constantly the status of the vital body signs, which can give a comprehensive overview of the health of an individual. Hence, these health monitoring systems based on wireless sensor technology will be able to decrease the costs of health monitoring leading to

T. Das (✉) · P. P. Kalita
Department of Information Technology, Gauhati University, Guwahati, Assam, India
e-mail: tanujadas55@gmail.com

R. Saha
School of Computing Science and Engineering, VIT Bhopal University, Bhopal, Madhya Pradesh, India

N. Das
B.Sc Nursing College, Silchar, Assam, India

the improvement of the quality of life (Lymberis and Gatzoulis, 2006). Monitoring of the vital body signs has been made possible due to the significant enhancement of the relevant technologies. In this chapter, some of the critical facets for the monitoring systems for vital body signs have been summarized, along with the architecture of some of the most advanced wearable vital signs technologies developed so far. Here, first a target has been made to provide the background study essential for the understanding of the basic vital body signs like electrocardiogram, heart rate, blood pressure, respiration rate, blood oxygen saturation and body temperature, etc. extracted from non-invasive wearable health devices. Then a review on the effect and monitoring needs for each of the vital sign is made in order to understand the starting point of intervention for the individual vital body signs. Finally, a detailed description on the current technological advancements on the health monitoring systems based on the vital body parameters is presented.

Keywords Internet of things · Wireless networks · Wearable sensor technology · Health monitoring systems · Vital signs · Disease prediction

This book chapter contains the following sections:

1. Introduction to the need for generalized IOT healthcare paradigm.
2. Role of body vitals monitoring system for disease prediction in IOT healthcare.
3. Valuable vital signs and their need to be monitored.
4. A review on the recent technological advances in the remote healthcare monitoring systems.

1 Introduction to the Need for Generalized IOT Healthcare Paradigm

The present world is burdened with the rampant cost of the healthcare services with uncountable amount of the population facing age-related as well as chronic conditions (Mathur et al., 2015). With the rapid development of technology, the everyone is looking forward to a world where every individual will be able afford the basic healthcare facilities (Okpala, 2018) in an effective manner. Although the technology still cannot eradicate each and every disease or prevent the population from aging, it can at least make the basic healthcare facilities pocket friendly and affordable. Also, technology can change the conventional health checkups from hospital-centric to home-centric and with the correct diagnosis, can also reduce the need for hospitalization (Zhou et al., 2019).

Today the regime of the internet of things (IoT) has provided a prospect of better functioning of medical centers and thereby contributing to the improved treatment of the patients (Mutlag et al., 2019). In simple words, IoT can be defined as machines communicating to each other and taking decisions autonomously (Hassan et al., 2019). IoT has the potential in improving access to quality healthcare and also reduces the cost endured in monitoring and analyzing the patients (Okpala, 2018). Extending the healthcare services using IoT in homes has already made it possible to collect data and track wellness, which is changing the management of chronic conditions and many other diseases (Alansari et al., 2018a).

The application of smart technology in healthcare makes the system more efficient and effective (Chau et al., 2019). The way healthcare is provided, is also changing due to the presence of autonomous and intelligent devices. Seamless data transmission using devices embedded with artificial intelligence (AI) makes it possible to collect real-time data and diagnose the diseases from the symptoms extracted from the sensor data (Banerjee et al., 2020).

Numerous medical emergencies (Ko et al., 2010) like heart failure, diabetes, asthma attacks etc., can be prevented by taking advantage of the sensor data generated by the autonomous IoT devices (Petrakis et al., 2018). Using an intelligent IoT device linked to a smartphone, real-time data can be generated and then can be sent to the respective medical server. As patients connect more with these embedded devices and generate more data, it becomes convenient for the physicians to identify and address their needs more efficiently (Petrakis et al., 2020).

Although IoT is considered as the new revolution in the healthcare industry, seamless data transfer with no or least data loss and traffic-free transmission with cost efficiency are some of the major challenges in the fourth generation healthcare systems (Bhoyar et al., 2019). Autonomous and remote surgeries need an ultra-low latency internet network with extremely high availability, reliability, and security for human to machine or machine to machine (M2M) or device to device (D2D) communication (Chakraborty and Rodrigues, 2020).

IoT sensors can collect data like blood oxygen level (SpO2), blood pressure level, ECG data, body mass index (BMI), etc. (Kalaivaani and Krishnamoorthi, 2020). These data can be transferred and stored into central servers or the cloud and can be shared between the authorized entities (Li et al., 2020). This makes it possible to monitor the patient regularly. Furthermore, with deep learning and artificial intelligence, we can extract new features from these generated data that can help in early detection and finding a cure (Philip et al., 2020). For example, people who have diabetes may have an insulin pump that can change autonomously because sensors that detect blood sugar levels periodically change it based on the body's sugar level (Sriram and Reddy, 2020).

The various IoT devices have the potential to automate the entire patient monitoring system and thus take the healthcare system to the next-level (Mistry et al., 2020). ZigBee, Bluetooth, Extensible Messaging and Presence Protocol (XMPP), Data-Distribution Service (DDS), Advanced Message Queuing Protocol (AMQP), Lightweight M2M (LwM2M) and other advance connectivity IoT protocols change the way of transferring information in the area of healthcare (Sultanow and Chircu, 2019). These connected healthcare devices and virtual infrastructure not only make the infrastructure precise and better but also enhance the quality of living for the patients (Islam et al., 2020).

For persons having critical diseases like heart or blood pressure anomaly, timely warning is important in any life-threatening situation. AI embedded with IoT systems can collect human vital data and analyze them, while leaving key aspects and messages needed to the patient in emergency situations via smartphones or any personal assistant devices (Greco et al., 2020). Regardless of the time and place, these early warnings can provide help in analyzing the state of a patient and thus give timely medical attention.

These smart embedded devices can also notify the physician early in emergency situations, through which any hospital can estimate its initial emergency traffic before the start of the day. This will help patients move faster through the hospital system, allowing hospitals to see more patients than usual. Therefore, by processing software real-time data on entry time, vapor time, transfers and discharges, we can not only be limited to finding the problem, but also give care in a new form (Mišić et al., 2020).

In this contemporary time of advanced technologies, artificial intelligence has a substantial task in the detection and diagnosis of chronic diseases, which is now an extensive field of study. But to train such complex and intensive machine learning algorithms and to extract any information from the attributes, we need huge amounts of data, which is not possible if we have to gather them manually. In this case, IoT enables us to collect a large amount of data about the patient's disease that will otherwise take many years to collect manually, which by itself is a huge area of study in terms of secure, energy-efficient, and seamless data transfer (Alansari et al., 2018b).

2 Role of Body Vital Monitoring System for Disease Prediction in IOT Healthcare

Human health varies with each individual and a "normal" body state for an individual may not be similar to another. Various internal and external conditions play a very different role in one's body state. Also, some conditions may also be acquired genetically.

The major spreading of chronic diseases is a growing concern in every corner of the world. Chronic diseases are everywhere and are not subjective to any one group. The conditions of chronic diseases are also unwaveringly growing, and the effects of these diseases may appear in the most unexpected places. Continuous monitoring is one of the best ways by which we can detect disease early and is the best possible way to prevent the rise of chronic diseases. The most common chronic diseases include heart diseases, cancer, and diabetes. Drug abuse, lack of exercise, unhealthy diet are major contributors to most chronic diseases (Min et al., 2018).

While traditional medical systems focus on one disease at a time, we need a comprehensive system that can continuously monitor multiple diseases at the same time to prevent the rise of chronic diseases. Continuous monitoring system also helps us tracking the patient health having chronic diseases in real time (Shin et al., 2019).

Remote health monitoring (RHM) (Brown, 2001), as shown in Fig. 1, is a system in which patients are monitored outside the current clinical environment. It serves

Fig. 1 Remote Health
Monitoring System (Patel
et al., 2012)

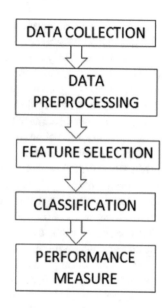

as a bridge to the close cooperation between many entities such as physicians, policymakers, researchers, and patients. RHM can continuously monitor and analyze several vital attributes like heartbeats, ECG data, Blood pressure level, BMI index, etc. at a single time. Nowadays, RHM can be implemented via wearable devices, smartphone apps, communication systems such as Radio Frequency Identification, Lora/Bluetooth, ZigBee, etc. (Majumder et al., 2017).

Now AI integrated with IoT has already started making changes in various areas of healthcare (Shah and Chircu, 2018). Areas like in radiology (Singla, 2020), dermatology (Eapen, 2020), oncology (Dubovitskaya et al., 2020), cardiology (Zagan et al., 2020), etc. deep learning neural algorithms have started beating physicians in terms of detecting diseases. Today's AI is now acting as a second reader on behalf of physicians where it can monitor multiple patients and provide medication simultaneously and may be tomorrow's AI is able to properly investigate and diagnose diseases where we are still lacking in terms of finding the exact cause.

Revolutionary researches are underway to reduce the cost, power consumption, and size of IoT devices without affecting quality services. Researches on various protocols are ongoing to increase the data transfer rate and size of the network (Hao and Foster, 2008). These wireless wearable devices can improve the healthcare network system by providing greater mobility and lowering the cost.

The remote monitoring system can monitor and track patients anywhere, regardless of their current locations. It allows the patients to perform their normal day-to-day work without risking their lives in a common danger. Fundamentally, the idea is about building wearable devices with wireless body sensors that can connect patients and physicians with a common integrated platform. It will help the clinicians in continuous monitoring of the patients. Then by artificial intelligence embedded in it, we can construct it as an autonomous and alternative recommendation unit in the absence of a physician (Albahri et al., 2018).

Smart healthcare system is a network of wireless health sensors and mobile devices connected to a central station with AI (Chen et al., 2018). These wearable devices capture a steady stream of patient data from body sensors and automatically transfer it to the patient's Electronic Medical Records (EMR). This new environment will not only track the health of the patient but will periodically remind various entities(doctor, patient, family, etc.) about the health status of the patient.

Thus, wearable healthcare devices (WHDs) bring new ways to track a person's prosperity during their day-to-day life or in any critical environment by continuously monitoring vital body signs while reducing their discomforts and without interrupting their social lives. It can help us track the health of soldiers who are doing duty here in remote locations and borders, from where even daily data collection is not possible. This opens up various avenues for treatment in villages far from developed areas of the country, where there is no physician to monitor them at all times.

This digitization of vital data of the human body will help us fight chronic diseases, and with enough data in the future, we can solve many chronic diseases by analyzing the expressions of their genomes and performing big data analysis. These give us hope to prevent diseases like cancer, AIDS, diabetes, etc., which are highly dependent on the expressions of the genome.

3   Valuable Vital Signs and Their Need to Be Monitored

The performance of any health monitoring system depends on the quality and information about the data collected. Information about the data, i.e., metadata plays a very important role in order to deal with the various stages of the processing of the data, viz. pre-processing, transformation, data mining and visualization and also adjusting to new challenges.

The various physiological signs present in the human body provide a very good understanding of the condition of the human body. Prior to knowing the way in which these bio-signals are obtained using the respective sensors, it is of foremost significance to have a awareness about how these different signals have an effect on the human body.

Numerous bio-signals can be acquired from the human body. But as it is not possible to include each and every one of them, we have particularly focused on those signals necessary for the detection of any anomaly present in the body. Those vital signs include the following: electrocardiogram (ECG), heart rate (HR), blood pressure (BP), respiratory rate (RR), blood oxygen saturation (SpO2) and body temperature.

The next sub-section discusses each of these signs, in terms of signal origin, medical and health importance and wearable sensors technology used.

3.1 Electrocardiogram (ECG)

Electrocardiogram (ECG/EKG) signal shows the electricity that flows through to our heart. The ECG signal is mainly consisting of P-wave, Q-wave, R-wave, S-wave and T-wave. By observing this P wave, QRS complex and T wave we can find the irregular rhythm of the ECG signal (Fig. 2). An ECG signal specially shows how the depolarization wave moves during each heartbeat, which is due to a wave of positive charge. Due to this reason, the consequent R-peaks (R-R interval) in a QRS complex are used to measure the heart cycles (Saritha et al., 2008).

The standard 12-lead ECG system typically gives a 3D view of our heart in both vertical and horizontal planes. The 12-lead ECG system is also divided into three sub-divisions: three bipolar limb leads system (lead I, II and III), three augmented limb leads systems(AVR, AVL and AVF), six precordial chest leads systems(V1, V2, V3, V4, V5 and V6) (Saritha et al., 2008).

The three bipolar limb leads and three augmented limb leads give us the frontal plane view of our heart, while six anterior chest lead systems see our heart in a horizontal plane. In three bipolar limb lead system, lead I see the electrical activity of the heart at the left/lateral side of the heart. Lead II and lead III to look at the inferior side of the heart at different angles. Like that in three augmented limb leads, AVR looks at the right sight of the heart, AVL looks at the left/lateral side and AVF looks at the inferior side of the heart. While the 6 precordial chest leads (V1, V2, V3, V4, V5 and V6) look at the hearts horizontal plane. These assessments play a major role

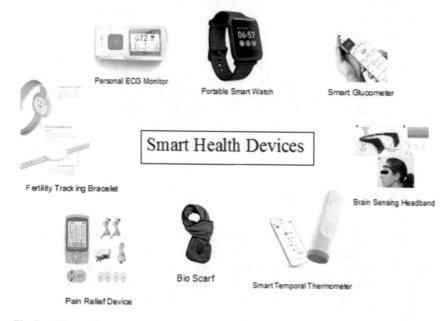

Fig. 2 ECG waveform

in the diagnosis of cardiovascular diseases (CVD), such as atrial fibrillation, angina, atherosclerosis, cardiac dysrhythmia, congestive heart failure (CHF), coronary artery disease, heart attack, bradycardia, and tachycardia (Saritha et al., 2008; Xu et al., 2008).

3.2   Heart Rate (HR)

Heart rate is another fundamental parameter that is used to measure the state of our body. This helps us detect an abnormal heart rhythm. Heart rate is the number of one's heartbeat per minute and varies from one person to another. It measures in beats per second(bpm). A normal heart rate is between 60 and 80 bpm (Ahmed et al., 2014). However, the female resting heart rate is faster than men. In addition, the heart rate varies according to the environment in which one lives, for example, the heart rate of people living at high altitudes increases compared to normal people. The heart rate also changes when one is exercising, under stress, exercising, walking, etc.

Heart rate depends on various physiological parameters like the age of a person, body condition, current fitness level, etc. There are various ways to monitor or calculate a person's heart rate; Usually, doctors count the number of pulse signals on the arm to calculate the heartbeat. We can also calculate heart rate from an electrocardiogram, with the marker method we can calculate heart rate by multiplying the number of QRS complexes during 6 s with 10 (Zhang and Bae, 2012). Besides, there are also methods such as the square counting method through which we can count the heartbeat by calculating the square between two QRS complexes.

Ballistocardiography is another method that reads ballistic forces on the heart (Sadek and Biswas, 2019). However, in today's scenario, photoplethysmography (PPG) (Charlton et al., 2020) is the most widely used method used in most fitness bands that track many vital signals, including the heartbeat. PPG is a non-invasive way to measure health data. It uses an optical sensor that shoots a light onto the skin, some amount of light is reflected back when it collides with blood vessels in our body. Capturing this reflected light with a photodetector allows us to record various vital signals of our body like heart rate, BP, Spo2, etc.

3.3   Blood Pressure (BP)

Blood pressure (BP) is the pressure exerted by blood on the muscular wall of blood vessels. The blood pressure reading is highest during systole. At the time when the heart is resting, the blood pressure level drops which is called diastolic pressure. A healthy person has systolic pressure reading somewhere between 90 and 120 mm Hg and diastolic pressure between 60 and 80 mm Hg (Elliott and Coventry, 2012; Turner et al., 2015).

Blood traces the landscape of the body through the circulatory system, and there are a lot of factors such as the properties of body fluids that pass through the circulatory pipes, narrow pipes, excess body fluids, etc., which affect the blood pressure of the body. Complex blood pressure monitoring has been in place for years involving instruments involving techniques and calculations. In general, physicians use a blood pressure cuff to measure a person's blood pressure, but this is not the best method for continuous monitoring. Continuous monitoring through blood pressure cuff can have major side effects, including skin irritation, sleep disruption, and an increase in stress level (Augusto et al., 2012).

Since hypertension is a silent killer, continuous monitoring is the only way to tackle this chronic disease. This is the area where wearable wireless devices play an important role for measuring the blood pressure level (Yilmaz et al., 2010). The new motion analysis system, PPG, and ECG are the newly emerging techniques through which we can calculate blood pressure (Puke et al., 2013). These techniques measure pulse wave velocity and with proper math calculations that give us an accurate blood pressure level (Appelboom et al., 2014). The PPG technique uses a red light beam to continuously monitor BP levels that penetrate deep into the skin which gives us a deeper inside of our body (Yilmaz et al., 2010). Many other technique have been developed for the same using various IoT-based devices (Hsu and Young, 2014; Woo et al., 2014).

3.4   Respiration Rate

Respiratory rate (RR) is the most common vital signs most physicians look for to track any abnormalities. It is the number of breaths a person takes per minute (Elliott and Coventry, 2012). Pair of each raise and fall of the patient's chest in normal condition is count as one breath. Normally, physicans count the breaths to half a minute and then multiply it with two to calculate the value of RR (Elliott and Coventry, 2012). Also, the way the patient breaths are also recorded, whether the breaths are deep or sallow. In an adult, the normal respiratory rate is between 12 and 20 bpm. The respiration rate provides a measure of any abnormalities found in the respiratory functions of a subject (Elliott and Coventry, 2012).

The RR increases when exercising or if we have a fever or in a particular type of pain. RR more than 20 breaths per minute is called tachypnea, which can be caused by acute or chronic conditions like asthma, lung disease, anxiety, fever, heart failure, etc. (Elliott and Coventry, 2012; Chan et al., 2012). On the other hand, RR less than 12 is called bradypnea, which mostly caused due to factors like overuse of narcotics, brain disorder, and hypothyroidism (Teng et al., 2008).

Nowadays, with the help of efficient motion sensors and ECGs, we can continuously monitor patient RR wirelessly (Kim et al., 2007). It can be calculated by quite a straightforward method using the R wave in the QRS signal. Similarly, many other techniques exist for the estimation of respiratory rate (Charlton et al., 2017; L'Her et al., 2019; Shen et al., 2017; Fusco et al., 2015).

3.5 Blood Oxygen Saturation (SpO2)

Saturation pressure of oxygen in blood (SpO2) gives us oxygen saturation levels in the blood. This parameter gives us knowledge about hypoxemia, which means that it can predict abnormalities in vital organs such as lung infections and heart diseases (Verhoeven et al., 2009). This can be measured with a multipara monitor as well as with a fingertip pulse oximeter. Its normal range should be between 95 and 100%. So on an average day, if the SpO2 level body is below 90% and is not being paid any attention, that means the body tissues such as brain tissue, heart tissue, and lung tissue are being damaged inadvertently. The ones who have moderate and chronic diseases require oxygen at different levels in which SpO2 reading can act as an alarm.

However, several different non-invasive methods have been proposed by researchers. But in the field of health and fitness science, photoplethysmography is the most accepted method when it comes to measuring the blood saturation level (Tamura et al., 2014). And as we have already noted in PPG (Sola et al., 2006), an optical sensor shoots a ray of light into the skin and calculates SpO2 levels by measuring the intensity of reflected light from blood vessels. In the current scenario, there are mostly fit bands and smartwatches that use this technology to collect body vital information such as heart rate and SpO2 level. Researchers are working hard to build and develop noise-free sensors that can measure oxygen levels in various body organs (Mendelson et al., 2013; Chen et al., 2014).

3.6 Body Temperature

Body temperature is a vital body sign in that it can provide early warnings before the body starts de-functioning due to high temperatures (Teng et al., 2008). Two types of body temperatures can be extracted from the body, namely, core temperature (CT) and skin temperature. In case of wearable health devices, skin temperatures are the most widely used and is used for monitoring a range of body conditions (Gaura et al., 2013; Buller et al., 2010, 2013). Body temperature is greatly affected by various factors such as, air circulation, ambient temperature and humidity (Gaura et al., 2013; Buller et al., 2010).

To accurately determine the body temperature, various wearable devices have been built by many researchers (Popovic et al., 2014; Boano et al., 2011; Webb et al., 2013), the most promising one being utilizing the a battery-less RFID thermometer (Miozzi et al., 2017). As it is quite complicated to determine core temperature using non-invasive methods, many techniques have been developed to simplify the process and yet to maintain the level of accuracy as well (Looney et al., 2018).

4 Review on the Recent Technological Advances in the Remote Healthcare Monitoring System

Smart wearable health equipment (SWHD) gives the whole world a new way of looking at its old health system (Sow et al., 2013). It is a new solution to many chronic diseases with frequent monitoring and self-help programs. In the coming years, we are expecting a more generalized healthcare system at a lower cost. People can take health benefits with proper diagnosis irrespective of their living places, which means a person in a remote village can also get a high-quality health assessment as the ones who live in a city area. These devices will also change the field of fitness science. With the help of continuous monitoring, athletes will be able to track their different body vital activities at the time of their training sessions.

The theory of Body Area Network (BAN) plays a very important role in the collection of the vital signs in the field of wearable health devices (Arefin et al., 2017) using different communication protocols (Khan and Pathan, 2018). The only major drawback of such sensors is limited memory and computing capacity. Overcoming these two drawbacks, the most commonly utilized tracking device for health monitoring consists of mobile phones. For example, many Android-based smartphones (Pigadas et al., 2011; Pirani et al., 2016) have been used by many researchers for such purposes utilizing the user's behavior pattern.

Numerous vital signs can be acquired using sensor and sensor networks and then transmitted to a central server for further processing (Kafalı et al., 2013). With the recent advancement of cloud computing (Verma et al., 2018; Sareen et al., 2018), the sensor data can be directly transmitted to a cloud server (Xia et al., 2015, 2017); authorized users can access the data with any Internet-enabled devices at any time from anywhere (Xiong et al., 2012). For example, Pigadas et al. (Yang et al., 2016) present an IoT cloud-based ECG monitoring system, where the sensed data are transmitted to the cloud sever via WiFi directly. The patients, doctors and family members can access the data via either the web or a mobile application.

Nowadays, smart wristwatches have become an addition to many health conscious people. AMON (Lukowicz et al., 2002) was one of the earliest devices of this kind and can successfully transfer three of the vital signs namely, heart rate, blood oxygen saturation and skin temperature. With the development of new technologies, like PulseO (Withings, 2020), Moov (MOOV, 2020) and PEAK (BASIS, 2020), it has become possible for real-time monitoring of many vital signs (Bieber et al., 2013). The most significant development in the field of wearable devices is the Google eye lens (Appelboom et al., 2014), which is due to the customization of the size of the devices.

Due to the advancement of smart electronics, textile industry has also started amalgamating the electronics into its environment (Presti et al., 2017). The concept of textrodes (Datta et al., 2019) is of importance in this matter, which is basically integrating smart textile with wearable health devices, for the purpose of collecting vital body signs. This concept has been utilized heavily by the industries based on lifestyle and sports monitoring (Andreoni et al., 2016). Examples include monitoring of the heart rate for persons involved in sports (Syduzzaman et al., 2015; Andreoni et al., 2016).

The process of integrating and developing wearable health devices is a challenging task, especially optimizing the size of the device containing the various sensors. Many attempts have been made in order to optimize the size without compromising the quality of the device using various methods (Georgia Tech Wearable MotherboardTM, 2020). Georgia Tech Wearable MotherboardTM (Gopalsamy et al., 1999) is worth mentioning here which has the capacity of transmitting in real time the three vital body signs of temperature, heart rate and respiration rate.

A garment named Sensing Shirt can collect the fundamental vital signs (Zhang et al., 2011) in a micro SD memory card while a multi-parameter shirt is capable of monitoring the ECG signal, heart rate and respiratory rate (Sardini et al., 2011), with a communication channel for remote assistance. One of the recent works on wearable devices includes LOBIN (Custodio et al., 2012), which is capable of accumulating as well as transmitting real-time vital data of the subjects within the vicinity of the hospital (Custodio et al., 2012). Then from the medical server, it is possible to monitor the various conditions of the subjects in real time.

A device named SQUID was proposed for real-time monitoring of the subjects requiring supervision from a hospital (Farjadian et al., 2013). Based on the analysis, a subject can be provided with the required advice from the medical expert. Along with the ability to monitor the heart rate, a smart t-shirt named MyWear (Cafagna et al., 2014) also combines a technology based on PolyPower for measuring the respiration rate.

A device named MIMS (Abbate et al., 2011) is capable of providing comprehensive and customizable real-time health monitoring services for aging persons utilizing the state-of-the-art smart systems. Another real-time monitoring system uses robust algorithms to track the subject's condition continuously (Duarte et al., 2015) to detect any early signs of any health-related issue. Similar works have been undertaken for subjects having chronic conditions requiring long-term therapy (Majeed et al., 2015). In order to handle and monitor stress, a smart system utilizes the subjects psychological stress data (Zhang et al., 2012) and then a feedback is then created for providing the respective therapy.

5 Summary

Undertaking development of smart wearable healthcare devices to create a globally integrated platform with inbuilt automation and as a medium of the interaction of different healthcare entities, we all are going on our way to achieving our upcoming future. But at present, the key interest is on integrated different wireless body sensors in a single device that can be wearable. On the other hand, communication between the different wireless biosensors requires a low latency bandwidth to communicate and to transfer data from one end to the other, which is a major challenge in developing counties and even in some developed countries like France as reported in the literature (Chan et al., 2012). Privacy of the health data is also one of the big ethical hurdles in this scenario. The solution is that companies have to engage patients for privacy discussions and part of keeping their data secure (Paiva et al., 2017). Empowering patient is one of the core principles in the digital healthcare system and updating regulations to empower patients with their health data should go in hand to hand with protecting what's important to them.

Healthcare culture is also changing in the present world with technology, now people want to connect with new technologies. Nowadays, people do not shy away from sharing information about their chronic diseases, which are now empowered with new technologies. People can measure their vital readings by themselves at home with digital health care and sensors. In the field of health care sensors, there are mainly three aspects that matter the most: long-term stability, resilience, and bio-strength. Tiny diagnostic devices and gadgets measuring vital signs is an important requirement to increase the functionality and portability of wearable devices. Designing textile healthcare devices with high water resistance and long-term stability is another important area to work on. Bio-compatibility needs to be highly considerate, covering the sensor with an antimicrobial or protective coating, preventing any possible toxicity of nanomaterials (Bandodkar and Wang, 2014).

Digital healthcare is the new start trend and tech giants like Google, Apple, or Amazon, who are now taking a more active role in healthcare sector. Each company pours money into medical projects and uses its unique strengths to make the healthcare system more effective. Many large car companies also join the race by planning to build their own cars with biosensors that will monitor the health of the driver. They all want to keep an eye on important information like stress level, respiratory rate, BP, heart rate, Spo2 level, etc. and are trying to extract meaningful information from it (Pantelopoulos and Bourbakis, 2009; Chan et al., 2012; Bandodkar and Wang, 2014). Determining the appropriate approach is worth investing in and adaption to changes is often hard. However, numerous healthcare issues can be eliminated or reduced if these investigations can be efficiently integrated.

Acknowledgements This research activity is a portion of the TEQIP Collaborative Research Scheme (CRS) project entitled, "Seamless Health Monitoring and Analysis of soldier using Machine Learning Approach" [CRS ID 1-5763896131]. The authors would like to thank NPIU, Government of India.

References

Abbate, S., Avvenuti, M., & Light, J. (2011). MIMS: A minimally invasive monitoring sensor platform. *IEEE Sensors Journal, 12*(3), 677–684.

Ahmed, W., Capodilupo, J., & Nicolae, A. (2014). Systems, devices and methods for continuous heart rate monitoring and interpretation. U.S. Patent Application (14/018), 262.

Alansari, Z., Soomro, S., Belgaum, M. R., & Shamshirband, S. (2018a). The rise of Internet of Things (IoT) in big healthcare data: review and open research issues. In: *Progress in advanced computing and intelligent engineering.* Springer.

Alansari, Z., Soomro, S., Belgaum, M. R., & Shamshirband, S. (2018b). The rise of Internet of Things (IoT) in big healthcare data: review and open research issues (pp. 675–685). Springer.

Albahri, O. S., et al. (2018). Systematic review of real-time remote health monitoring system in triage and priority-based sensor technology: Taxonomy, open challenges, motivation and recommendations. *Journal of Medical Systems,42*(5), 80.

Andreoni, G., Standoli, C. E., & Perego, P. (2016). Defining requirements and related methods for designing sensorized garments. *Sensors, 16*(6), 769.

Appelboom, G., Camacho, E., Abraham, M. E., Bruce, S. S., Dumont, E. L., Zacharia, B. E., et al. (2014). Smart wearable body sensors for patient self-assessment and monitoring. *Archives of Public Health, 72*(1), 1–9.

Arefin, M. T., Ali, M. H., & Haque, A. F. (2017). Wireless body area network: An overview and various applications. *Journal of Computer and Communications, 5*(7), 53–64.

Augusto, J. F., Teboul, J. L., Radermacher, P., & Asfar, P. (2012). Interpretation of blood pressure signal: Physiological bases, clinical relevance, and objectives during shock states. In *Applied Physiology in Intensive Care Medicine* (Vol. 2). Springer.

Bandodkar, A. J., & Wang, J. (2014). Non-invasive wearable electrochemical sensors: A review. *Trends in Biotechnology, 32*(7), 363–371.

Banerjee, A., Chakraborty, C., Kumar, A., & Biswas, D. (2020). Emerging trends in IoT and big data analytics for biomedical and health care technologies. In *Handbook of data science approaches for biomedical engineering.* Elsevier.

BASIS. (n.d.). PEAK—The ultimate fitness and sleep tracker. Retrieved November 15, 2020.

Bhoyar, P., Sahare, P., Dhok, S., & Deshmukh, R. (2019). Communication technologies and security challenges for internet of things: A comprehensive review. *AEU-International Journal of Electronics and Communications, 99*, 81–99.

Bieber, G., Haescher, M., & Vahl, M. (2013). Sensor requirements for activity recognition on smart watches. In *Proceedings of the 6th International Conference on Pervasive Technologies Related to Assistive Environments.*

Boano, C. A., Lasagni, M., Romer, K. & Lange, T. (2011). Accurate temperature measurements for medical research using body sensor networks. In *2011 14th IEEE International Symposium on Object/Component/Service-Oriented Real-Time Distributed Computing Workshops.* IEEE.

Bonato, P. (2003). Wearable sensors/systems and their impact on biomedical engineering. *IEEE Engineering in Medicine and Biology Magazine, 22*(3), 18–20.

Brown, S. J. (2001). Remote health monitoring and maintenance system, US Patent 6,168,563. Google Patents.

Buller, M. J., Tharion, W. J., Hoyt, R. W. & Jenkins, O. C. (2010). Estimation of human internal temperature from wearable physiological sensors. In *Iaai.*

Buller, M. J., Tharion, W. J., Cheuvront, S. N., Montain, S. J., Kenefick, R. W., Castellani, J., Latzka, W. A., Roberts, W. S., Richter, M., Jenkins, O. C., et al. (2013). Estimation of human core temperature from sequential heart rate observations. *Physiological Measurement,34*(7), 781.

Cafagna, C., Diterlizzi, A., & Voorhorst, F. (2014). MyWear: Customized green, safe, healthy and smart work-and sports-wear. In *2014 International Conference on Engineering, Technology and Innovation (ICE).* IEEE.

Chakraborty, C., & Rodrigues, J. J. (2020). A comprehensive review on device-to-device communication paradigm: trends, challenges and applications. *Wireless Personal Communications,* 1–23.

Chan, M., Estéve, D., Fourniols, J. Y., Escriba, C., & Campo, E. (2012). Smart wearable systems: Current status and future challenges. *Artificial Intelligence in Medicine, 56*(3), 137–156.

Charlton, P. H., Birrenkott, D. A., Bonnici, T., Pimentel, M. A., Johnson, A. E., Alastruey, J., et al. (2017). Breathing rate estimation from the electrocardiogram and photoplethysmogram: A review. *IEEE Reviews in Biomedical Engineering, 11*, 2–20.

Charlton, P. H., Kyriacou, P., Mant, J., & Alastruey, J. (2020). Acquiring wearable photoplethys-mography data in daily life: The PPG diary pilot study. *Multidisciplinary Digital Publishing Institute, 2*(1), 80.

Chau, K. Y., Lam, M. H. S.., Cheung, M. L., Tso, E. K. H., Flint, S. W., Broom, D. R., Tse, G., & Lee, K. Y. (2019). Smart technology for healthcare: Exploring the antecedents of adoption intention of healthcare wearable technology. *Health Psychology Research, 7*(1).

Chen, C. M., Kwasnicki, R., Lo, B., & Yang, G. Z. (2014). Wearable tissue oxygenation monitoring sensor and a forearm vascular phantom design for data validation. In *2014 11th International Conference on Wearable and Implantable Body Sensor Networks*. IEEE.

Chen, M., Li, W., Hao, Y., Qian, Y., & Humar, I. (2018). Edge cognitive computing based smart healthcare system. *Future Generation Computer Systems, 86,* 403–411.

Custodio, V., Herrera, F. J., López, G., & Moreno, J. I. (2012). A review on architectures and communications technologies for wearable health-monitoring systems. *Sensors, 12*(10), 13907–13946.

Datta, D., Banerjee, R., & Kamalesh, S. (2019). Wearable health monitoring fabric. US Patent App. 16/105,196. Google Patents.

Duarte, J. M., Cerqueira, E., & Villas, L. A. (2015). Indoor patient monitoring through Wi-Fi and mobile computing. In *2015 7th international conference on New Technologies, Mobility and Security (NTMS)*. IEEE.

Dubovitskaya, A., Novotny, P., Xu, Z., & Wang, F. (2020). Applications of blockchain technology for data-sharing in oncology: Results from a systematic literature review. *Oncology, 98*(6), 74–82.

Eapen, B. R. (2020). Artificial intelligence in dermatology: A practical introduction to a paradigm shift. *Indian Dermatology Online Journal, 11*(6), 881.

Elliott, M., & Coventry, A. (2012). Critical care: The eight vital signs of patient monitoring. *British Journal of Nursing, 21*(10), 621–625.

Farjadian, A. B., Sivak, M. L., & Mavroidis, C. (2013). SQUID: Sensorized shirt with smartphone interface for exercise monitoring and home rehabilitation. In *2013 IEEE 13th International Conference on Rehabilitation Robotics (ICORR)*. IEEE.

Fusco, A., Locatelli, D., Onorati, F., Durelli, G. C., & Santambrogio, M. D. (2015). On how to extract breathing rate from PPG signal using wearable devices. In *2015 IEEE Biomedical Circuits and Systems Conference (BioCAS)*. IEEE.

Gaura, E., Kemp, J., & Brusey, J. (2013). Leveraging knowledge from physiological data: On-body heat stress risk prediction with sensor networks. *IEEE Transactions on Biomedical Circuits and Systems, 7*(6), 861–870.

Georgia Tech Wearable MotherboardTM. (n.d.). The Intelligent Garment for the 21st Century. Retrieved October 15, 2020.

Gopalsamy, C., Park, S., Rajamanickam, R., & Jayaraman, S. (1999). The Wearable Motherboard: The First generation of adaptive and responsive textile structures (ARTS) for medical applications. *Virtual Reality, 4*(3), 152–168.

Greco, L., Percannella, G., Ritrovato, P., Tortorella, F., & Vento, M. (2020). Trends in iot based solutions for health care: Moving ai to the edge. *Pattern Recognition Letters*.

Hao, Y., & Foster, R. (2008). Wireless body sensor networks for healthmonitoring applications. *Physiological measurement, 29*(11), R27.

Hassan, W. H., et al. (2019). Current research on Internet of Things (IoT) security: A survey. *Computer Networks, 148,* 283–294.

Hsu, Y. P., & Young, D. J. (2014). Skin-coupled personal wearable ambulatory pulse wave velocity monitoring system using microelectromechanical sensors. *IEEE Sensors Journal, 14*(10), 3490–3497.

Islam, M. S., Humaira, F., & Nur, F. N. (2020). Healthcare applications in iot. *Global Journal Medical Research: (B) Pharma, Drug, Discovery, Toxicology, Medicine, 20,* 1–3.

Kafalı, Ö., Bromuri, S., Sindlar, M., van der Weide, T., Aguilar Pelaez, E., Schaechtle, U., et al. (2013). Commodity 12: A smart e-health environment for diabetes management. *Journal of Ambient Intelligence and Smart Environments, 5*(5), 479–502.

Kalaivaani, P., & Krishnamoorthi, R. (2020). Design and implementation of low power bio signal sensors for wireless body sensing network applications. *Microprocessors and Microsystems, 79,* 103271.

Khan, R. A., & Pathan, A. S. K. (2018). The state-of-the-art wireless body area sensor networks: A survey. *International Journal of Distributed Sensor Networks, 14*(4), 1550147718768994.

Kim, J., Hong, J., Kim, N., Cha, E., & Lee, T. S. (2007). Two algorithms for detecting respiratory rate from ecg signal. In *World Congress on Medical Physics and Biomedical Engineering 2006.* Springer.

Ko, J., Lim, J. H., Chen, Y., Musvaloiu-E, R., Terzis, A., Masson, G. M., et al. (2010). MEDiSN: Medical emergency detection in sensor networks. *ACM Transactions on Embedded Computing Systems (TECS), 10*(1), 1–29.

L'Her, E., N'Guyen, Q. T., Pateau, V., Bodenes, L., & Lellouche, F. (2019). Photoplethysmographic determination of the respiratory rate in acutely ill patients: Validation of a new algorithm and implementation into a biomedical device. *Annals of Intensive Care, 9*(1), 11.

Li, M., Enkoji, A., Key, M., Marroquin, A., & Prabhakaran, B. (2020). BSNCloud: Cloud-centered wireless body sensor data collection, streaming, and analytics system. In *EAI International Conference on Body Area Networks.* Springer.

Looney, D. P., Buller, M. J., Gribok, A. V., Leger, J. L., Potter, A. W., Rumpler, W. V., et al. (2018). Estimating resting core temperature using heart rate. *Journal for the Measurement of Physical Behaviour, 1*(2), 79–86.

Lukowicz, P., Anliker, U., Ward, J., Troster, G., Hirt, E., & Neufelt, C. (2002). AMON: a wearable medical computer for high risk patients. In *Proceedings of the Sixth International Symposium on Wearable Computers.* IEEE.

Lymberis, A., & Gatzoulis, L. (2006). Wearable health systems: From smart technologies to real apdplications. In *2006 International Conference of the IEEE Engineering in Medicine and Biology Society.* IEEE.

Majeed, Q., Hbail, H., & Chalechale, A. (2015). A comprehensive mobile ehealthcare system. In *2015 7th Conference on Information and Knowledge Technology (IKT).* IEEE.

Majumder, S., Mondal, T., & Deen, M. J. (2017). Wearable sensors for remote health monitoring. *Sensors, 17*(1), 130.

Mathur, P., Srivastava, S., & Mehta, J. L. (2015). High cost of healthcare in the United States-a manifestation of corporate greed. *Journal of Forensic Medicine, 1*(1), 1000103.

Mei, Q., & Gül, M. (2019). A crowdsourcing-based methodology using smartphones for bridge health monitoring. *Structural Health Monitoring, 18*(5–6), 1602–1619.

Mendelson, Y., Dao, D., & Chon, K. H. (2013). Multi-channel pulse oximetry for wearable physiological monitoring. In: *2013 IEEE International Conference on Body Sensor Networks.* IEEE.

Min, J., Zhao, Y., Slivka, L., & Wang, Y. (2018). Double burden of diseases worldwide: Coexistence of undernutrition and overnutrition-related noncommunicable chronic diseases. *Multidisciplinary Digital Publishing Institute, 19*(1), 49–61.

Miozzi, C., Amendola, S., Bergamini, A., & Marrocco, G. (2017). Reliability of a re-usable wireless epidermal temperature sensor in real conditions. In *2017 IEEE 14th International Conference on Wearable and Implantable Body Sensor Networks (BSN).* IEEE.

Mišić, V. V., Gabel, E., Hofer, I., Rajaram, K., & Mahajan, A. (2020). Machine learning prediction of postoperative emergency department hospital readmission. *Anesthesiology: The Journal of the American Society of Anesthesiologists, 132*(5), 968–980.

Mistry, I., Tanwar, S., Tyagi, S., & Kumar, N. (2020). Blockchain for 5G-enabled IoT for industrial automation: A systematic review, solutions, and challenges. *Mechanical Systems and Signal Processing, 135,* 106382.

MOOV, M. (n.d.). NOW. Retrieved October 15, 2020.

Mutlag, A. A., Abd Ghani, M. K., Arunkumar, Na., Mohammed, M. A., & Mohd, O. (2019). Enabling technologies for fog computing in healthcare IoT systems. *Future Generation Computer Systems, 90,* 62–78.

Okpala, P. (2018). Assessment of the influence of technology on the cost of healthcare service and patient's satisfaction. *International Journal of Healthcare Management, 11*(4), 351–355.

Paiva, J. S., Dias, D., & Cunha, J. P. (2017). Beat-ID: Towards a computationally low-cost single heartbeat biometric identity check system based on electrocardiogram wave morphology. *PloS One, 12*(7), e0180942.

Pantelopoulos, A., & Bourbakis, N. G. (2009). A survey on wearable sensorbased systems for health monitoring and prognosis. *IEEE Transactions on Systems, Man, and Cybernetics, Part C (Applications and Reviews), 40*(1), 1–12.

Patel, S., Park, H., Bonato, P., Chan, L., & Rodgers, M. (2012). A review of wearable sensors and systems with application in rehabilitation. *Journal of Neuroengineering and Rehabilitation, 9*(1), 1–17.

Pateraki, M., Fysarakis, K., Sakkalis, V., Spanoudakis, G., Varlamis, I., Maniadakis, M., et al. (2020). Biosensors and Internet of Things in smart healthcare applications: Challenges and opportunities. In *Wearable and Implantable Medical Devices*. Elsevier.

Petrakis, E. G., Sotiriadis, S., Soultanopoulos, T., Renta, P. T., Buyya, R., & Bessis, N. (2018). Internet of Things as a Service (iTaaS): Challenges and solutions for management of sensor data on the cloud and the fog. *Internet of Things, 3,* 156–174.

Philip, J. M., Durga, S., & Esther, D. (2020). Deep learning application in IoT health care: A survey. In *Intelligence in Big Data Technologies\Beyond the Hype*. Springer.

Pigadas, V., Doukas, C., Plagianakos, V. P., & Maglogiannis, I. (2011). Enabling constant monitoring of chronic patient using android smart phones. In *Proceedings of the 4th International Conference on Pervasive Technologies Related to Assistive Environments*.

Pirani, E. Z., Bulakiwala, F., Kagalwala, M., Kalolwala, M., & Raina, S. (2016). Android based assistive toolkit for alzheimer. *Procedia Computer Science, 79,* 143–151.

Popovic, Z., Momenroodaki, P., & Scheeler, R. (2014). Toward wearable wireless thermometers for internal body temperature measurements. *IEEE Communications Magazine, 52*(10), 118–125.

Presti, D. L., Massaroni, C., Formica, D., Saccomandi, P., Giurazza, F., Caponero, M. A., & Schena, E. (2017). Smart textile based on 12 Fiber Bragg gratings array for vital signs monitoring. *IEEE Sensors Journal, 17*(18), 6037–6043.

Puke, S., Suzuki, T., Nakayama, K., Tanaka, H., & Minami, S. (2013). Blood pressure estimation from pulse wave velocity measured on the chest. In *2013 35th Annual International Conference of the IEEE Engineering in Medicine and Biology Society (EMBC)*. IEEE.

Sadek, I., & Biswas, J. (2019). Nonintrusive heart rate measurement using ballistocardiogram signals: A comparative study. *Signal, Image and Video Processing, 13*(3), 475–482.

Sardini, E., Serpelloni, M., & Ometto, M. (2011). Multi-parameters wireless shirt for physiological monitoring. In *2011 IEEE International Symposium on Medical Measurements and Applications*. IEEE.

Sareen, S., Sood, S. K., & Gupta, S. K. (2018). IoT-based cloud framework to control Ebola virus outbreak. *Journal of Ambient Intelligence and Humanized Computing, 9*(3), 459–476.

Saritha, C., Sukanya, V., & Murthy, Y. N. (2008). ECG signal analysis using wavelet transforms. *Bulgarian Journal of Physics, 35*(1), 68–77.

Shah, R., & Chircu, A. (2018). IOT and AI in healthcare: A systematic literature review. *Issues in Information Systems, 19*(3).

Shen, C. L., Huang, T. H., Hsu, P. C., Ko, Y. C., Chen, F. L., Wang, W. C., et al. (2017). Respiratory rate estimation by using ECG, impedance, and motion sensing in smart clothing. *Journal of Medical and Biological Engineering, 37*(6), 826–842.

Shin, J., Yan, Y., Bai, W., Xue, Y., Gamble, P., Tian, L., & Kandela, I. (2019). Bioresorbable pressure sensors protected with thermally grown silicon dioxide for the monitoring of chronic diseases and healing processes. *Multidisciplinary Digital Publishing Institute, 3*(1), 37–46.

Singla, S. (2020). AI and IoT in healthcare. In *Internet of things use cases for the healthcare industry*. Springer.

Sola, J., Castoldi, S., Chetelat, O., Correvon, M., Dasen, S., Droz, S., Jacob, N., Kormann, R., Neumann, V., Perrenoud, A., et al. (2006). SpO2 sensor embedded in a finger ring: Design and implementation. In *2006 International Conference of the IEEE Engineering in Medicine and Biology Society*. IEEE.

Sow, D., Turaga, D. S., & Schmidt, M. (2013). *Mining of sensor data in health-care: A survey* (1st ed.). Boston MA, Springer.

Sriram, R. D., & Reddy, S. S. K. (2020). Artificial intelligence and digital tools: Future of diabetes care. *Clinics in Geriatric Medicine, 36*(3), 513–525.

Sultanow, E., & Chircu, A. (2019). A review of iot technologies, standards, tools, frameworks and platforms. In *The internet of things in the industrial sector*. Springer.

Syduzzaman, M., Patwary, S. U., Farhana, K., & Ahmed, S. (2015). Smart textiles and nanotechnology: A general overview. *Journal of Textile Science and Engineering, 5,* 1000181.

Tamura, T., Maeda, Y., Sekine, M., & Yoshida, M. (2014). Wearable photoplethysmographic sensors|past and present. *Electronics, 3*(2), 282–302.

Teng, X. F., Zhang, Y. T., Poon, C. C., & Bonato, P. (2008). Wearable medical systems for p-health. *IEEE Reviews in Biomedical Engineering, 1,* 62–74.

Tokognon, C. A., Gao, B., Tian, G. Y., & Yan, Y. (2017). Structural health monitoring framework based on Internet of Things: A survey. *IEEE Internet of Things Journal, 4*(3), 619–635.

Turner, J. R., Viera, A. J., & Shimbo, D. (2015). Ambulatory blood pressure monitoring in clinical practice: A review. *The American Journal of Medicine, 128*(1), 14–20.

Verhoeven, D., Teijaro, J. R., & Farber, D. L. (2009). Pulse-oximetry accurately predicts lung pathology and the immune response during in uenza infection. *Virology, 390*(2), 151–156.

Verma, P., Sood, S. K., & Kalra, S. (2018). Cloud-centric IoT based student healthcare monitoring framework. *Journal of Ambient Intelligence and Humanized Computing, 9*(5), 1293–1309.

Webb, R. C., Bonifas, A. P., Behnaz, A., Zhang, Y., Yu, K. J., Cheng, H., et al. (2013). Ultrathin conformal devices for precise and continuous thermal characterization of human skin. *Nature Materials, 12*(10), 938–944.

Withings. (n.d.). Inspire Health Pulse Ox|Track. Improve. Retrieved October 15, 2020.

Woo, S. H., Choi, Y. Y., Kim, D. J., Bien, F., & Kim, J. J. (2014). Tissue-informative mechanism for wearable non-invasive continuous blood pressure monitoring. *Scientific Reports, 4,* 6618.

Wu, F., Wu, T., & Yuce, M. R. (2019). An internet-of-things (iot) network system for connected safety and health monitoring applications. *Sensors, 19*(1), 21.

Xia, Z., Zhu, Y., Sun, X., Qin, Z., & Ren, K. (2015). Towards privacy-preserving content-based image retrieval in cloud computing. *IEEE Transactions on Cloud Computing, 6*(1), 276–286.

Xia, Z., Xiong, N. N., Vasilakos, A. V., & Sun, X. (2017). EPCBIR: An efficient and privacy-preserving content-based image retrieval scheme in cloud computing. *Information Sciences, 387,* 195–204.

Xiong, N., Han, W., & Vandenberg, A. (2012). Green cloud computing schemes based on networks: A survey. *IET Communications, 6*(18), 3294–3300.

Xu, P., Zhang, H., & Tao, X. (2008). Textile-structured electrodes for electrocardiogram. *Textile Progress, 40*(4), 183–213.

Yang, Z., Zhou, Q., Lei, L., Zheng, K., & Xiang, W. (2016). An IoT-cloud based wearable ECG monitoring system for smart healthcare. *Journal of Medical Systems, 40*(12), 286.

Yilmaz, T., Foster, R., & Hao, Y. (2010). Detecting vital signs with wearable wireless sensors. *Sensors, 10*(12), 10837–10862.

Zagan, I., Gheorghiţă Găitan, V., Petrariu, A. I., Iuga, N., & Brezulianu, A. (2020). Design, fabrication, and testing of an IoT healthcare cardiac monitoring device. *Computers, 9*(1), 15.

Zhang, J., Tang, H., Chen, D., & Zhang, Q. (2012). deStress: Mobile and remote stress monitoring, alleviation, and management platform, In *2012 IEEE Global Communications Conference (GLOBECOM)*. IEEE.

Zhang, C. F., & Bae, T. W. (2012). VLSI friendly ECG QRS complex detector for body sensor networks. *IEEE Journal on Emerging and Selected Topics in Circuits and Systems, 2*(1), 52–59.

Zhang, Z. B., Shen, Y. H., Wang, W. D., Wang, B. Q., & Zheng, J. W. (2011). Design and implementation of sensing shirt for ambulatory cardiopulmonary monitoring. *Journal of Medical and Biological Engineering, 31*(3), 207–215.

Zhou, H., Yang, G., Lv, H., Huang, X., Yang, H., & Pang, Z. (2019). IoT-enabled dual-arm motion capture and mapping for telerobotics in home care. *IEEE Journal of Biomedical and Health Informatics, 24*(6), 1541–1549.

Review of Body Vitals Monitoring Systems for Disease Prediction

Srabani Patikar, Priyanka Saha, Sarmistha Neogy, and Chandreyee Chowdhury

Abstract With the increasing population and diverse environment, health care data prediction plays an important role. The goal of the work is to build a system that predicts a disease accurately based on basic knowledge. With the advancement of ICT-based Healthcare systems, Wearable smart devices (WSD) play an important role in monitoring body vitals and helps in taking proper decisions regarding one's health. The role of smart and developed systems as WSD helps tremendously to keep check all vital attributes of a patient and thus controlling their conditions accordingly. WSDs have significant potential to detect any abnormal occurrence of events in a patient such as a sudden drop of blood pressure, decrease oxygen saturation, monitoring blood glucose level, decreasing pulse rate which can help in proper decision making in time thus saving lives. In the last few years, monitoring body vitals has become an intensively researched area and several studies have been done for analyzing these signs so that any further casualty can be detected early. So a real-time health monitoring system with WSDs helps in cost-effective, accurate, and easy to apply secured data analysis. Today WSDs are available in many forms like smartwatches, smart jewelry, smart clothing, different fitness tracker, smart glasses are available to help monitor one's health vitals by themselves. This work presents a comprehensive review of this emerging field of research.

Keywords Wearable smart devices · Healthcare system · Body vitals monitoring · Machine learning approaches · Prediction

S. Patikar (✉) · P. Saha · S. Neogy · C. Chowdhury
Jadavpur University, Kolkata, India
e-mail: srabanipatikar@gmail.com

© The Author(s), under exclusive license to Springer Nature Singapore Pte Ltd. 2022   197
S. Biswas et al. (eds.), *Internet of Things Based Smart Healthcare*, Smart Computing and Intelligence, https://doi.org/10.1007/978-981-19-1408-9_9

1 Introduction

Body vital monitoring system is an emerging solution that helps to monitor our vital signs daily with minimum interference and can be done with little attention. It helps to self-monitor our health status. Regular monitoring of body vitals helps to find any clinical condition if there is any, and early diagnosis will help further treatment. Wearable Health Devices are the most popular techniques when it comes to personal Healthcare Monitoring systems. Vital signs are considered as a person's baseline indicator of health status. Depending on these signs, many diseases can be predicted early with proper treatment. The main vital signs of monitoring are Pulse Rate, Body Temperature, Respiration Rate, and finally Blood Pressure. Other important vital signs are heart rate, Oxygen saturation, Capillary Refill Time, Respiratory Effort. Wearable Health Devices (WHD) (Wang et al. 2018) are easily accessible, can be worn comfortably, regardless of the hardware and sensors that are small. Significant advancement in the field of wireless communication, biomedical science (Comroe and Dripps 1978) and information technology, medical telemetry has seen a tremendous advancement in terms of diagnosis and treatment. Medical telemetry helps in a new level of personalization along with a body vital monitoring system. As monitoring system provides data on a fixed interval basis, huge data is being generated regularly which should be stored and processed securely. For this purpose, WBAN (Wireless Body Area Network) (Khan and Yuce 2010) is an attempt to provide data encryption, mobility, and authentication. WBAN is one of the most helpful and suitable technology for building robust and suitable wearable health monitoring systems. Applications of WBAN are in Electromyography, Electrocardiogram, Electroencephalogram, capsule endoscope, An Accelerometer used for motion capture, etc. (Yuce 2010; Jovanov et al. 2005; Kang et al. 2015).

The first step of the work is the collection of records on which a system can be made. The main challenge of this work is to deal with real-life data based on data history. There are several types of data and sometimes those are not structured. Data is collected from different electronic devices and sensors. For different diseases, different parameters are gathered. This work is done by medical experts or doctors. Then data is processed through some data analysis techniques which go through some steps like Dimensionality reduction, Data preprocessing, and Classification (Li et al. 2016). Figure 1 shows the basic steps of the healthcare data prediction.

Three techniques (Dhillon and Singh 2019) are mainly used for disease prediction, namely, Supervised learning (Zhu and Goldberg 2009; Hastie et al. 2009), Unsupervised learning (Ghahramani 2003; Dayan et al. 1999; Figueiredo and Jain 2002) and Reinforcement learning (Sutton and Barto 2018; Barto 1997). The ground truth for the datasets for disease prediction are obtained from the health experts. Performance of the Machine learning techniques can be shown using confusion matrix, which divides the prediction in four parts on true and false prediction.

Prediction depends on some factors, those are the size of the data, types of training data, the behavior of the data. There is no specific model which suits every case so different models may vary for different diseases, geographical areas, age groups, etc.

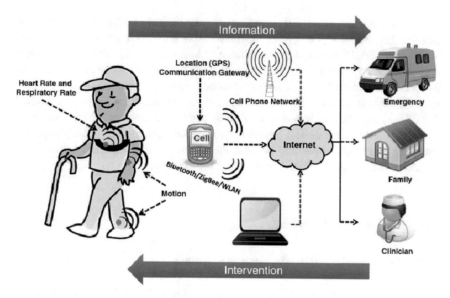

Fig. 1 General steps of data analysis

A study on relevant works in this field could be found in the next section. Section 2 mentions the open research issues of this emerging research direction. The subsequent section discusses the applications of smart devices. Security measures are discussed in Sect. 5. The technical analysis steps are highlighted in Sect. 6 followed by our conclusion in Sect. 7.

2 Relevant Works

Related work consists of mainly two parts. One is Data collection and second one is analysis techniques.

2.1 Data Collection

Data is collected from different sensor sources. Data is of different types like numeric, image, sound, text data, etc. These can be collected from different data repositories or IoT devices.

Tayyab et al. (2017) reported the design of a device that can monitor pulmonary edema. They try to capture the radio frequency using a fabric like an element. Chen et al. (2017) built a healthcare system which is a washable smart cloth, consisting of all the electronic elements like electrodes, sensors, and wires. It worked with Psychological data. Allison et al. (2017) created devices that have active layer morphology and stability. Focusing on coating they make fiber and fabric-based devices. Shahbakhti et al. (2022) proposed an algorithm on a kurtosis-based strategy. Their motive is to manage and stop successive decomposition at the optimal level. Performance has been calculated for two databases and one comparative study is made on Automatic Wavelet Independent Component Analysis (AWICA) and Enhanced AWICA (EAWICA) algorithms. Baldo et al. (2020) performed one comparative study on sensors. These sensors collect pressure, temperature, and humidity. They deployed smart sensors in the shoes and observe the difference that from the conventional thermometer. Humidity difference is shown for the two legs.

2.2 Analysis Techniques

2.2.1 Feature Extraction and Feature Selection

In this study, correlation methods are used for feature selection. Liu et al. (2020) applied Pearson correlation in activity data, where the data is numeric. The linear correlation method is used with the covariance of x and y divided by the multiplication of their variance. Sadiqi et al. used Spearman correlation as the feature selection mechanism for the Dutch version of AOSpine PROST (Patient Reported Outcome Spine Trauma) (Sadiqi et al. 2020). Here the coefficient values are chosen from -1 to $+1$. The threshold of correlation is taken greater than 0.70. Martis et al. (2013) work with Electrocardiogram signals. This study is used to detect the problems of the heart. Dimensionality extraction techniques PCA, LDA is used here. Tominaga (1999) performed an analysis in different databases like chemotherapeutic agents, antibacterials, antineoplastics, and antifungals. PCA-LDA (Chen et al. 2005; López et al. 2009; Giri et al. 2013) is used to model the data.

2.2.2 Learning Approaches

Most of the works reported applied supervised learning approaches for disease detection. Naïve Bayes, Decision tree, and neural network classifier are used to detect heart disease in Palaniappan and Awang (2008). Here the class is defined by the concern of doctors. The main purpose of this work is to design a system that can predict Heart disease.

Vitola et al. (2017) described the damage of piezoelectric sensor network and machine learning approach. The best-performed machine learning algorithms are fine KNN and weighted KNN as reported by the authors.

Khalilia et al. (2011) worked with National Inpatient Sample (NIS) data. This data is imbalanced and is predicted using ensemble learning. They also compared support vector machine (SVM), bagging, boosting, and Random forest.

Caruana et al. (2015) predicts the pneumonia risk by several models like boosted trees, random forests, neural network, logistic regression, naive-Bayes, and single decision trees (Kaur and Wasan 2006).

Deepa et al. (2020) Collected data from an AI-based system. The prediction is done on diabetes data. They proposed a Stochastic Gradient Descent classifier for prediction and to prevent shrinkage.

Stack generalized method is built along with weights as discussed by Nandy et al. (2020). Here prediction and weights are stacked together. Weights are calculated using a neural network with one hidden layer. This work is done on activity data. The data is collected from different wearable and smartphone sensors (Mohd and Mohamed 2005).

In Saha et al. (2018), the authors proposed a two-phase ensemble classifier where the base classifiers are selected through their performance. Here, the weights are calculated by dividing accuracy by average accuracy. The sensor data of smartphones is collected for activity recognition (Sellappan and Chua 2005).

3 Open Research Issues

Body Vital monitoring systems generally refer to low-cost, wireless IoT based Madakam et al. (2015), Yeole and Kalbande (2016), Islam et al. (2015) patient monitoring system (Dicks et al. 2012; Brown 2010; Vegesna et al. 2017 that is developed for remote patient monitoring at low cost. Using only minimal IT infrastructure, Healthcare Industries using these systems can be able to deploy care setting efficiently (Wang et al. 2014). As the system generates continuous data, a doctor or clinicians can detect any changes if there are any, and take immediate action. This provides a great impact and accuracy while minimizing the error rate. Below are some important factors that are getting benefitted from Body Vital Monitoring System rather from Wearable Health Devices.

- Body vital monitoring system helps in activity areas such as fitness, wellness, non-medical applications, and self-monitoring. It helps in the prediction of events that have not occurred yet, thus providing medical information to help in the prevention of further chronic diseases and support disease detection.
- Telemetry is often used for providing continuous support for at-risk patients. But in some places, where health infrastructure is not stable to provide enough assistance, the body vital monitoring system provides huge support for clinically ill patients and can detect early signs. In case of any cardiac emergency, a patient can show symptoms of cardiac emergency before 8 hours. With the help of these Wearable Health Devices, it is possible to trace the abnormalities.

– It reduces the workload of the healthcare professionals and doctors. It is quite tough for a doctor or clinician to constantly monitor a few numbers of patients those are in critical condition. But using this body vital monitoring system, one could get constant details of vital of a clinically ill patient and can act accordingly if anything wrong is seen. This is particularly useful for the treatment as well as containment of contagious diseases, such as, Covid-19.

4 Applications of Smart Devices

A smart device is an electronic device that is connected via other devices or networks through some protocols such as Bluetooth, Wi-fi, 5G, ZigBee that can work independently and contact other devices. Smart devices can be designed from a variety of factors and can be used in the physical world, human-centered environment, and distributed computing environment. Smart devices are composed of three layers hardware layer, network layer, and application layer. Portable health gadgets or smart devices help in monitoring body vitals. Some devices are connected to smartphones that helps to stay fit and may encourage to start and maintain a healthier lifestyle (Dias et al. 2018). Some devices can manage chronic situations and quietly can change the way of life. Below some smart devices used are shown in Fig. 2 for patient monitoring are discussed.

Fig. 2 Smart health devices

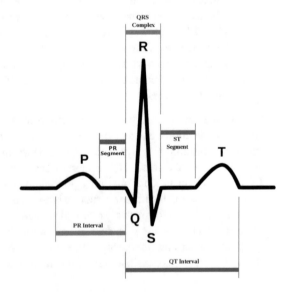

4.1 Personal ECG Monitor

These devices allow one to track health conditions anytime anywhere and provides a medical grade eco cardiogram in the smartphone in just a few seconds. These devices use wireless Bluetooth and are splash, rain-resistant so that one can wear them daily. Using these devices doctors or healthcare professionals can access accurate medical data remotely (Tan et al. 2008). These devices are clinically accurate and validate data and analyze overall heart performance in real-time.

4.2 Portable Smart Watch

Portable smartwatches are the most advanced smartwatches for regular use. Its design is incorporated with state-of-the art-medical technology which can measure blood pressure, oxygen saturation, pulse rate (Saleem et al. 2022). It can also connect to smartphones via Bluetooth and can send all the data collected to smartphones at a regular interval. All smartwatches are waterproof and force resistant so can be worn regularly.

4.3 Smart Glucometer

This wireless smart glucose monitoring system measures the glucose level promptly and sends data to smartphones. It is a portable solution for diabetic people to keep track of its glucose label. These devices are sleek, fashionable, and portable for daily use Jain et al. (2019).

4.4 Brain Sensing Headband

It is one of the most portable and smart solutions of an EEG device. Equipped with all 7 electroencephalography sensors, it does help to reduce stress, a real-time tool to monitor the brain's functionality, and can teach to be calm and stress-free. Connected via Wi-Fi or Bluetooth, a doctor or other healthcare professional can keep track of a person's health status remotely (Lin et al. 2018).

4.5   Smart Temporal Thermometer

One of the easiest and fastest ways to measure one's temperature is to use these smart infrared-based temporal thermometers. Just place the thermometer in one's temple, press the button, and temperature will show on its LED display within few seconds. These devices are so fast and equipped with multiple infrared sensors that they can measure body temperature thousands of times within seconds. Paired up with smartphones via Bluetooth or Wi-Fi, one can keep a record of his feverish symptoms (Tamura et al. 2018).

4.6   Fertility Tracking Bracelet

Fertility Tracking devices are becoming a true companion for tracing fertility stage (Shilaih et al. 2018). It uses body temperature, breathing rate, resting pulse rate to decide the fertility window. One can wear it while sleeping and synchronize with its respective smart app and it will provide a fertility window accurately.

4.7   Pain Relief Device

These devices are useful solutions for people suffering from arthritis, sciatica, or carpal tunnel pain. It delivers low voltage pulses to the skin to stimulate nerve fibers which block pain signals to the brain. It is equipped with some preprogrammed modes which one can operate according to their requirement.

4.8   Bio Scarf

A smart alternative to traditional air pollution-resistant masks, these smart scarfs are warm and comfortable fashion accessories with automatic air filtration devices that lower the risk of respiratory health problems. It is effective against pollutants, viruses, allergens. It has a capacity of N-95 air filtration and purifies contaminated air (https://www.springwise.com 2022).

5   Data Security

Information that is retrieved from the Wearable Health Devices should maintain some privacy and security protocols because of patient confidentiality (Selvaraj and Doraikannan 2019). So, data security is an important aspect for better disease prediction from undistorted data collected from patient monitoring systems. Thus, securing the devices is very important. When connections are made through Bluetooth, Wifi, or through wire then there is a chance of data leakage and data manipulation. To ensure the safety of patient monitoring system:

1. Data Freshness: Wearable Health Devices produce real-time data, and all these data should be processed and transferred securely. As a small change in health data could be alarming, data available for analysis to doctors or clinicians should be always fresh.
2. Data Confidentiality: It is of utmost importance for data to be protected from unofficial access and the devices that are collecting data should be secured. If any security hole is present while collecting data and transferring data to other locations, it is necessary to maintain the data confidentiality of every device.
3. Data Authentication: During data transfer from WHD to the remote server, it must be known that data must be from a trusted and known authority. So data must be transferred from trustworthy sources.

Confidentiality, integrity, and availability are the main elements of data security. Confidentiality maintains the authorized access. Integrity ensures accurate access to data. Availability means losing no data for security. Data should be accessible in such a way that can avoid potential breaches. If these data can be maintained in real-time then the loss, alteration, data disclosure can be prevented. Along with access control, the data and activity should be monitored continuously as the health data is maintained for immediate care and actions. Data security is maintained by some important techniques like sensitive pieces of information are encrypted, keep backups and ensure security levels.

Data encryption plays an important role in health data. Sometimes with health data, some private pieces of information are also attached, so here data encryption is needed. Data encryption is a process of translating data in such a way that it only be accessible using a password or key. After encryption data is called Ciphertext. There are several algorithms are available for data encryption. Those are like TripleDES, Twofish encryption algorithm, Blowfish encryption algorithm, Advanced Encryption Standard (AES), IDEA encryption algorithm, MD5 encryption algorithm, HMAC encryption algorithm, RSA security. Broadly, two main cryptography techniques are available Public Key Cryptography and Private Key Cryptography.

Wireless Body area networks (WBANs) (Roy et al. 2020) collect data from the human body using biosensors and send them to the medical servers through wireless channels. These data are crucial for human health monitoring, as these data communicate through wireless channels so there is the possibility of security attacks. These attacks can happen in three tiers like for first-tier PAN (Personal Area Network), for second-tier LAN (Local Area Network), and third-tier WAN (Wide Area Network). In different areas like sensor nodes, medical servers, and channels, different types of attacks such as fabrication attack, masquerade attack, eavesdropping, modification attack, denial of service (DoS), jamming, and tunneling attacks are shown. The methods of WBANs that depend on the cloud perform better but the risk of attack is also high. Wireless Sensor Network (WSN) (Vyas and Pal 2020) collects information from physical or environmental states. The application of WSN is WBAN, the architecture is related. The data is collected on scattered sensors in a zone and send to the sink and user by multi-hop framework. In different network-layer, different threat attacks have appeared. There are some security structures like IEEE 802.11 security solutions, IEEE 802.15.6 security solutions, IEEE 802.15.4 security solutions, etc. are used.

6 Technical Analysis

Technical analysis is broadly divided into two parts. The first part consists of applying different classification and clustering techniques to see the nature of the data and which mathematical formulae suit a particular data. The second part is used to see the performance of the data in a specific setup. Data preprocessing, Feature extraction, Feature selection, Data processing, and classification or clustering fall under the first step. On the other hand second step consists of the confusion matrix and the performances. These methods are elaborately described below.

6.1 Data Preprocessing

Data preprocessing is performed after collecting raw data. Data cleaning is performed first after data acquisition. Data cleaning is performed mainly in three ways. These are handling missing values, removal of inconsistent values, and removal of dupli-cate values. Missing value can be removed by dropping that particular instance and replacing the value by mean or the value whose probability of occurrence is high (Song and Shepperd 2007). Health data may contain an inconsistent value. These inconsistent values, treated as outliers can confuse the classifiers in identifying the distinguishing patterns present in the dataset and thus a data can be wrongly pre-dicted. Overfitting may occur for the duplicate instances, which are also removed for correct prediction (Elmagarmid et al. 2006).

Healthcare data is collected from different devices. So data integration is needed to place the data in a single frame. Otherwise, it is difficult to process the whole data together (Lenzerini 2002). Data is collected from different files and databases. In different databases data is in a structured, unstructured, and semi-structured format. Data may contain same data types as well as different data types. Data integration also includes some problems like representation of the same attributes but in a different name, matrices representation can be different for the same data, duplicate features can occur while collecting data. As a result of data, integration data need to be transformed. Data transformation is performed by normalization or aggregation, concerning data.

Data is collected from different healthcare centers, which are very large. Data is sliced into small parts, the number of attributes is reduced to perform data reduction (Bevington and Robinson 2003). Sometimes, to reduce the storage large data is compressed.

6.2 Feature Extraction

Feature extraction generally applies statistical methods to extract the distinguishing temporal or spatial relationship of the data attributes. To some extent, domain knowledge is required to extract effective features from data. Recently, deep learning techniques such as convolutional neural networks are reported to be applied that can extract high dimensional features. However, the effectiveness of such techniques depends on the availability of sufficiently large well-balanced datasets. Feature extraction improves performance, increases training speed, extendibility is increased. Feature Selection techniques are used to reduce the dimension of the data to make it easily interpretable, avoid overfitting, and remove those features which have less impact on the classification process (Saeys et al. 2008). There are a few techniques available for feature selection. Those are Principle Component Analysis (PCA), Independent Component Analysis (ICA), Linear Discriminant Analysis (LDA), and Locally Linear Embedding (LLE).

Principle Component Analysis is a dimensionality reduction method that depends on variation and pairwise distances between features (Kuncheva and and Faithfull 2013). PCA reduces the error for reconstruction as well as increases the variance. It takes original data as input and returns dimensionally reduced data.

Independent Component Analysis separates the data mixture (Lee et al. 2000) into independent elements. This method is mainly used for detaching the signals which come from EEG and MRI. Features are independent if the linear and nonlinear dependency between features is zero.

Linear Discriminant Analysis minimizes the scattering by separating the mean of each class. It depends upon the labels of instances (Huang et al. 2002). Only where the data follows Gaussian distribution, LDA performs better as it follows the Gaussian method.

Locally Linear Embedding (LLE) is the process of combining sets of PCA to solve the nonlinear problem. Like PCA, it also accounts for distances with the local instances. LLE reduces the unwanted dimensions and places them into lower-dimensional space.

Three types of feature selection methods are commonly used in machine learning-based patient monitoring systems. Those are Filter Method, Wrapper Method, and Embedded Method.

Filter method does not depend upon any machine learning technique. Here features are selected on tests based on some statistical methods. The filter method can be applied in different ways, which depends on the data. These methods are Information gain, Chi-square test, and Correlation coefficient, etc. (Rachburee and Punlumjeak

2015). Information gain depends on the class label. It calculates the entropy-based on the output class. The Chi-square test finds the score for the feature and the corresponding class value. That method is applicable for categorical values. Correlation deals with numerical values. It is a process of finding the relationships between variables. It checks if two or more features are correlated to each other or not. The correlation coefficient lies between -1 to 1. A negative correlation means one feature decreases with the increasing of another feature, positive correlation infers that two features increase and decrease together and the Correlation coefficient is zero means features or attributes are not correlated to each other. There are three types of correlation measures, namely, Pearson, Kendall, and Spearman correlation (Puth et al. 2015). Pearson product-moment correlation is used to find the relation between the linear variables. Kendall rank correlation is a non-parametric process of ranking by quantities. Spearman rank correlation tries to find out two variables are directly proportional or inversely proportional.

Wrapper Method breaks the problem space into subsets and trains each subset on different machine learning models. All possible combinations are evaluated using a greedy approach. There are mainly four types of wrapper methods available. The Forward Feature Selection method adds dimensions in each step of the iteration, when the performance starts falling by adding new features then those features are discarded (Das 2001). The backward Feature Elimination method starts with all the features, then each stage evaluates the performance (Kohavi and Sommerfield 1995). Then, features are gradually eliminated at each step until stable performance is achieved. The exhaustive Feature Selection method gathers all possible mixture of features. The cluster which performed well is selected. The recursive Feature elimination method searches for a subset of features recursively which performs better. It also preserves ranks based on the deletion of features.

Embedded Method is the combination of filter and wrapper method (Hameed et al. 2018). In each step, it tries to find out those attributes which can train better using the model training process. It can be implemented mainly in two ways. Those are Lasso regression and Ridge regression (Ranstam and Cook 2018).

6.3 Learning Approaches

Learning algorithms help to create an environment that can interact with a human being. In the patient monitoring context, the machine learning approaches can be described in mainly three ways. Those are Supervised Learning, Unsupervised Learning, and Reinforcement Learning.

6.3.1 Supervised Learning

Supervised learning is a two-step process where the prediction algorithms are trained with previous experience (data with labels). When a new test data instance is fed to the algorithm, it predicts one of the labels based on its previous knowledge. There are two types of Supervised learning, those are Classification and Regression. Classification is a process to find the class or label of data. On the other hand, Regression tries to find out the particular value. Some supervised learning techniques are described below.

Linear regression finds the relationship between output and input variables. It is differentiated in two ways namely, Simple and Multiple. Simple linear regression tries to find out the relationship between two variables in such a way that that one variable can be determined by other variables. Multiple linear regression tries to find out the relation between multiple variables with dependent variables. Our target is to find out the Hypothesis which is nearer the target value (Huo and Huang 2017).

Gradient descent always tries to find out minimum gradient in each iteration in such a way it can proceed nearer to the target value. Learning rate plays an important role in gradient descent. If we take the value of the learning rate too high then it will not cover all points, there is a probability of missing the optimum point. On the other hand, if we put the learning rate too small then the process becomes more time-consuming. Three types of Gradient descent methods are used. Those are Batch Gradient Descent, Mini-batch Gradient Descent, and Stochastic Gradient Descent. Batch Gradient descent utilizes a set of data in each step. It takes much time for a huge dataset but it gives stable output. Stochastic Gradient Descent uses only one instance and the decision is based on that. A small set of data is applied in Mini batch Gradient Descent for training.

Logistic regression convert probabilistic value into class value (Morrison 2013). It can be Binary or Multiclass. It restricts the hypothesis between 0 and 1. It is represented as a sigmoid function.

Decision tree is based on a tree data structure that is used to classify a new instance. A decision tree (Aljaaf et al. 2015; Habibi et al. 2015) is made by divide and conquer approach applied on the dataset. Leaf nodes indicate the class of the instance. For different outcomes, an instance is partitioned. The class of the subsets depends on heuristics like the Gini index of diversity or information gain ratio. There is a probability of overfitting in the decision tree. To solve this problem pruning is applied to make the accuracy stable (Safavian and Landgrebe 1991; Zhang et al. 2019).

K Nearest Neighbor tries to find out the distance from train data and take the decision on the distance measured. Distances are calculated using different methods like Euclidean, Manhattan, and Minkowski. KNN (Alotaiby et al. 2017; Venkatesan et al. 2018) can also be clubbed with Fuzzy membership functions (Patikar et al. 2020). The value of the K should be greater than 3. K denotes the number of observations (Zhang et al. 2017).

Naïve Bayes classification is based on Bayes Theorem. It tries to find out conditional independence between two attributes. Naïve Bayes works efficiently in spam filtering and grouping of documents. That is combined with several kernel formulae like Gaussian, Multinomial, Complement, and Bernoulli Kelly and Johnson (2021) etc.

Support Vector Machine (SVM) is a "supervised machine learning algorithm". The classification is implemented by finding the hyper-plane that differentiates the classes (Keerthi et al. 2001; Graf et al. 2004; Cao et al. 2006). The margin between classes are maximized using standard Quadratic equation. When the data is not separated by a linear line, different types of kernel can be chosen such as, Gaussian and sigmoid etc. (Chang et al. 2005). To decrease the computational cost kernel methods are used where dimension is high. Support vector machine breaks the training data to reduce memory space, these points are called support vectors (Vishwanathan and Murty 2002).

Random forest was proposed by Breiman Lawrence et al. (2006). It adds a separate layer of randomness to bootstrap aggregation where the number of features are more. Random forest is a collection of tree classifiers. A vote is generated for each tree for the maximum occurred class. To classify an instance a new data instance is passed to each sub trees and one class is generated for each case, the class which gets maximum vote is considered. Random forest reduces the pruning problem which is an advantage over Decision tree.

6.3.2 Unsupervised learning

Unsupervised learning tries to find out the class of data without the previous learning step. The main objective of Unsupervised learning is to find out the hidden pattern of a particular set of data. Unsupervised learning is broadly differentiated in two ways, those are Clustering and Association. Clustering tries to break data into smaller parts. Association tries to find out the connection in large datasets.

K means clustering divides the data into smaller parts in such a way that the similarities in the groups are stronger than in other groups. It starts with the random points and ends up when the points become stable. In each iteration, the centroid is calculated. Like KNN it also tries to find out the distance from each point to the centroids (Fahim et al. 2006).

Hierarchical clustering is to join the nearest clusters into a cluster. This iteration ends when the single cluster is formed. It can be calculated by observing the distance.

6.3.3 Reinforcement Learning

Reinforcement learning takes action immediately in a situation. Here Agent, Environment, Reward, State, Policy, and value play important roles to take decisions instantly (Woergoetter and Porr 2008). It is popularly used by recommendation systems as through the exploration and exploitation of the state-space, reinforcement learning techniques can adapt dynamically to the incoming data and hence can figure out the optimal action to be taken.

6.4   Performance Measure

Performance is calculated using some statistical methods. Depends on the methods of learning different evaluation techniques are used. These techniques are used to evaluate as well as select the suitable method for a particular scenario. The evaluation methods are Classification Accuracy, Logarithmic Loss, Confusion Matrix, Mean Absolute Error and Mean Squared Error.

Classification Accuracy is the rightly predicted samples on all data samples. On the occurrence of classes, the training accuracy is calculated. Test accuracy decides the true prediction of test data. The accuracy difference can measure the performance of a particular setup.

Logarithmic Loss is beneficial for multiclass problems. It calculates a logarithmic value for all samples and all classes. The range of the logarithmic Loss is from 0 to infinity Alankar et al. (2022).

Confusion Matrix shows all the possibilities of a prediction. The possibilities can be classified in four ways. Those are True positive, False positive, True Negative, and False Negative. True Positive and False positive both are predicted as true on the other hand True negative and False-negative both are predicted as false. Based on confusion matrix (Chang et al. 2005) some different measures is been calculated. Sensitivity is the truly predicted true values concerning all true data samples. It is also called Recall. Specificity is the falsely predicted true values concerning all false data samples. Precision is true results for predicted true results. F1 score is the Harmonic mean of Precision and Recall. It lies between 0 and 1 (Karunachandra 2008).

Mean Absolute Error is the average deviation of actual value and predicted value. It works effectively for regression problems.

Mean Squared Error is based on large problems. It calculates the square of the differences except for absolute difference Al-Janabi et al. (2018).

7   Conclusion

Body vital monitoring system consists of three different parts. The first part describes how health sensations are transformed into electronic data, the second part is about making a monitoring system that works independently and finally taking actions. The data which are collected are numeric, image, sound, and text. Raw data is collected in different forms, and they are sometimes grouped. For different problems, different sensors are deployed in the body. Data from different devices are collected and collaborated to predict diseases. Devices are attached to the body to collect the data. Smart devices are designed in such a way that they can be carried easily, cost-effective, secure, and incur low power consumption. Machine learning and Deep learning approaches are used to make the system ready for work alone. Then finally a system is installed in such a way that can work appropriately. These machine learning algorithms work on statistical methods. Performances are calculated on the learning techniques. In body vital monitoring system the main challenges are the data which is produced from electronic devices, are very big, Data cannot be in the fixed format for a specific disease or scenario. The prediction rules are suitable for a particular situation or a particular set of data. Not only traditional Machine learning algorithms are used nowadays some embedded methods are also used. In this study, some applications are discussed as well as some device descriptions are given which are used in the Body vital monitoring system. Data analysis techniques like feature extraction, feature selection, data preprocessing, learning approaches are described. In this body, vital monitoring system response plays a vital role. The function of storing the data and processing of data happens simultaneously. Otherwise, the response can not be made immediately. Delay in response can be a reason for fatal damage. Some data security threats are also discussed along with data analysis. In the healthcare industry, body vital monitoring systems are becoming the most important element.

References

Alankar, B. A., Hannan, G. A., Nitin, D. Y., & Ali, M. (2022) A survey on machine learning algorithms.

Aljaaf, A. J., Al-Jumeily, D., Hussain, A. J., Dawson, T., Fergus, P., & Al-Jumaily, M. (2015). Predicting the likelihood of heart failure with a multi level risk assessment using decision tree. In *2015 Third International Conference on Technological Advances in Electrical, Electronics and Computer Engineering (TAEECE)* (pp. 101–106). IEEE.

Al-Janabi, S., Salman, M. A., & Fanfakh, A. (2018). Recommendation system to improve time management for people in. *Journal of Engineering and Applied Sciences, 13*(24), 10182–10193.

Allison, L., Hoxie, S., & Andrew, T. L. (2017). Towards seamlessly-integrated textile electronics: methods to coat fabrics and fibers with conducting polymers for electronic applications. *Chemical Communications, 53*(53), 7182–7193.

Alotaiby, T. N., Alrshoud, S. R., Alshebeili, S. A., Alhumaid, M. H., & Alsabhan, W. M. (2017). Epileptic MEG spike detection using statistical features and genetic programming with KNN. *Journal of Healthcare Engineering*

Baldo, T. A., de Lima, L. F., Mendes, L. F., de Araujo, W. R., Paixao, T. R., & Coltro, W. K. (2020). Wearable and Biodegradable Sensors for Clinical and Environmental Applications. *ACS Applied Electronic Materials*

Barto, A. G. (1997). Reinforcement learning. In *Neural systems for control* (pp. 7–30). Academic Press.

Bevington, P. R., & Robinson, D. K. (2003). *Data reduction and error analysis.* New York: McGraw-Hill.

Brown, S. J., Health Hero Network Inc. (2010). Patient control of health-related data in a remote patient monitoring system. U.S. Patent 7,827,040.

Cao, Y., Xu, J., Liu, T. Y., Li, H., Huang, Y., & Hon, H. W. (2006). Adapting ranking SVM to document retrieval. In *Proceedings of the 29th Annual International ACM SIGIR Conference on Research and Development in Information* (pp. 186–193).

Caruana, R., Lou, Y., Gehrke, J., Koch, P., Sturm, M., & Elhadad, N. (2015). Intelligible models for healthcare: Predicting pneumonia risk and hospital 30-day readmission. In *Proceedings of the 21th ACM SIGKDD International Conference on Knowledge Discovery and Data Mining* (pp. 1721–1730).

Chang, Q., Chen, Q., & Wang, X. (2005). Scaling Gaussian RBF kernel width to improve SVM classification. In *2005 International Conference on Neural Networks and Brain* (Vol. 1, pp. 19–22). IEEE.

Chen, M., Ma, Y., Li, Y., Wu, D., Zhang, Y., & Youn, C. (2017). Wearable 2.0: Enabling human-cloud integration in next generation healthcare systems. *IEEE Communications Magazine, 55*(1), 54–61. https://doi.org/10.1109/MCOM.2017.1600410CM.

Chen, W., Er, M. J., & Wu, S. (2005). PCA and LDA in DCT domain. *Pattern Recognition Letters, 26*(15), 2474–2482.

Comroe, J. H., & Dripps, R. D. (1978). Scientific basis for the support of biomedical science. In *Biomedical Scientists and Public Policy* (pp. 15–33). Springer, Boston, MA.

Das, S. (2001). Filters, wrappers and a boosting-based hybrid for feature selection. In *Icml* (Vol. 1, pp. 74–81).

Dayan, P., Sahani, M., & Deback, G. (1999). Unsupervised learning. *The MIT Encyclopedia of the Cognitive Sciences*, 857–859.

Deepa, N., Prabadevi, B., Maddikunta, P. K., Gadekallu, T. R., Baker, T., Khan, M. A., & Tariq, U. (2020). An AI based intelligent system for healthcare analysis using ridge adaline stochastic gradient descent classifier. *Journal of Supercomputing*.

Dhillon, A., & Singh, A. (2019). Machine learning in healthcare data analysis: A survey. *Journal of Biology and Today's World, 8*(6), 1–10.

Dias, D., & Paulo Silva Cunha, J. (2018). Wearable health devices-vital sign monitoring, systems and technologies. *Sensors, 18*(8), 2414.

Dicks, K., Kent, R., Crosley, T., Bartlett, T., & MedApps Inc. (2012). Systems and methods for remote patient monitoring and user interface. U.S. Patent 8,126,735.

Elmagarmid, A. K., Ipeirotis, P. G., & Verykios, V. S. (2006). Duplicate record detection: A survey. *IEEE Transactions on Knowledge and Data Engineering, 19*(1), 1–16.

Fahim, A. M., Salem, A. M., Torkey, F. A., & Ramadan, M. (2006). An efficient enhanced k-means clustering algorithm. *Journal of Zhejiang University-Science A, 7*(10), 1626–1633.

Figueiredo, M. A. T., & Jain, A. K. (2002). Unsupervised learning of finite mixture models. *IEEE Transactions on Pattern Analysis and Machine Intelligence, 24*(3), 381–396.

Ghahramani, Z. (2003). Unsupervised learning. In *Summer school on machine learning* (pp. 72–112). Springer, Berlin, Heidelberg.

Giri, D., Acharya, U. R., Martis, R. J., Sree, S. V., Lim, T. C., VI, T. A. & Suri, J. S. (2013). Automated diagnosis of coronary artery disease affected patients using LDA, PCA, ICA and discrete wavelet transform. *Knowledge-Based Systems, 37*, 274–282.

Graf, H., Cosatto, E., Bottou, L., Dourdanovic, I., & Vapnik, V. (2004). Parallel support vector machines: The cascade svm. *Advances in Neural Information Processing Systems, 17*, 521–528.

Habibi, S., Ahmadi, M., & Alizadeh, S. (2015). Type 2 diabetes mellitus screening and risk factors using decision tree: Results of data mining. *Global Journal of Health Science, 7*(5), 304.

Hameed, S. S., Petinrin, O. O., Osman, A., & Hashi, F. S. (2018). Filter-wrapper combination and embedded feature selection for gene expression data. *International Journal of Advance Soft Computing Applications, 10*(1).

Hastie, T., Tibshirani, R., & Friedman, J. (2009). Overview of supervised learning. In *The elements of statistical learning* (pp. 9–41). Springer, New York, NY.

https://www.springwise.com/scarf-with-built-in-air-pollution-protection/.

Huang, R., Liu, Q., Lu, H., & Ma, S. (2002). Solving the small sample size problem of LDA. In *Object recognition supported by user interaction for service robots* (Vol. 3, pp. 29–32). IEEE.

Huo, Z., & Huang, H. (2017). Asynchronous mini-batch gradient descent with variance reduction for non-convex optimization. In *Thirty-First AAAI Conference on Artificial Intelligence (AAAI 2017)*.

Islam, S. R., Kwak, D., Kabir, M. H., Hossain, M., & Kwak, K. S. (2015). The internet of things for health care: A comprehensive survey. *IEEE Access, 3*, 678–708.

Jain, P., Joshi, A. M., & Mohanty, S. P. (2019). iGLU: An intelligent device for accurate noninvasive blood glucose-level monitoring in smart healthcare. *IEEE Consumer Electronics Magazine, 9*(1), 35–42.

Jovanov, E., Milenkovic, A., Otto, C., & De Groen, P. C. (2005). A wireless body area network of intelligent motion sensors for computer assisted physical rehabilitation. *Journal of Neuroengineering and Rehabilitation, 2*(1), 1–10.

Kang, J., & Adibi, S. (2015). A review of security protocols in mHealth wireless body area networks (WBAN). In *International Conference on Future Network Systems and Security* (pp. 61–83). Springer, Cham.

Karunachandra, K. N. N. (2008). Oral health care needs among pregnant women in the Divulapitiya MOH area, Doctoral dissertation.

Kaur, H., & Wasan, S. K. (2006). Empirical study on applications of data mining techniques in healthcare. *Journal of Computer Science, 2*(2), 194–200.

Keerthi, S. S., Shevade, S. K., Bhattacharyya, C., & Murthy, K. R. K. (2001). Improvements to Platt's SMO algorithm for SVM classifier design. *Neural Computation, 13*(3), 637–649.

Kelly, A., & Johnson, M. A. (2021). Investigating the statistical assumptions of Naïve Bayes classifiers. In *2021 55th Annual Conference on Information Sciences and Systems (CISS)* (pp. 1–6). IEEE.

Khalilia, M., Chakraborty, S., & Popescu, M. (2011). Predicting disease risks from highly imbalanced data using random forest. *BMC Medical Informatics and Decision Making, 11*(1), 51.

Khan, J. Y., & Yuce, M. R. (2010). Wireless body area network (WBAN) for medical applications. *New Developments in Biomedical Engineering, 31*, 591–627.

Kohavi, R., & Sommerfield, D. (1995). Feature subset selection using the wrapper method: Overfitting and dynamic search space topology. In *KDD* (pp. 192–197).

Kuncheva, L. I., & Faithfull, W. J. (2013). PCA feature extraction for change detection in multidimensional unlabeled data. *IEEE Transactions on Neural Networks and Learning Systems, 25*(1), 69–80.

Lawrence, R. L., Wood, S. D., & Sheley, R. L. (2006). Mapping invasive plants using hyperspectral imagery and Breiman Cutler classifications (RandomForest). *Remote Sensing of Environment, 100*(3), 356–362.

Lee, T. W., Lewicki, M. S., & Sejnowski, T. J. (2000). ICA mixture models for unsupervised classification of non-Gaussian classes and automatic context switching in blind signal separation. *IEEE Transactions on Pattern Analysis and Machine Intelligence, 22*(10), 1078–1089.

Lenzerini, M. (2002). Data integration: A theoretical perspective. In *Proceedings of the Twenty-first ACM SIGMOD-SIGACT-SIGART Symposium on Principles of Database Systems* (pp. 233–246).

Li, Q., Liu, C., Oster, J., & Clifford, G. D. (2016). Signal processing and feature selection preprocessing for classification in noisy healthcare data. *Machine Learning for Healthcare Technologies, 2*(33), 2016.

Lin, S. K., Wang, L. C., Lin, C. Y., & Chiueh, H. (2018). An ultra-low power smart headband for real-time epileptic seizure detection. *IEEE Journal of Translational Engineering in Health and Medicine, 6*, 1–10.

Liu, Y., Mu, Y., Chen, K., Li, Y., Guo, J. (2020). Daily activity feature selection in smart homes based on Pearson correlation coefficient. *Neural Processing Letters*, 1–17.

López, M. M., RamÁrez, J., Górriz, J. M., Álvarez, I., Salas-Gonzalez, D., Segovia, F., & Chaves, R. (2009). SVM-based CAD system for early detection of the Alzheimer's disease using kernel PCA and LDA. *Neuroscience Letters, 464*(3), 233–238.

Madakam, S., Lake, V., Lake, V., & Lake, V. (2015). Internet of things (IoT): A literature review. *Journal of Computer and Communications, 3*(05), 164.

Martis, R. J., Acharya, U. R., & Min, L. C. (2013). ECG beat classification using PCA, LDA, ICA and discrete wavelet transform. *Biomedical Signal Processing and Control, 8*(5), 437–448.

Mohd, H., & Mohamed, S. H. S. (2005). Acceptance model of electronic medical record. *Journal of Advancing Information and Management Studies, 2*(1), 75–92.

Morrison, G. S. (2013). Tutorial on logistic-regression calibration and fusion: Converting a score to a likelihood ratio. *Australian Journal of Forensic Sciences, 45*(2), 173–197.

Nandy, A., Saha, J., & Chowdhury, C. (2020). Novel features for intensive human activity recognition based on wearable and smartphone sensors. *Microsystem Technologies*, 1–15.

Palaniappan, S., & Awang, R. (2008). Intelligent heart disease prediction system using data mining techniques. In *2008 IEEE/ACS International Conference on Computer Systems and Applications* (pp. 108–115). IEEE.

Patikar, S., Saha, P., Neogy, S., & Chowdhury, C. (2020). An approach towards prediction of diabetes using modified fuzzy K nearest neighbor. In *2020 IEEE International Conference on Computing, Power and Communication Technologies (GUCON)* (pp. 73–76). IEEE.

Puth, M. T., Neuhäuser, M., & Ruxton, G. D. (2015). Effective use of Spearman's and Kendall's correlation coefficients for association between two measured traits. *Animal Behaviour, 102,* 77–84.

Rachburee, N., & Punlumjeak, W. (2015). A comparison of feature selection approach between greedy, IG-ratio, Chi-square, and mRMR in educational mining. In *2015 7th International Conference on Information Technology and Electrical Engineering (ICITEE)* (pp. 420–424). IEEE.

Ranstam, J., & Cook, J. A. (2018). LASSO regression. *Journal of British Surgery, 105*(10), 1348–1348.

Roy, M., Chowdhury, C., & Aslam, N. (2020). Security and privacy issues in wireless sensor and body area networks. In *Handbook of Computer Networks and Cyber Security* (pp. 173–200). Springer, Cham.

Sadiqi, S., Post, M. W., Hosman, A. J., Dvorak, M. F., Chapman, J. R., Benneker, L. M., Kandziora, F., Rajasekaran, S., Schnake, K. J., Vaccaro, A. R., & Oner, F. C. (2020). Reliability, validity and responsiveness of the Dutch version of the AOSpine PROST (Patient Reported Outcome Spine Trauma). *European Spine Journal*, 1–14.

Saeys, Y., Abeel, T., & Van de Peer, Y. (2008). Robust feature selection using ensemble feature selection techniques. In *Joint European Conference on Machine Learning and Knowledge Discovery in Databases* (pp. 313–325). Springer, Berlin, Heidelberg.

Safavian, S. R., & Landgrebe, D. (1991). A survey of decision tree classifier methodology. *IEEE Transactions on Systems, Man, and Cybernetics, 21*(3), 660–674.

Saha, J., Chowdhury, C., & Biswas, S. (2018). Two phase ensemble classifier for smartphone based human activity recognition independent of hardware configuration and usage behaviour. *Microsystem Technologies, 24*(6), 2737–2752.

Saleem, N., Rahman, A., Rizwan, M., Naseem, S., & Ahmad, F. (2022). Enhancing security of android operating system based phones using quantum key distribution.

Sellappan, P., & Chua, S. L. (2005). Model-based healthcare decision support system. In *Proceedings of International Conference on Information Technology in Asia CITA'05* (pp. 45–50). Kuching, Sarawak, Malaysia.

Selvaraj, P., & Doraikannan, S. (2019). Privacy and security issues on wireless body area and IoT for remote healthcare monitoring. *Intelligent Pervasive Computing Systems for Smarter Healthcare*, 227–253.

Shahbakhti, M., Rodrigues, A.S., Augustyniak, P., Broniec-Wójcik, A., Sološenko, A., Beiramvand, M., & Marozas, V. (2022). SWT-kurtosis based algorithm for elimination of electrical shift and linear trend from EEG signals. *Biomedical Signal Processing and Control, 65*, 102373.

Shilaih, M., Goodale, B. M., Falco, L., Kübler, F., De Clerck, V., & Leeners, B. (2018). Modern fertility awareness methods: Wrist wearables capture the changes in temperature associated with the menstrual cycle. *Bioscience Reports, 38*(6).

Song, Q., & Shepperd, M. (2007). Missing data imputation techniques. *International Journal of Business Intelligence and Data Mining, 2*(3), 261–291.

Sutton, R. S., & Barto, A. G. (2018). *Reinforcement learning: An introduction.* MIT Press.

Tamura, T., Huang, M., & Togawa, T. (2018). Current developments in wearable thermometers. *Advanced Biomedical Engineering, 7,* 88–99.

Tan, T. H., Chang, C. S., Chen, Y. F., & Lee, C. (2008). Implementation of a portable personal EKG signal monitoring system. In *International Conference on Medical Biometrics* (pp. 122–128). Springer, Berlin, Heidelberg.

Tayyab, M., Sharawi, M. S., Shamim, A., & "A wearable RF sensor on fabric substrate for pulmonary edema monitoring. (2017). Sensors networks smart and emerging technologies (SENSET). *Beirut,2017*, 1–4. https://doi.org/10.1109/SENSET.2017.8125007.

Tominaga, Y. (1999). Comparative study of class data analysis with PCA-LDA, SIMCA, PLS, ANNs, and k-NN. *Chemometrics and Intelligent Laboratory Systems, 49*(1), 105–115.

Vegesna, A., Tran, M., Angelaccio, M., & Arcona, S. (2017). Remote patient monitoring via non-invasive digital technologies: A systematic review. *Telemedicine and e-Health, 23*(1), 3–17.

Venkatesan, C., Karthigaikumar, P., Paul, A., Satheeskumaran, S., & Kumar, R. J. I. A. (2018). ECG signal preprocessing and SVM classifier-based abnormality detection in remote healthcare applications. *IEEE Access, 6,* 9767–9773.

Vishwanathan, S. V. M., & Murty, M. N. (2002). SSVM: A simple SVM algorithm. In: *Proceedings of the 2002 International Joint Conference on Neural Networks, IJCNN'02* (Cat. No. 02CH37290) (Vol. 3, pp. 2393–2398). IEEE.

Vitola, J., Pozo, F., Tibaduiza, D. A., & Anaya, M. (2017). A sensor data fusion system based on k-nearest neighbor pattern classification for structural health monitoring applications. *Sensors, 17*(2), 417.

Vyas, A., & Pal, S. (2020). Preventing security and privacy attacks in WBANs. In *Handbook of Computer Networks and Cyber Security* (pp. 201–225). Springer, Cham.

Wang, Z., Zhao, C., & Qiu, S. (2014). A system of human vital signs monitoring and activity recognition based on body sensor network. *Sensor Review*.

Wang, D., Li, D., Zhao, M., Xu, Y., & Wei, Q. (2018). Multifunctional wearable smart device based on conductive reduced graphene oxide/polyester fabric. *Applied Surface Science, 454,* 218–226.

Woergoetter, F., & Porr, B. (2008). Reinforcement learning. *Scholarpedia, 3*(3), 1448.

Yeole, A. S., & Kalbande, D. R. (2016). Use of internet of things (IoT) in healthcare: A survey. In *Proceedings of the ACM Symposium on Women in Research 2016* (pp. 71–76).

Yuce, M. R. (2010). Implementation of wireless body area networks for healthcare systems. *Sensors and Actuators, A: Physical, 162*(1), 116–129.

Zhang, S., Li, X., Zong, M., Zhu, X., & Cheng, D. (2017). Learning k for KNN classification. *ACM Transactions on Intelligent Systems and Technology (TIST), 8*(3), 1–19.

Zhang, B., Ren, J., Cheng, Y., Wang, B., & Wei, Z. (2019). Health data driven on continuous blood pressure prediction based on gradient boosting decision tree algorithm. *IEEE Access, 7,* 32423–32433.

Zhu, X., & Goldberg, A. B. (2009). Introduction to semi-supervised learning. *Synthesis Lectures on Artificial Intelligence and Machine Learning, 3*(1), 1–130.

Quantitative Assessment of Smartphone Usage in College Students—A Digital Phenotyping Approach

Kalyan Sasidhar

Abstract Community-related health monitoring and prediction have become the focal points of research and development in the last decade. Health care particularly garnered much interest from the research fraternity. With powerful sensing capabilities, smartphones have become the de-facto measurement platforms. Digital phenotype is a new paradigm that aims at exploring and quantifying individual-level human behavior characteristics through an in-situ method of data collection primarily from personal digital devices such as smartphones and wearable sensors. Various works have attempted digital phenotype on different scales for varied populations to study user behavior across three dimensions, namely physical (motor activities performed, device usage styles,); social (online and offline interaction); and mental (psychological behavioral aspects). In this work, we conduct a behavioral sensing experiment through digital phenotype on a cohort of 47 college students over one and half months at our institute. We quantify the total time spent on physical activity, social interaction, and sleep. We also quantify the smartphone usage duration per day and discuss the potential impact of phone use on student life behavior and health. Our findings indicated that most students seem to be on the idle side of the physical activity spectrum, are sleeping less and are using their smartphones for a wide range of purposes and for extended hours.

Keywords Mobile sensing · Smartphones · Activity · Sleep

1 Introduction

The major invention that the human race witnessed in the past decade has been the smartphone and the hardware and software technological developments associated with it. Coupled with these is the proliferation of digital platforms, solutions, and applications blurring the line between real and virtual life. Smartphones with built-in

K. Sasidhar (✉)
Dhirubhai Ambani Institute of Information and Communication Technology, Gandhinagar, Gujarat, India
e-mail: Kalyan_sasidhar@daiict.ac.in

© The Author(s), under exclusive license to Springer Nature Singapore Pte Ltd. 2022   217
S. Biswas et al. (eds.), *Internet of Things Based Smart Healthcare*, Smart Computing and Intelligence, https://doi.org/10.1007/978-981-19-1408-9_10

networking and communication technology have broken geographical boundaries, making lives more comfortable but at the same time impacting human behavior. Reduction in physical and sleep activities is manifested due to extensive use of social media, games, entertainment, and even mindless scrolling of applications on phones.

Researchers discovered that the built-in sensors in smartphones could be used for sensing purposes, and coined the term mobile sensing which essentially involves sensing various physical quantities such as motion, orientation, ambient sound, light, etc., and extracting useful information from that data to study behavioral patterns (Lane et al., 2010). Digital phenotyping an extension of mobile sensing quantifies behavior on the individual-level phenotype through in-situ sensing. Applications include health (Marsch, 2021), social science (Raento et al., 2009), mental health (Servia-Rodríguez et al., 2017), psychiatry (Melcher et al., 2020), (Liang et al., 2019; Insel and TR, 2020), and psychology (Chein et al., 2017). The phenotype-based study's motivation is the ease in data collection facilitated through the wide availability of smartphones with users ranging across all age groups. With Android and iOS mobile operating systems' evolution, young adults seem to be the significant users and contributors to mobile applications (Statistica, 2013) and (TCS, 2013).

Most studies on phone use by students in India followed a qualitative assessment method through questionnaires (Subba et al., 2013), (Davey, 2014), (Bisen et al., 2016) and interviews (Dixit et al., 2010). The studies compiled information on the brand of phone preferred, type of applications installed and used, and the psychological feeling of losing a phone. Responses for such methods may not be accurate since it is difficult to recall actions or events of the past. For instance, one may not remember accurately his/her phone usage duration in the past week. This could lead to incorrect responses or even personal bias (Vaizman et al., 2017), potentially producing skewed conclusions. In contrast, exhaustive work on mobile sensing methods has shown to be reliable and complement qualitative data (Lane et al., 2010).

Our study aimed to quantify smartphone usage behavior and its impact on health. Daily routine activities of people include work, regular physical exercise, sleep habits, and socializing. Sudden changes in such behaviors could show adverse effects on health. Research shows that some kind of physical activity on a regular basis is critical (Maher et al., 2013). Research also says that gradual reduction in physical activity has a profound impact on the muscle strength irrespective of the age(Liberman et al., 2017) and (Laforest et al., 1990). Similarly, inadequate sleep over the long term affects the biological clock and health of a person (Rod et al., 2018). With the advent of social media, there seems to be more online presence of oneself than offline interaction. Having a healthy socializing routine has shown positive outcomes of removing loneliness in people (Cohen, 2004). Student life particularly poses challenges such as handling academic stress, language or cultural barriers for social interaction leading to loneliness, depression, and other mental health issues (Douglas et al., 1997). Mobile-health (mHealth) applications and interventions are already being applied (Gowin et al., 2015; Lathia et al., 2013).

Hence, understanding how much time students spend on physical activity, sleep, and sociability is imperative. Therefore, utilizing the smartphone as a platform, we conducted an experiment-based study for 45 days to assess students' behavioral trends and health impact. For understanding the effect on health, we detect and quantify in hours per day the activity type (idle or moving or sleeping), the social interaction levels, and the mobility patterns on campus. Our study consisted of the following research questions:

- What is the total duration of smartphone usage?
- What is the total time students spend on physical activity such as walking?
- What are the sleep patterns of these students?
- How much time is being spent for face-to-face social interaction as opposed to online interaction?
- As a group, which location or areas on campus do students prefer to visit and how much time do they spend in those locations?

Our study resulted in the following findings:

1. Students were physically active for 4 ± 1.5 hours on average.
2. Smartphone usage was on average 6.7 ± 3.5 hours.
3. The sleep hours were on average 5.5 ± 2 hours.
4. Students had a healthy face-to-face interaction of 4 hours on average.
5. 40% of the students spent an average of 7 ± 1.5 hours in their dorm rooms.

This book chapter consists of ten sections. In Sect. 2, we present the methodology of our experiment wherein we discuss the study procedure, the data collection mechanism, and other logistics. Following this in Sect. 3, we introduce the readers to smartphone technology and its growth over the years. We further throw light on the embedded sensors, the working of the accelerometer and its application to activity recognition. The next three sections comprise of the results of our study. We start with activity recognition in Sect. 4, followed by sleep detection in Sect. 5, sociability analysis in Sect. 6, and analysis of mobility patterns in Sect. 7. Finally, we conclude with some discussions in Sect. 8 followed by Acknowledgments.

2 Experiment and Study Design

2.1 Study Procedure

The entire study consisted of student orientation, data collection, analysis, and presentation of results. The participants were primarily our own undergraduate students. Among the 48 students who completed the study, ten were from the final year, 20 were from the third year, ten from the second, and eight from the first year. We informed all participants what data we were going to collect and how the app works. The students signed a consent form agreeing to the data collection mechanism and the privacy policies. We showed how to install the mobile application. We also requested the students to fill in a survey form providing their demographic information, personality traits, and current smartphone usage preferences.

The students followed their regular routine of attending classes, hanging out during breaks, moving between multiple locations, etc. At the end of 24 hours, the app automatically transferred the data to a local server. Two research fellows interacted with each student twice a week to gather responses related to their daily routine which included mobility on campus, places frequently visited, physical exercising preferences, sleep routines, and socializing.

2.2 Incentives and Privacy Considerations

As an incentive, we paid each student INR 3000. We received around 990 hours of data for the entire study duration. To protect participants' personal information, anonymity of student's identity was maintained. We clarified that we collected and inferred only the type of applications used and not the content.

2.3 Data Collection

The data collection phase lasted for 45 days during the Autumn semester. We developed a mobile app that activates each of the sensors through Sensor managers provided by Android. The sensors respond to change in the physical quantity. After analog to digital conversions (ADC), a digital value is stored in array format and later written to a csv file. Figure 1 shows the interface of the mobile app.

The app was programmed to automatically collect accelerometer, proximity, microphone, light sensor data, location (Wi-Fi), and application usage. Using the data, we inferred (a) activity (stationary, non-stationary, i.e., walking or running or cycling), (b) sleep duration, (c) social interactions, (d) mobility patterns, and (e) overall smartphone usage hours. In the next section, we introduce the reader to smartphone technology and discuss aspects related to the operating system, the built-in sensors, and their use.

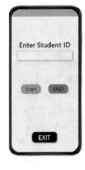

Fig. 1 The interface shows a textbox to enter student ID and a start and stop button for data collection. Once the student enters the ID and touches the Start button, the data collection starts and the app runs in the background. The Stop button is provided to stop the application if required

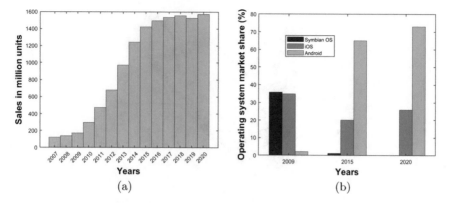

Fig. 2 **a** Mobile phone shipment sales increased by 196% between 2007 and 2020 **b** The rise in Android- based phones from 2009 to 2020 is around 188%, while Symbian OS-based phones and iOS-based phones show 196% and 26% decrease in sales

3 Smartphone Technology

The first smartphone was the LG G1 with a single core Qualcomm MSM7201A (528MHz CPU clock) processor, 192 MB RAM, and 256MB storage running on Android 1.1 operating system. The phone was embedded with a three axis accelerometer, magnetometer, and a microphone along with Bluetooth 2.0 and Wi-Fi radios. Fast forward to 2020, the latest phones contain six to eight cores Qualcomm Snapdragon 855 (2GHz clock) processor, 8GB RAM, and 128GB storage space running on Android 10. Embedded sensors include optical fingerprint, accelerometer, gyroscope, proximity, compass, and barometer. The built-in sensors when compared with sensors in a wireless sensor network are different in the fact that they are independent of each other and do not require any protocols to enable interaction or dependency. Below in Fig. 2, we visually illustrate the various statistics[1] pertaining to smartphone growth over the years in terms of smartphone shipments and operating system popularity.

We now discuss the working of an accelerometer.

3.1 Working of an Accelerometer

The accelerometer, in the context of a smartphone, measures the amount of force applied on the three axes x, y, and z. The sensor has a mass with comb-like protrusions and a capacitance associated with each pair of protrusions. Depending on the force, the capacitance changes which changes the voltage. The change in voltage is mapped to force values. The units are g force(1g, 2g, etc) or m/s^2, where 1g is equivalent to

---

[1] All stats obtained from https://gs.statcounter.com/.

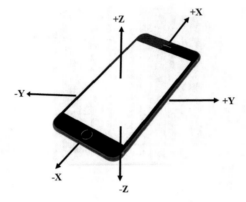

Fig. 3 The figure shows the x axis corresponds to the direction of travel, the y axis represents the horizontal axis movement and the z axis represents the vertical movement, i.e., measuring gravitational force. Any movement on the device applies force on the sensor which causes variations in the magnitudes on three axes. A static position captures only the gravitational forces across the z axis

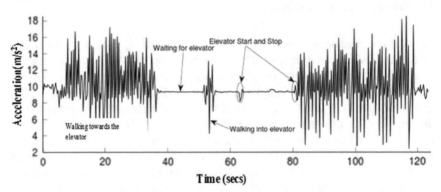

Fig. 4 The rhythmic movement of the legs causes the phone to move exerting forces on the x and y axes. When the user is idle, only gravitational force is exerted. Hence, the amplitude of idle activity varies around $9.8m/s^2$ when compared with highs and lows of walking. The intra-sample variance computed was also higher for walking than that of idle activity. This is a differentiating feature of both these activities. The small changes in the z axis were triggered by the elevator start and stop action

$9.8m/s^2$. Figure 3 shows the three axes along the phone and how the positive and negative directions of the axes are interpreted.

Figure 4 explains the variations in force exerted by human activity (walking or idle) along the three axes.

Apart from just detecting the type of activity, the three axes sensor data can also be used to interpret walking activity with more granularity. For instance, as listed in Table 1 (Kalyan Pathapati Subbu, 2011), changes in x axis mean taking turns while walking, whereas changes in y axis mean walking straight and so on.

Table 1 Interpretation of data from three axes

Axis	Direction	Walking mode
x	Left/Right	Taking turns
y	Front/Rear	Walking straight
z	Up/Down	Upstairs or Downstairs

In the next section, we discuss how we applied this concept in detecting activity type among students, what inferences were made pertaining to idle, non-idle, and sleep activity, and present the other major findings of the study.

4 Activity Detection

For recognizing the activity (walking, running, standing or sitting), a characteristic feature has to be selected. We chose the variance as explained in Sect. 3. This feature was then given as input to three classification algorithms, namely Support Vector Machine(SVM), Random Forest(RF), and Logistic Regression(LR) algorithms. SVM creates an optimally separating line (hyperplane) to distinguish samples into multiple classes. Random forests are multilevel decision trees and logistic regression tries to fit data to a certain curve (linear,quadratic) and create a model.

We labeled our initial data consisting of 10,000 data points using the variance feature. We then trained the classifiers on the data , tested the unlabeled data and computed the classification accuracy using F-score given by $F_{score} = \frac{2.precision.recall}{precision+recall}$. However, not satisfied with the classification accuracies, we applied co-training principle which is a semi-supervised approach. Here, a small set of labeled data is used to train and test with a larger set of unlabeled data. The prediction rates were improved by combining two independent and different classifiers (Radu et al., 2014). Figure 5 shows the improvement in accuracy after applying co-training.

From the non-idle class samples, we computed the time in hours for each student. This was repeated for the idle class. Figure 6 illustrates a sample trend of student activity hours for the entire 45 days.

To summarize the numbers, students were idle for 13 hrs/day(excluding sleep hours) on average and active for 4 ± 1.5 hrs/day on average. The average error between ground truth (where we asked the students to estimate the number of hours of physical activity) and phone-based estimation across all students was 10.5 ± 2 hours for idle and 3 ± 2 hours for non-idle. We use a box plot, Fig. 7, to illustrate statistically the variations between the two activity states.

Curious to find out more from students about their low levels of physical activity, we inquired about their interest and preference in exercising. Out of 45 days, only 10% of the days, students claimed to exercise. Only three students exercised every

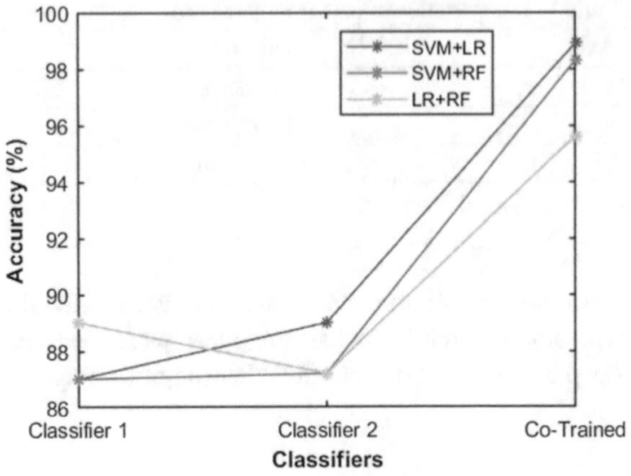

Fig. 5 The legend shows how for each pair of technique (SVM, LR or SVM, RF or LR, RF), co-training improved the accuracy when compared over that obtained when independently the techniques were applied

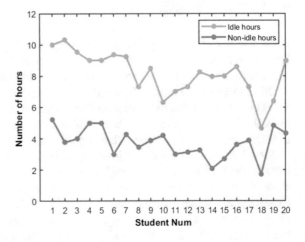

Fig. 6 The graph shows the average idle and non-idle activity hours trend. The idle hours are overwhelmingly higher than the non-idle hours

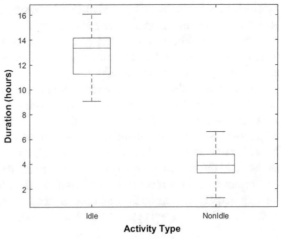

Fig. 7 The plot shows the median values and inter-quartile ranges for both idle and non-idle activities. The idle hours are overwhelmingly larger than the non-idle

day, whereas 18 exercised once in three days. The remaining 26 students did not prefer exercising. All of these results tied together strengthen the general belief or hypothesis that the sedentary levels of the younger generation are on the rise.

5 Sleep Detection

Sleep is a vital aspect of human health and sleep routines vary between individuals. However, disruption of sleep occasionally or continuously for prolonged periods does have detrimental effects on future health (Rod et al., 2011; Cappuccio et al., 2010). Human sleep continuously goes through a cycle of stages starting from rapid eye movement (REM) to non-REM and finally to the deepest stage called slow-wave sleep. The duration of sleep cycle usually lasts anywhere between 90–110 minutes (Lockley, 2018).

Existing research has started to focus on assessing technology, or to be precise, smartphone impact on sleep duration and sleep quality (Rod et al., 2018). However, most works look at the impact through qualitative methods. We, on the other hand, use mobile sensors inside the phone. We detected the sleep activity by considering the following features. The user activity state, ambient light and noise levels(low), and phone screen status (locked or unlocked). A decision tree predicts the activity state as sleep if the student, i.e., the phone is idle, the screen is locked, and the light and noise levels are low continuously for a minimum of 30 minutes. We borrow this idea from (Chen et al., 2013). Figure 8 depicts the frequency of sleeping hours of students.

From Fig. 8, we can conclude that higher number of students (35.9% of students) averaged five to six hours of sleep. Only one student had more than seven hours of sleep time (2.6% of students). An average error of 55 ± 10 minutes was obtained between the ground truth (student recorded sleep and wake times) and sensor estimated.

Fig. 8 Sleep hours distribution: The pie chart shows the distribution of students according to their sleep hours. Majority of the students (27) slept for less than six hours and this routine was observed from their data for close to 18 days

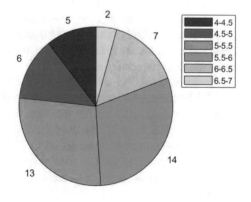

■	4–4.5
■	4.5–5
■	5–5.5
☐	5.5–6
☐	6–6.5
☐	6.5–7

In Sect. 8, we compare this finding with the sleep quality responded by students. In the next section, we move on to discussing the location preferences on campus and the mobility patterns of students

6 Sociability

Sociability means preference for being and interacting with some company (a group of friends, close aides, etc.,). Most existing studies on sociability of students use self-reporting methods to questions such as who they like to be with, how many people do they like being with, and so on. The gap in such works was the accuracy in estimating the actual duration of interaction.

For understanding sociability, we consider the duration of interaction students have on campus with peers. This involves quantifying their conversation levels. For this process, we utilized the microphone which records audio from various backgrounds including classrooms, lecture halls, cafeterias, libraries, and so on. The sensor samples every two minutes the amplitude value of the sound signal. In our earlier work (Subbu et al., 2009), we proposed a context-aware system by extracting some features from audio data to distinguish classes of background like silence, speech, and other environments. These features can be considered as elements of a multidimensional vector, and when trained on these features, classifiers can detect the environment present and provide contextual information. Borrowing the method in this work, we first classify the background between noisy and silent. Then we further extract speech from the noisy environment detected.

After data collection, preprocessing of data included sampling, segmenting the recordings into 256 samples, each of 30 ms duration audio files. We further labeled each sample according to the environment where they were captured. A Hamming windowing was applied on each frame to reduce discontinuities at the beginning and end of the signal pertaining to that frame. After this, a frequency domain analysis was conducted to obtain appropriate features for classification. However, before classification, feature extraction had to be performed. The power spectrum of the audio signal presents itself with features that were extracted in the form of amplitudes.

The human auditory system does not recognize audio with frequencies over 1KHz. Such audio signals are mapped to human audible frequencies on a scale called the mel scale. For frequencies below 1000 Hz, a linearly spaced filter is applied, whereas for those above 1000Hz, a logarithmic spacing is used. For details on filter banks and the Mel Frequency Cepstral Coefficients (MFCC) process, we urged the readers to refer to (MartInez, 2012). After this step, for the classification of the audio samples into vocal and non-vocal, we used the VQ method (Makhoul et al., 1985) due to its ease of implementation and accuracy. Figure 9 shows the interaction pattern of a sample of 20 students. We can see the variations for each student.

Figure 10 presents the distribution of students' conversation levels across different time slots.

Fig. 9 Total hours of social interaction are excluding interaction during class. The presence of the student or rather his phone at the classroom location was obtained from Wi-Fi data and those hours were deducted from the total conversation hours of the day

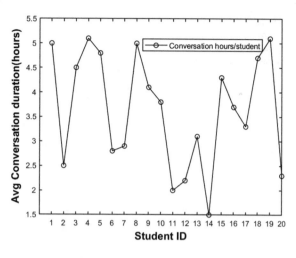

Fig. 10 The duration is split into two hour slots showing that a majority of the students had 4–5 hours/day of interactions with their friends which is a healthy sign

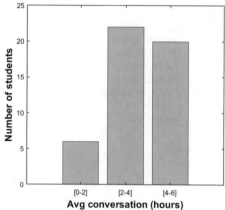

7 Location and Mobility Patterns

Mobility mainly includes extracting the various places/locations one visits, the frequency and duration of the visits. Existing research has shown that decreased mobility levels (i.e., moving around multiple locations) when combined with reduced sleep hours (Thomée et al., 2011) and excessive smartphone usage are associated with symptoms of depression. In other words, depressive people tend to confine themselves to one or two places only (say home or office) for a long term (months), are addicted to their phones (Aggarwal et al., 2012), and prefer not to interact with anyone. In some cases, if qualitative responses are biased or skewed towards lower scales, conclusions lead to false positives such as detecting depression in a person when he is otherwise not (Demasi et al., 2016).

Fig. 11 The box plot shows that most students preferred spending time in their hostel rooms, followed by cafeteria

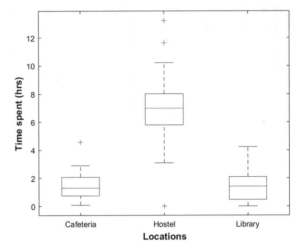

Fig. 12 a During this time slot (lunchtime), the density of student movement was high indicated by the red color near the cafeteria, whereas in **b**, there was no major movement, the reason being laboratory hours requiring presence of students

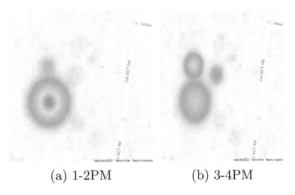

(a) 1-2PM   (b) 3-4PM

We have not delved into mental health specifically, but have looked at how physically active the students were and their mobility behavior inside the campus. The Wi-Fi access point ID was continuously logged by the mobile app every two minutes. Later, we mapped the access point data to human understandable location tag (library, classrooms, lab, hostel, cafeteria, etc.). For each student, we obtained a set of most visited locations on campus, by setting a threshold of at least 10 mins as stay time at a particular location. Figure 11 illustrates the distribution of the top three locations preferred by students.

A web-based interface showing the heat map of student movement Fig. 12 during different times of the day was also created as a byproduct of this analysis. Such information could help the administration in understanding the student movement for better campus crowd management.

7.1 Mobility Patterns

Now that the most common locations visited and the time spent at each location have been discussed, we now discuss students' mobility trends for the 45 day period. To understand the trend, we correlate it with the academic calendar on a week by week basis for roughly 7 weeks. The activity data in hours was averaged across all students per day and plotted to infer the movement activity on the campus. The academic calendar lists events such as examinations, cultural festivals, sports day, and other extracurricular activities that happen on the campus. Figure 13 illustrates the findings.

- Week 1: The mobility levels were average but gradually toward the third day of the week, the graph saw a rise as the weekend was approaching.
- Week 2: During the start of the week, a technical fest was organized. This created more movement around the campus as can be seen by the rise from the mid of the second week. Again, once the fest ended over the weekend, students stayed in their rooms as indicated by low mobility.
- Week 3: At the start of the week, their mobility levels were high but gradually reduced. As the semester progressed, the students were settling down, focusing on classes, visiting libraries, so they had low mobility.
- Week 4: Mobility levels were low at the start of the week after which we observed a gradual increase, the reason being the start of the sports fest at the campus.
- Week 5: This week did not see major ups and downs in the mobility.
- Week 6: This week was the mid-semester exam week. So, as natural behavior, the mobility started to decline.
- Week 7: Once the exams completed, the mobility started to increase.

Fig. 13 Mobility pattern trend of students for a period of 7 weeks

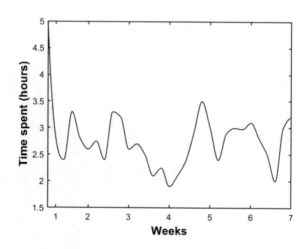

8 Discussions

In this section, we first present the overall mobile phone usage including the categories of apps used often. Following this, we discuss students' perception of sleep quality.

8.1 Smartphone Addiction: Mobile Usage Hours

As mentioned in the Sect. 2, our mobile app monitors the usage which includes the screen time, the type of app currently being used, and its duration. Figure 14 illustrates the overall usage distribution of smartphones across all students.

We also categorized the usage among entertainment apps, social media, gaming, education, and so on. Our other findings include the following:

- 70% (33 of 48) of students spent 4 hours/day on social media.
- 53% (25 of 48) of students spent 3.5 ± 1.5 hours on gaming apps.
- 20% (10 of 48) of students played PubG for close to two hours/day.
- 60% students preferred using their phones for not just communication and entertainment, but also for education.

Although the results resonate with most existing work in terms of excessive usage of phones, reduction in sleep and increasing levels of inactivity, we found some positive impacts too. For instance, as mentioned, many students used their smartphones for sharing educational materials, watching video lectures/tutorials, and using productivity apps. Even though this may have seemed unacceptable, the last few months have seen even greater usage of smartphones. The pandemic has forced education

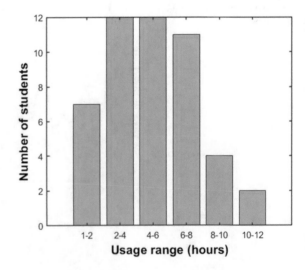

Fig. 14 The average mobile usage among the students was 6.87 hours per day on average. The skewness toward the right shows that a majority of the students' phone use was higher than average

to go online making humans even more dependent on phones, laptops, and other gadgets. To conclude, using technology for longer time periods now has become inevitable.

8.2 Sleep Quality Impact

Looking at the sleep duration results, we felt that students lacked the appropriate amount of sleep. To gauge the students' feelings about whether the reduced sleep routine impacted them, we asked them to rate the quality of their sleep on a scale of 1 to 5. with 1 being Very bad, 2—Fairly bad, 3—Fairly good, 4—Very good, and 5—Sound sleep. Figure 15 illustrates the distribution of sleep quality responses from students.

The students reported that, for almost 37 days of the study, they had good sleep. Only for seven to eight days (16%), some reported difficulty in sleeping. Our future work aims to analyze the subset of those who reported sleeping difficulties. To conclude, we can say that students managed to remain fresh without feeling fatigued with a sound sleep of five hours.

Overall, our study has highlighted how smartphone has impacted student behavior. This is a first of its kind study attempted on Indian students and some comparisons that can be drawn from the existing work is that students irrespective of the geographical location, spend major chunk of their time on smartphones. The activity and sleep duration also seem to be on the same lines. Other factors such as sociability and mobility were different. This could be due to the social background, personality

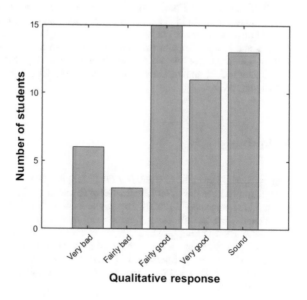

Fig. 15 A majority of them reported to have fairly good and very good sleep even though their average sleep hours were 5.5 h

types, and so on. On the bright side, education technology backed by companies like Google, Microsoft, Zoom, and others is banking on smartphones by developing apps such as Google meet, Teams, and Zoom.

9 Conclusions

Due to the digital era's tremendous growth, we witness how technology is becoming a dominant factor in our daily lives. Smartphone-based passive sensing has become an emerging technique to understand human life and behavior. This study presented a novel method, namely digital phenotype, to monitor and assess college students' health-related behaviors. The method attempted on a student cohort for the first time in India proved the viability of using smartphones and their embedded sensors as platforms for collecting, analyzing, and inferring behavior. This study provided trends on the physical activity, sleep, sociability, and mobility patterns of students while carrying out daily routines on campus during an academic term.

The activity levels indicate that students may be preferring a sedentary lifestyle; possible factors contributing to this behavior could be prolonged usage of smartphones, social media, gaming, and reduced sleep hours. Social interaction on the campus was healthy with no sign of deterioration even with increased use of mobile phones. Our future work, among many, plans to take up the mental health issue that is plaguing the student community and understand how smartphone technology can be used as an intervention platform.

Acknowledgements I would like to first and foremost thank the Indian Council for Social Science Research for funding this project and providing us the opportunity to explore and obtain interesting observations. Next, would like to thank my colleague and collaborating faculty Prof. Alka Parikh. I would also like to thank the M.Tech students: Dimple shah and Aswini, PhD students: Maitri Vaghela and Pramod Tripathi for working as research fellows. Thanks to all student volunteers without whom the work would not have been possible. Last but not least, i would like to thank the Director and the administrative department of DAIICT for providing all the required support to conduct this project.

References

Aggarwal, M., Grover, S., & Basu. D. (2012). Mobile phone use by resident doctors: Tendency to addiction-like behavior. *German Journal of Psychiatry, 15,* 50–55.

Bisen, S., & Deshpande, Y. (2016). An analytical study of smartphone addiction among engineering students: A gender differences. *International Journal of Indian Psychology, 4*(1).

Cappuccio, F. P., D'Elia, L., Strazzullo, P., & Miller, M. A. (2010). Sleep duration and all-cause mortality: A systematic review and meta-analysis of prospective studies. *Sleep, 33,* 585–592.

Chein, J., Wilmer, H., & Sherman, L. (2017). Smartphones and cognition: A review of research exploring the links between mobile technology habits and cognitive functioning. *Frontiers in Psychology, 8.*

Chen, Z., Lin, M., Chen, F., Lane, N. D., Cardone, G., Wang, R., Li, T., Chen, Y., Choudhury, T., & Campbell, A. T. (2013). Unobtrusive sleep monitoring using smartphones. 7th International Conference on Pervasive Computing Technologies for Healthcare and Workshops, pp. 145–152.

Cohen, S. (2004). Social relationships and health. *American Psychologist, 59,* 676–684.

Davey, A. (2014). Assessment of smartphone addiction in Indian adolescents: A mixed method study by systematic-review and meta-analysis approach. *International Journal of Preventive Medicine, 5,* 1500–1511.

Demasi, Aguilera, Recht. (2016). Detecting change in depressive symptoms from daily wellbeing questions, personality, and activity, IEEE Wireless Health.

Dixit, S., Shukla, H., Bhagwat, A., Bindal, A., Goyal, A., Zaidi, K. A., & Shrivastava, A. (2010). A study to evaluate mobile phone dependence among students of a medical college and associated hospital of central India. *Indian Journal of Community Medicine, 35,* 339–341.

Douglas, K. A., Collins, J. L., Warren, C., Kann, L., Gold, R., Clayton, S., Ross, J. G., & Kolbe, L. J. (1995). Results from the national college health risk behavior survey. *Journal of American College Health, 46,* 55–67.

Gowin, M., Cheney, M., Gwin, S., & Franklin Wann, T. (2015). Health and fitness app use in college students: A qualitative study. *American Journal of Health Education, 46,* 223–230.

Insel, T. R., & TR, I. (2020). Digital phenotyping: A global tool for psychiatry. *World Psychiatry: Official Journal of the World Psychiatric Association (WPA), 7,* 297–299.

PhD Dissertation. https://digital.library.unt.edu/ark:/67531/metadc103371/m2/1/high_res_d/dissertation.pdf.

Laforest, S., St-Pierre, D. M. M., Cyr, J., & Gayton, D. (1990). Effects of age and regular exercise on muscle strength and endurance. *European Journal of Applied Physiology and Occupational Physiology, 60,* 104–111.

Lane, N. D., Miluzzo, E., Lu, H., Peebles, D., Choudhury, T., & Campbell, A. T. (2010). A survey of mobile phone sensing. *IEEE Comm Mag, 48*(9), 140–150.

Lathia, N., Pejovic, V., Rachuri, K. K., Mascolo, C., Musolesi, M., & Rentfrow, P. J. (2013). Smartphones for large-scale behavior change interventions. *IEEE Pervasive Computing, 12,* 66–73.

Liang, Y., Zheng, X., & Zeng, D. D. (2019). A survey on big data-driven digital phenotyping of mental health. *Information Fusion, 52,* 290–307.

Liberman, K., Forti, L. N., Beyer, I., & Bautmans, I. (2017). The effects of exercise on muscle strength, body composition, physical functioning and the inflammatory profile of older adults. *Current Opinion in Clinical Nutrition & Metabolic Care, 20,* 30–53.

Lockley, S. W. (2018). Principles of sleep-wake regulation. Oxford University Press.

Maher, J. P., Doerksen, S. E., Elavsky, S., Hyde, A. L., Pincus, A. L., Ram, N., & Conroy, D. E. (2013). A daily analysis of physical activity and satisfaction with life in emerging adults. *Health Psychology, 32,* 647–656.

Marsch, L. A. (2021). Digital health data-driven approaches to understand human behavior. *Neuropsychopharmacology, 46*(1), 191–196.

Martinez, J., Perez, H., Escamilla, E., & Suzuki, M. M. (2012). Speaker recognition using Mel frequency Cepstral Coefficients (MFCC) and Vector quantization (VQ) techniques. 22nd International Conference on Electrical Communications and Computers, Cholula, Puebla, pp 248–251.

Mathur, A., Manasa Kalanadhabhatta, L., Majethia, R., & Kawsar, F. (2017). Moving beyond market research: Demystifying smartphone user behavior in India. *Proceedings of the ACM on Interactive, Mobile, Wearable and Ubiquitous Technologies, 1,* 1–27.

Makhoul, J., Roucos, S., & Gish, H. (1985). Vector quantization in speech coding. *Proceedings of the IEEE, 73*(11), 1551–1588.

Melcher, J., Hays, R., & Torous, J. (2020). Digital phenotyping for mental health of college students: A clinical review. *Evidence-Based Mental Health, 23*(4), 161–166

Radu, V., Katsikouli, P., Sarkar, R., & Marina, M. K. (2014). A semi-supervised learning approach for robust indoor-outdoor detection with smartphones. Proceedings of the 12th ACM Conference on Embedded Network Sensor Systems, pp. 280–294.

Raento, M., Oulasvirta, A., & Eagle, N. (2009). Smartphones: An emerging tool for social scientists. *Sociological Methods and Research, 37*, 426–454.

Rod, N. H., Vahtera, J., Westerlund, H., Kivimaki, M., Zins, M., Goldberg, M., & Lange, T. (2011). Sleep disturbances and cause-specific mortality: Results from the gazel cohort study. *American Journal of Epidemiology, 173*, 300–309.

Rod, N. H., Dissing, A. S., Clark, A., Gerds, T. A, & Lund, R. (2018). Overnight smartphone use: A new public health challenge? A novel study design based on high-resolution smartphone data. *PLOS ONE, 13*, 1–12.

Servia-Rodríguez, S., Rachuri, K. K., Mascolo, C., Rentfrow, P. J., Lathia, N., & Sandstrom, G. M. (2017). Mobile sensing at the service of mental well-being. Proceedings of the 26th International Conference on World Wide Web, ACM Press.

Statistica. (2013). Forecast of mobile phone users in India.

Subba, S., Mandelia, C., Pathak, V., Reddy, D., Goel, A., Tayal, A., Nair, S., & Nagaraj, K. (2013). Ringxiety and the mobile phone usage pattern among the students of a medical college in south India. *Journal of Clinical and Diagnostic Research, 7*, 205–209.

Subbu, K., Xu, N., & Dantu, R. (2009). iKnow Where You Are, IEEE International Conference on Computational Science and Engineering, pp. 469–474.

TCS Digital divide. http://tcs.com/digital-divide-closes-students-owning-smart-phones.

Thomée S, Härenstam, A., & Hagberg, M. (2011). Mobile phone use and stress, sleep disturbances, and symptoms of depression among young adults—a prospective cohort study. BMC Public Health.

Vaizman, Y., Ellis, K., & Lanckriet, G. (2017). Recognizing detailed human context in the wild from smartphones and smartwatches. *IEEE Pervasive Computing, 16*(4), 62–74.

Home Automation System Combining Internet-of-Things with Brain–Computer Interfacing

Sima Das and Sriparna Saha

Abstract The main aim of this chapter is to control home and healthcare appliances using two types of automation which are EEG based brain–computer interfaces and command-based using Telegram Bot. In the brain–computer interface, data are captured using EEG, and the bandpass filter is used for filtering data in the range between 12 to 100 Hz, artifact removal is done using independent component analysis, feature extraction and selection are done by Fast Fourier theorem, and then translation by command recognition. After optimizing all steps command send to the microcontroller, where the circuit is designed using ESP8266 Node MCU and Relay. Another process is to control home automation using Telegram Bot, this process is for physically fit people, they will use the Telegram Bot to control home automation at low cost. The objective of this chapter is to control home applications using EEG and BCI that could help to support old and paralyzed people to be independent in their daily life. So, this system fulfilled the expectations of home automation in two different ways that can hugely impact society in day-to-day life.

Keywords Electroencephalogram · Brain–computer interface · Machine learning · Internet-of-Things · ThingSpeak · TalkBack · Telegram Bot · Home automation

1 Introduction

In this era, the number of disabling and old people increases day by day (Dommaraju, 2017). Disability is a health problem in India (Desai et al., 2017). For different kinds of diseases like amyotrophic lateral sclerosis, brain stroke, paralysis, old people are challenged for performing mundane activities in their daily life (Transactions et al., 2003). Scientists have tried to overcome this problem of handicapped and old people in their daily routine by the latest communication technology interfacing with the human brain to facilitate a smart home system. Brain–computer interface is the technique that converts brain activity into a digital form such that it can be used to

S. Das · S. Saha (✉)
Department of Computer Science and Engineering, Maulana Abul Kalam Azad University of
Technology, West Bengal, Haringhata, India
e-mail: sahasriparna@gmail.com

© The Author(s), under exclusive license to Springer Nature Singapore Pte Ltd. 2022
S. Biswas et al. (eds.), *Internet of Things Based Smart Healthcare*, Smart Computing
and Intelligence, https://doi.org/10.1007/978-981-19-1408-9_11

read the user's mind and do the designated task without moving the body parts. An electroencephalogram is a system in which electrodes are attached to the user's scalp that receives brain signals. The brain signal fetched by the EEG acquisition system is transmitted over the Wi-Fi using the ESP8266 microcontroller. Instructions on how to handle the data received are flashed inside the memory of the microcontroller. A smart home is a technology using a network and artificial intelligence for a better quality of living. All electronic gadgets have become smart such that the entire home system can be controlled automatically. Home automation system uses a brain–computer interface, specially designed for the needy people whose body part has got damaged or paralyzed that's why they can't move from one place to another to control the various electrical equipment. The chapter depicts EEG-based smart home control techniques using IoT, machine learning, and Telegram Bot that can easily be handled by a normal as well as a paralyzed person.

The rest of the chapters are as follows. Section 2 discusses the literature survey, section 3 discusses the proposed work of the current system, section 4 discusses the conclusion and future direction, and section 5 discusses the experimental setup and the result part of the proposed work.

1.1 The Application of Smart Health Care

Smart health care consists of multiple members like a patient, doctor, hospital environments, disease diagnosis, nurse, etc. The technologies construct using IoT, smartphone, cloud computing, big data, electronics components, 5G technologies, biotechnologies, wearable devices, etc., for good and smart health care in the least time. Through the employment of these technologies, good health care will effectively scale back the price and improves the use of the potency of medical resources. Presently, in some regions, telemedicine and self-service medical aid are established. The technologies target good health care in the following 3 categories, those are: hospital or scientific analysis, telemedicine establishments, and health care at home. Nowadays using smart healthcare, medical treatments are more reliable (Tian et al., 2019). Based on the needs, the smart healthcare can be used for:

- Diagnose and treatment
- Disease preventing
- Health management
- Health monitoring
- Virtual assistant using speech recognitions
- Smart hospitals
- Smart home
- Assist for drug research

1.2 Home Automation Related to Health Care

The aged populace over the age of sixty-five is predicted to be doubled from 375 million in the year 1990 to 761 million in 2025 (Lee, Chuah, et al., 2013). Smart home-based health care technology allows the user to access home automation remotely along with health care facility (Kurti & Ph, 2014). In the healthcare system, the system can automatically predict human activities by reading their mind using EEG. EEG measures the human brain's cognitive function and as an output gives them a familiar environment. This is a hazardless technology mainly built for old age and paralyzed people which facilitate automatic home control and send messages to the nearest people if they have any health-related problem. A house or habitation with a group of network sensors and gadgets that stretch the functionality of the house by enumerating intelligence devices, manage, mechanization, discourse awareness, and practically every part remotely activate within the region, the smart healthcare occupants and helping within the delivery of aid services. Omnipresent is an associate degree progressively setting out to enter the user's electronic house in its most up-to-date type beneath the term IoT, network, sensors, and computers to make sensible home automation (Bennett et al., 2017).

1.3 Human Brain

The brain is an important part of the human and animal neurotic organization (Hagan et al., 2012), the link between brain system construction and its performance could be centralized, neuro-science research reflects the interplay of a minimum of three kinds of functions, they are: (1) physiology connectedness, (2) static and dynamic activity management, and (3) indirect connections of non-stationary topographical alignment of brain indicator (Rudrauf et al., 2014). The human brain (Fig. 1) is complex in nature that analysis structure and communicates with its function (Batista-garc & Ivette, 2018). Mostly, brain weights depend on the body height, weight, and age, but brain weights less affected by gender (Dekaban & Sadowsky, 1978). Maximum human brain is contained in different types of mosaic, but 'male' and 'female' brain is not different in nature (Joel et al., 2018).

Some parts of the human brain and its functions are explained below

1.3.1 Pons

The pons (Shao et al., 2016) or pons Varolii is a component of the brain stem, in humans and different bipeds lies inferior to the midbrain, supercilious to the medulla oblonga and former to the cerebellum. The pons Varolii is also known as the "bridge of varolius", and this region of the brain stem facilitates neural pathways by carrying olfactive signals into the thalamus. The pons varollii is within the brain stem located

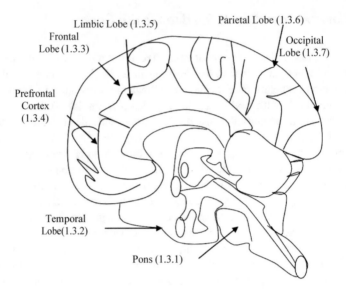

Fig. 1 Human brain

in between the midbrain and medulla and frontal of the cerebellum. A separating groove in between the pons varolii, and therefore, the medulla is the inferior pontine sulcus. The pons varolii is loosely divided into 2 parts: the basilary a part of the pons varolii, and therefore, the pontine tegmentum. Running down the midplane of the ventral surface is the basilar artery, most of the pons varolii are equipped by the pontine arteries, that emerge from the arteria. A smaller portion of the pons varolii is equipped by the anterior and posterior inferior cerebellar arteries. The pons Varolii in human measures concerning 2.5 centimetres (Storm et al., 2003).

1.3.2 Temporal Lobe

The temporal lobe (Kiernan, 2012) is one of the four major lobes of the cerebral mantle within the brain of mammals. The lobe is found below the lateral fissure on each cerebral hemisphere of the class brain, and the lobe is concerned in process sensory input into derived meaning for the acceptable retention of optical memory, terminology, and feeling association.

1.3.3 Frontal Lobe

The frontal lobe (Souza et al., 2014) is the greatest of the four major lobes of the brain in mammals, and is found at the leading of every hemisphere. The lobe is roofed by the frontal area. The frontal area includes the premotor cortex, and therefore, the primary cortical area, motor cortex.

1.3.4   Prefrontal Cortex

The prefrontal cortex (PFC) (Lara & Wallis, 2015), is the cerebral mantle that wraps the forepart of the frontal lobe. This cortex can measure personality and also the functions of the anterior cortex. This brain region has been concerned with designing complicated psychological feature behavior, temperament expression, higher cognitive process, analgesic social behavior, and analgesic sure aspects of speech and languages, the fundamental activity of this brain region is taken into account to be an interpretation of intuition and behavior in accordingly with internal intentions.

1.3.5   Limbic Lobe

The anatomical structure of the limbic lobe (Pessoa & Hof, 2500) is an associate arc-shaped region of cortex on the medial surface of every hemisphere of the class brain, consisting of components of the frontal, temporal, and parietal lobes. The term is ambiguous, with some authors together with the Para terminal body structure, the subcallosal space, the cingulate gyrus, the Para-hippocampal gyrus, the dentate gyrus, hippocampus, and subiculum, whereas the Terminologia Anatomica includes cingulate sulcus and gyrus and omits the hippocampus.

1.3.6   Parietal Lobe

The parietal lobe (Cappelletti et al., 2009) is one in each of the 4 major lobes of the cerebral cortex within the brain of mammals. The lobe is situated on the top of the temporal lobe and beside the frontal lobe and central sulcus. The lobe combined sensory data among numerous modalities, as well as special sense and navigation. The most important sensory inputs from the skin surface relay through the thalamus to the lobe.

1.3.7   Occipital Lobe

The occipital lobe is one in each of the 4 major lobes of the cerebral cortex within the brain of mammals. This lobe is the visual process centre of the class brain containing the anatomical area of the visual region.

1.4   Electrode Placement in Human Brain

German psychiatrist Hans Berger invented electroencephalogram (EEG) (Rümeysa et al., 2020). Electrodes are placed on the scalp for acquiring electrical signals from Nasion to Inion (vertically) and another one from the ear to the tip of another ear

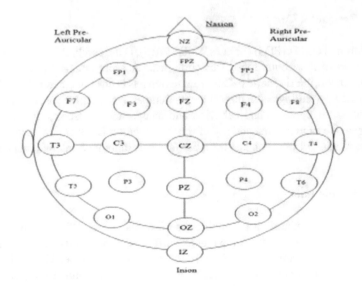

Fig. 2 Standard 10–20 electrode placement with pre-auricular setup

(horizontally) followed by a 10–20 International standards system (in Fig. 2). In the Standard 10–20 system, electrodes cover 10 or 20% distance of nearby electrodes of the front-back and left-right distances of the entire scalp. The positions of electrodes are classified into 6 main markers, they are: Parietal (P), Frontal (F), Prefrontal (PF), Temporal (T), Occipital (O), and Central (C). The placing of electrodes on the left side of the brain is of odd ranges, they are FP1, F7, T3, T5, O1, C3, F3, P3, etc. The electrodes which are placed on the right side of the brain scalp are of even ranges, they are: are FP2, F8, T4, T6, O2, C4, F4, P4, FPZ, FZ, CZ, PZ that are placed on the midline of the scalp with 10%, 20%, 20%, 10%, 10% intervals (Wan et al., 2019).

1.5 Brain–Computer Interface

Brain–computer interfaces (Fig. 3) acquire brain signals, analyze the signal, and then convert them into commands that measure to output devices that do desired actions. BCIs don't use traditional contractile organ output pathways. A BCI may be a computer-based system that obtains brain signals, examines them, and interprets them into instruction that is relayed to produce output to hold the desired action.

1.5.1 Device Setup

In brain–computer interfacing is a setup where computer is connected to the elec-troencephalogram devices. The EEG is placed on the human brain scalp. Brain signal

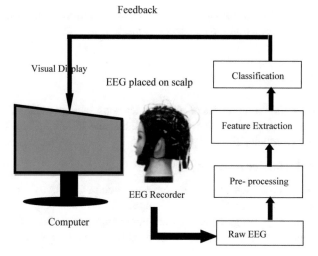

Fig. 3 Block diagram of brain–computer interface

passes as electrical signal and captured by EEG devices and stored in the computer as numerical form.

1.5.2 Dataset Collection

During data collection of EEG, electrodes were allotted on the scalp to follow the distance 10–20% international standards rule. The electrodes are placed on the scalp using conductive gel or electrode cap. The EEG dataset is stored in the computer as numeric values in excel format. The raw dataset collects and further processes to get the output.

1.5.3 Preprocessing

Preprocessing is done by two sub-methods, they are filtering and artifact removing. Filtering is the process designed for filtering high and low-pass amplifiers as user requirement. During signal acquisition, some unwanted and noisy signals are caught, this is called artifacts. Reasons for some common artifacts that occur are: when electrodes are not in specific positions, not cleaned properly, some problem with equipment's power line interference, etc. Another types of artifacts occurs for human activating during data acquisition they are: eye blinking, muscles pain, ocular artifacts, cardiac artifacts, etc. For better results, dataset is cleaned to remove any noise, which might be accumulated while capturing EEG signals.

Feature Extraction: In machine learning, feature extraction is a process that reduces the dimension of raw data to remove the unwanted dataset. In this step, vital features are selected from the input dataset that determines and contain relevant information, transformed into the reduced dataset.

1.5.4 Classification

Classification is the vital process of machine learning which predicts the class after given the dataset. In machine learning algorithms, the following types of learning techniques are (Ayodele, 2014) available:

- **Supervised machine learning**

In supervised machine learning, there have a predefined target dataset, that maps into the input dataset and give desired outputs. The name "supervised learning" came from, learning with guidance or learn under supervisor. Example of these type of learning algorithms are: Support vector machine, Linear regression and Random forest, etc.

- **Unsupervised machine learning**

In the unsupervised machine learning (Sathya & Abraham, 2013) algorithm, there is no predefined value set previously. In supervised learning, classification is done by the given set of inputs, that's why it is also called self-organization learning. Apriori and k- means clustering are examples of the unsupervised machine learning algorithm.

- **Semi-supervised machine learning**

In semi-supervised (Pulabaigari, 2018) algorithm, some datasets are labeled and the rest of the datasets are unlabeled that's why it is a combination of supervised and unsupervised techniques.

- **Reinforcement learning**

In the reinforcement technique, the rule learns a way to act after the measurement of the dataset. After observation of the environment, the technique provides a feedback that guides the procedure to predict the output.

1.5.5 Result/Output

After all steps, it's time to show the desired output. It is the last but not the least step that directly communicate with the human. The final step generates the human-understandable result according to the given input dataset.

1.6 Electroencephalogram Using Machine Learning

Electroencephalography (EEG) is an associate degree electro-physiological observation methodology to record the electrical activity of the brain. Electroencephalogram could be a complicated signal and might need many years of training to understand it properly. In recent times, machine learning (ML) has shown vast promise in serving to be of encephalogram signals, it's smart features representations from dataset. Whether or not decilitre represents benefits as correlated to a lot of ancient encephalogram process approaches.

ML algorithms build a model supported by a sample information, called "training data", based on which a model is created, this in turns help in predictions. Email filtering and vision are examples of machine learning techniques. A set of machine learning is closely associated with machine statistics, which focuses on creating predictions victimizations computers, however, not all machine learning is applied to math learning. The study of mathematical improvement delivers strategies, theory, and application domains to the sphere of machine learning. Data processing could be a connected field of study, that specializes in explorative information analysis through unattended learning. In its application across business issues, machine learning is additionally spoken of as prognostic analysis. Machine learning may be a basic idea within the field of progressive science. Over the past 20 years, this domain evolved a lot and currently been utilized wildly in several fields. In drugs, the widespread usage of machine learning has been determined in recent years.

1.7 Internet-of-Things Devices and Technologies

Internet-of-Things describe the network of physical objects—that is "things" connected with different types of sensors and technology and software for the aim of interacting and transferring information with different gadgets (devices, machines) and systems over the web. There are varieties of big issues regarding dangers within the growth of Internet-of-Things, particularly within the field of privacy and security trade. Now-a-days government begins to handle these issues as well as certain international standards are also present. IoT devices supported the enlargement of web association on the far side commonplace of the specific standard devices.

1.7.1 How Will IoT Work?

It essentially depends on 2 things to rework a standard device into IoT sensible device. They are: (a) The device that has the potential to attach to the web in any approach, (b) the device that is embedded with technology and useful software package. Some constitutional device that support internet associate and conjointly sensors. Each functions are integrated with associated IoT devices. The marketplace for IoT technology is increasing quickly day-to-day and changing into an acceptable one for a variety of users.

1.7.2 IoT Life Cycle

IoT contains a terribly straightforward lifecycle of growth. Implement followed by observation, manipulation, and services that proceeded from daily updates at the tip. In this section, we have discussed the IoT life cycle (in Fig. 4), the IoT life cycles depend on each other and the following steps are: construction, development, installation, operation, decommission, and updating or re-constructions. The steps are discussed below:

- **Construction**

Construction is the first step of Internet-of-Things life cycle. In this specific design, the implementation phase is compromised with initial softwares and hardwares.

- **Development**

In this stage, device hardware is associated with an appropriate software.

- **Installation**

The softwares are installed in the hardware and connected to the network. Starts configuring to the system components. Configures operational components, and performs bootstrapping.

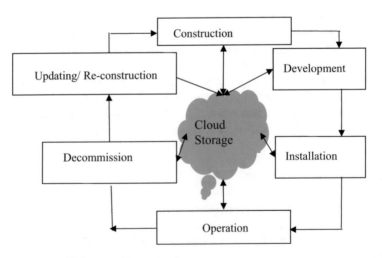

Fig. 4 Internet-of-Things life cycle

- **Operation**

In this phase, device components are connected with IoT applications. The phase is used to execute and monitor the function.

- **Decommissioning**

Decommissioning phase deals with any fault like factory reset, unwanted physical components that can be removed. The device gets disconnected from the servers, and closed down, this means the system has reached its end of life.

- **Updating/Re-construction**

When different types of problems arrive in the software, the need to update the software or re-construction is needed. Service deployment, termination, re-configuration is done in the updating phase. Re-construction is the phase where new developments are added into the system, softwares and firmwares are updated.

1.7.3 Advantages of IoT Devices

IoT encourages the interaction with different types of devices known as machine to machine communication, it provides smart automation and management, embeds with additional technical information, enables IoT devices with sturdy watching features, reduces the manual task, produces time and cost savings, gives smart automatic standard of living. The IoT devices are smart options to build and improve the quality of life.

Novelty of this system:

1. Home automation can be accessed by using Telegram Bot.
2. Home automation by using Brain–Computer Interface (BCI) will be very helpful for the old aged people and persons with disability.
3. 5v Relay, ThingSpeak cloud platform reduced the manufacturing cost and maintenance cost drastically.
4. We can control the home automation system from anywhere inside or outside of the home using Telegram Bot.
5. Overall energy consumption of the house will be reduced drastically because the user can control off and on the applications as needed.
6. Most importantly, it saves the time of the user.

1.7.4 Limitation of IoT Devices

Though there are many blessings in this area, the area has some limitations too. The limitations are: IoT devices don't have any standard compatibility, and some extremely complicated devices lead to failure. The devices could get stricken by privacy.

2 Literature Survey

The author Lee et al., used EEG non-invasive technique to the emotive panel using a mouse emulator and emokey to produce mouse click signal via 8051 microcontroller and RS232 USB cable for control smart home (Lee, Nisar, et al., 2013). Pushpa S et al. used the NeuroSky brainwave sensor to sense eye blink and brain signal that interfaces with the ARM7 processor and send the result to the relay for switching on or off the home appliances. Adams et al. used brain–computer interface-based Steady-State Visually Evoked potential, the system is designed to control the whole house through online (Adams et al., 2019). Alrajhi et al. used a brain–computer interface-based smart home system designed for people suffering from quadriplegia disease to open and close doors, cognitive and facial expressive suite detection using Emotiv, EPOC+ used for brain signal detection. Bhemjibhaih et al. used a brain–computer interface with the home application using image acquisition, calculating user viewing angle, and capturing EEG signals (Bhemjibhaih et al., 2018). In (Murthy et al., 2017), Murthy et al., designed the circuit using Raspberry Pi with IoT and Telegram Bot to control the home application with a fingertip. In (Anvekar, 2017), Anvekar et al., have used Rasberry Pi with IoT and Telegram for home automation along with a USB webcam for image capturing and it was used for home security. In (Salvi et al., 2019), Salvi et al., built a smart home assistant using google dialog flow and Telegram.

3 Proposed Work

The proposed work (in Fig. 5) is based on two types of home automation techniques: (1) Brain–computer interfaces using EEG and another is (2) Message-based Telegram Bot.

The first method of the proposed work is given in Figs. 5, 6, and 7 of the system, which is based on brain–computer interface, where the data acquisition takes place from the human scalp and converts the electrical signal to the numerical value using Brain Tech Traveler system and sends to NodeMCU and then stores it in a storage device. Filtering is done by bandpass filter; artifacts are removed using Independent component analysis, feature extraction is done by fast Fourier theorem, the signal is translated and sent to the application device control system using ThingSpeak Talk-Back App. The transmitter and receiver communicate with each other and are finally applied to the home application. The second method is based on instant messaging

Fig. 5 Home automation system using Brain–computer interface and telegram bot

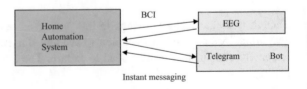

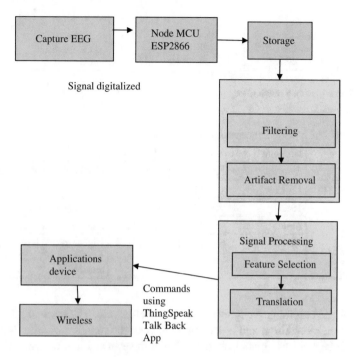

Fig. 6 Transmitter circuit for home automation system using brain–computer interface

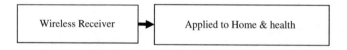

Fig. 7 Receiver circuit for home automation system using BCI

using a smartphone and Telegram Bot for two-way communication between sender and receiver.

3.1 Electrode Placement and Data Acquisition

To capture the electrical signal that occurs in the brain with every thought, the current system has used non-invasive method of electroencephalogram (EEG) device along with Brain Tech Travelers acquisition system, which converts electrical value into a numerical value. We have followed the method of 10–20 system of electrode placement on the brain. The pre-frontal cortex is situated at front of the brain in the cortex where high thought, emotions, and concentrations take place. This is why we have chosen this area for electrode placement. Electrodes are placed on the temporal lobe because it is used to recognize primary auditory perception. The frontal lobe is used

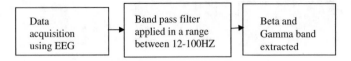

Fig. 8 Filtering using a notch filter

Table 1 Different types of frequencies and mental states

References	Different types of brainwaves and their ranges		
	frequency range (Hz)	Type of brainwave	Condition of mental states
Joel et al. (2018)	12–15	Low range beta	Relaxed, focused
	16–20	Mid-range Beta	Thinking, aware
	21–30	High range beta	Agitation, alertness
	30–100	Gamma	Higher mental activity occurs when suddenly a new situation arrived

for planning, reasoning, recognition, motor function, etc. The parietal lobe is used for sensation recognition and association between the function of other lobes. The occipital lobe receives inputs from the retina of the eye, and it is known as the visual cortex. The reference was placed for reducing environmental noise.

3.2 Preprocessing

The preprocessing is done by 2 sub-processes; they are described below:

3.2.1 Filtering

A filter is used for removing electrical noise (in Fig. 8), in this case, we are using a bandpass filter with range of 12–100 HZ (Table 1).

3.2.2 Artifact Removing

When we collect data from EEG, there are many artifacts. Artifacts (in Fig. 9) can be effective to recognize actual commands which came from the brain through an electrical signal. After removing electrical noise from the raw dataset, the next step is to clean muscles and pulse artifacts.

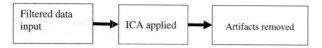

Fig. 9 Artifact removing using ICA

3.3 Signal Processing

Signal processing is done by the following steps:

3.3.1 Feature Selection

After filtering and artifact removal, the next step is feature selection (in Fig. 10). The system is based on brain–computer interface, that's why after capturing the brain signal, it's essential to understand its actual meaning. Eye blinking, emotion and state of mind, and detection range are the features that are selected during the process. Root mean square (RMS), Average power spectrum (APS) is applied for feature selection.

$$F(S) = \frac{1}{R} \sum_{x=0}^{x=R-1} f(x) \exp\left[-\frac{2\Pi Sx}{R}\right] \tag{1}$$

$$\text{Root Mean Square Feature} = \frac{\sqrt{\left(\sum_{j=1}^{R} s_j^2\right)}}{R} \tag{2}$$

here R is a row vector that indicates the Root mean square levels of the column of S in the frequency domain, and S_j is the jth component of the signal.

Fig. 10 Feature selection using FFT and Windows Hamming method

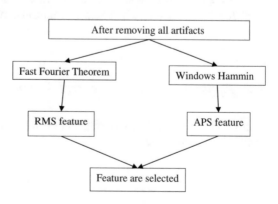

$$\text{Average Power Spectrum Feature} = 10x \log\left(\frac{W(m)}{2}\right) \tag{3}$$

where

$$W(m) = 0.54 - 0.46 \cos\left(\frac{2\Pi m}{R}\right) \tag{4}$$

here $0 \le m \le R - 1$.

$W(m)$ is the window hamming method.

3.3.2 Translate

After features are selected, the next step is to translate the signal to the command. The Brain–computer interface is trained to the user's brain. BCI technique is used for acquisition of data from the human brain and the data is interfaced by the Brain-Tech Traveler system. Programs are written in ThingSpeak Cloud Platform using MATLAB, and after processing all the steps, the signal generated is sent back to the ESP8266 Wi-Fi module using ThingSpeak TalkBack in the form of a command that is previously declared in the ThingSpeak TalkBack App in the ThingSpeak Cloud.

3.3.3 Storage and Software Used

For further processing, the data is required to be stored. We have used MATLAB software for programming. From brain sensor, 179 bytes of data will be received and this data is sent to the ThingSpeak platform's MATLAB for further processing. The eye blink, attention send to the hardware. The Arduino software deals with hardware and software communication. After processing of the data is sent to the ESP8266 NODE MCU. The control commands are transmitted and based on that home appliances are managed.

3.4 Application Device Control System

In this section, we have discussed about the different types of IoT devices and their applications in this system.

Fig. 11 ESP8266 node MCU

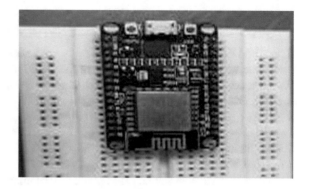

3.4.1 Node MCU ESP8266 Board with Arduino

Node MCU (as shown in Fig. 11) is low cost firmware and it is open source IoT platform runs on the ESP2866 Wi-Fi System-on-a-chip (SoC). In SoC, all circuits and components are integrated in a single chip. Microcontroller is a chip combined with a single metal-oxide-semiconductor and integrated circuit. A microcontroller can contain one or more processor cores that attached with memory and input-output devices. Microcontroller used as embedded system that automatically controls devices based on the coding stored into its memory. Node MCU ESP266 can communicate with the internet through the Wi-Fi router to which it is connected.

3.4.2 Relay

A relay (as shown in Fig. 12) is electrically operated switch that can also be operated electromechanically. Relay consists of a set of inputs and operating terminals that can be used where low power signal is required. It can be used as a signal repeater. A traditional electromagnetic relay is structured as a coil wrapped around soft iron core. In this chapter, we have used relay to automatically turn on and off the power supply of an electrical gadget depending on the signal from the microcontroller.

Fig. 12 Relay

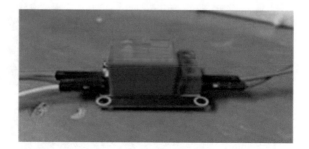

3.4.3 Telegram *Bot*

Telegram Bot is a Cloud based service, APIs can be used at free of cost. Number of hits to the server against a single Bot is limited to 30 per second. This Telegram Bot has been used in the current system to control the devices and get notification from the system.

3.4.4 ThingSpeak

ThingSpeak is an open source cloud platform that interfaces with Internet-of-Thing and API to store the data and retrieve the data using hypertext transfer protocol (HTTP) and messaging protocol via internet. ThingSpeak has support for MATLAB software that analyzes and visualizes big data without the purchase of MATLAB license. In this chapter, we have used ThingSpeak platform for reducing system cost.

3.4.5 Device Setup

Node MCU ESP8266 board with Arduino connected with relay, Telegram bot and ThingSpeak (as shown is Fig. 13). Node MCU ESP266 can communicate with the internet through the Wi-Fi router, relay is automatically turned on or off whenever needed and ThingSpeak is a opensource cloud platform that interfaces with Internet-of-Thing and API to store the data and retrieve the data using hypertext transfer protocol and Telegram Bot has been used in current system to control the devices and get notification from the system. After connection, all devices of the home and health care automation setup can be controlled by the human brain. In Fig. 14, we can see howthe EEG dataset is collected using brain–computer interface. In Fig. 15, there is a block diagram for Home and healthcare automation system that uses Internet-of-Things and Bot for intelligent home care and health care. The second method of the proposed work given in Fig. 14, which is based on instant messaging using smart phone and Telegram Bot used for two-way communication between sender and receiver.

Fig. 13 Device set up

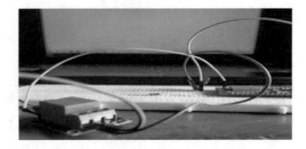

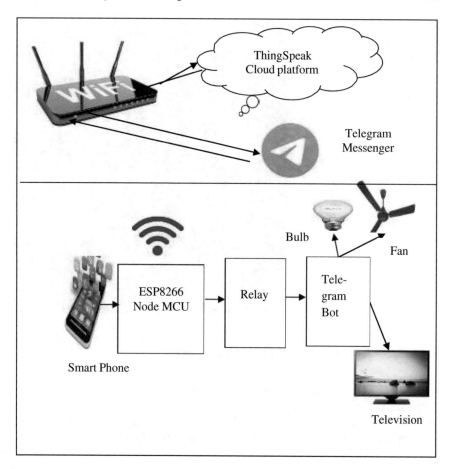

Fig. 14 Block diagram of home automation system using IoT

4 Results

4.1 Experimental Setup

The experiment is applied to 15 subjects who have different categories: (i) 5 physically fit, (ii) 5 old, and (iii) 5 physically challenged participants. For this experiment, we choose 15 mentally fit persons who participated with their wish. The participant's were seated on a comfortable chair and the 10–20 system with 21 electrodes are placed on the participant's scalp and the end Braintech Traveler (Fig. 15) is connected.

Fig. 15 Experimental set up and data acquisition using Braintech traveler system

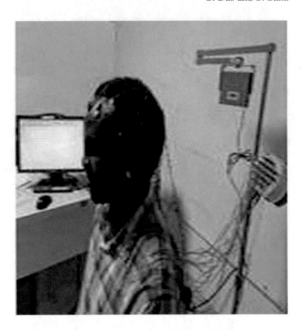

4.2 EEG Recording and Data Collection

The 10–20 system 21 electrodes are placed on the system scalp (as shown in Fig. 16). These are prefrontal (FP1-FP2), frontal (F3-F4-F7-F8), temporal (T3-T4-T5-T6), occipital (O1-O2), parietal (P3-P4), reference electrodes (A1-A2), primary motor cortex (C3-C4), ground or common reference points (FZ, CZ, PZ) (Tables 2 and 3).

Fig. 16. 10–20 system of 21 electrodes placement

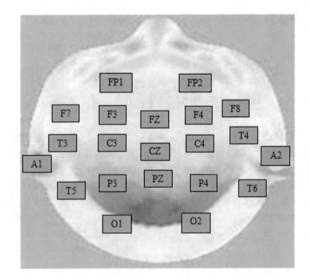

Table 2 Home automation system using EEG and BCI

Task	Home automation system using brain–computer interface	
	brain–computer interfaces	Device
Light is on using brain–computer interface		
light is off using brain–computer interface		

In this experiment, we have chosen 15 participants from different categories as shown in Table 4. Here Subject-1, Subject-2, Subject-3, Subject-4, Subject-5 are physical challenged people, Subject-6, Subject-7, Subject-8, Subject-9, Subject-10 are the old aged people and the last category, Subject-11, Subject-12, Subject-13, Subject-14, Subject15 are physically fit people. It is interesting to compare and analyse the performance of different categories of people. The experiment is done 5 times on each people for different kind of home automation and observed that the mean accuracy is above 80%, that ensures the systems, applicability for a large group of people.

Table 3 Home automation system using telegram BOT

Task	Home automation system using brain–computer interface	
	Instant messaging	Device
Light is on using Telegram bot		
Light is off using Telegram bot		

5 Conclusion and Future Direction

The main goal of this chapter is to enroot and achieve home automation system in healthcare. The proposed system is designed in two-way—in first procedure, home and healthcare automation are done by EEG with brain–computer interface and the second one is developed using message based home automation that is done by Telegram Bot. The noninvasive BCI techniques are used to control home and health automation system using EEG-based brain signals. The electrodes are allotted on the cranium. The system is trained and tested by participants. This system controls physical devices through brain signal, and this can help the paralyzed or physically disabled. Through this device, the elderly people can independently do their work

Table 4 Performance analysis using BPNN

Category	Success rate of the 15 subjects		
	Subjects	Old aged (%)	Average (%)
Physically challenged	Subject-1	78.26	80.9
	Subject-2	80.3	
	Subject-3	79.6	
	Subject-4	81.5	
	Subject-5	85.3	
Old aged people	Subject-6	78	80.1
	Subject-7	81.2	
	Subject-8	80.3	
	Subject-9	82	
	Subject-10	79.3	
Physically fit	Subject-11	85.6	80.9
	Subject-12	82.6	
	Subject-13	76.9	
	Subject-14	78.5	
	Subject-15	81.2	
Average mean for all subjects			80.6

on their own. Another method is by Telegram Bot used for physically fit people to control entire home at low cost. The entire system is centrally operated by the bot technology using IoT and Node MCU. This system is implemented using IoT to automate the control of whole house using a finger.

In future, we want to integrate speech recognition system for better user operability and add home security feature.

Acknowledgements The work is funded by the university for providing research seed money, (File No.: 9.6/Regis./SD/Mn.(SS)/2019 dated 19.06.2019) and UGC Start-up Grant under the scheme of Basic Scientific Research (File No. F.30-449/2018(BSR) dated 21.11.2019). The work is approved by Institutional Ethics Committee, Ref. No.: MAKAUT:IEC-(18-19)/03.

References

Adams, M. et al. (2019). Towards an SSVEP-BCI controlled Smart Home, vol. 0, pp. 2737– 2742.
Anvekar, R. G. (2020). IoT application development: Home security system, no. Tiar 2017.
Ayodele, T. O. (2014). Types of machine learning algorithms, no. August.
Batista-garc, K., & Ivette, C. (2018). Behavioral sciences what we know about the brain structure— Function relationship.
Bennett, J., Rokas, O., & Chen, L. (2017). Healthcare in the smart home: A study of past, present and future, pp. 1–23.

Bhemjibhaih, D. P., Sanjay, G. D., Sreejith, V., & Prakash, B. (2018). Brain-computer interface based home automation system for paralysed people. In *2018 IEEE Recent Advances Intelligent Computational Systems*, pp. 230–233.

Cappelletti, M., Lee, H. L., Freeman, E. D., & Price, C. J. (2009). The role of right and left parietal lobes in the conceptual processing of numbers, pp. 331–346.

Dekaban, A. S., & Sadowsky, D. (1978). Changes in brain weights during the span of human life: Relation of brain weights to body heights and body weights.

Desai, S., Mantha, S. S., & Phalle, V. M. (2017). Advances in smart wheelchair technology.

Dommaraju, P. (2017). Perspectives on old age in India, no. November, pp. 0–21.

Hagan, C. E., Bolon, B., & Keene, C. D. (2012). *20. Nervous System*, First Edition. Elsevier Inc.

Joel, D. et al. (2018). Analysis of human brain structure reveals that the brain 'Types' typical of males are also typical of females, and vice versa, vol. 12, no. October, pp. 1–18.

Kiernan, J. A. (2012). Anatomy of the temporal lobe, vol. 2012.

Kurti, J., & Ph, D. (2014). Health care in home automation systems with speech recognition and mobile technology, no. 05, pp. 262–265.

Lara, A. H., & Wallis, J. D. (2015). The role of prefrontal cortex in working memory: A mini review, vol. 9, no. December, pp. 1–7.

Lee, J., Chuah, Y., & Chieng, K. T. H. (2013a). Smart elderly home monitoring system with an android phone, vol. 7, no. 3, pp. 17–32.

Lee, W. T., Nisar, H., Malik, A. S., Yeap, K. H., & Ieee, S. M. (2013b). A brain computer interface for smart home control, pp. 35–36.

Lv, S. et al., Uhylhz vflhqwlilf sdshu, vol. 29.

Murthy, P. N. V. S. N., Rao, S. T., & Rao, G. M. (2017). Home automation using telegram, vol. 6, no. 6, pp. 64–69.

Ouchi, H. (2019). Transductive learning of neural language models for syntactic and semantic analysis, pp. 3665–3671.

Pessoa, L., & Hof, P. R. (2015). From Paul Broca ' s Great limbic lobe to the limbic system, vol. 2500, pp. 2495–2500.

Pulabaigari, V. (2018). Semi-supervised learning: A brief review," no. July.

Rudrauf, D., Benali, H., & Marrelec, G. (2014). Relating structure and function in the human brain: Relative contributions of anatomy, stationary dynamics, and non- stationarities, vol. 10, no. 3.

Rümeysa, İ., Seda, S., & Sevmez, F. (2020). The inventor of electroencephalography (EEG): Hans.

Salvi, S., Geetha, V., & Jamura, S. K. S. (2019). A conversational smart home assistant built on telegram and google dialogflow. In *TENCON 2019—2019 IEEE Region 10 Conference*, pp. 1564–1571.

Sathya, R., & Abraham, A. (2013). Comparison of supervised and unsupervised learning algorithms for pattern classification, vol. 2, no. 2, pp. 1–38.

Shao, R., Keuper, K., Geng, X., & Lee, T. M. C. (2016). EBioMedicine pons to posterior cingulate functional projections predict affective processing changes in the elderly following eight weeks of meditation training. *EBIOM, 10*, 236–248.

de Souza, L. C. et al. (2014). Frontal lobe neurology and the creative mind Article type: Received on: Accepted on: Citation: Frontal lobe neurology and the creative mind 1. Neuropsychiatric Branch, Neurology Division, University Hospital, Universidade Federal de Minas Gerais, Belo Horizonte, MG, Brazil Corresponding author: ICM research center.

Storm, P. B., Ph, D., Johnson, R. M., & Ph, D., et al. (2003). A surgical technique for safely placing a drug delivery catheter into the pons of primates, vol. 52, no. 5, pp. 1169–1177.

Tian, S., et al. (2019). Smart healthcare: Making medical care more intelligent. *Global Health Journal, 3*(3), 62–65.

Transactions, I., Neural, O. N., & Engineering, R. (2003). Guest editorial brain—Computer interface technology: A review of the second international meeting, vol. 11, no. 2, pp. 94–109.

Wan, X. I. N., Zhang, K., Ramkumar, S., & Deny, J. (2019). A Review on electroencephalogram based brain computer interface for elderly disabled. *IEEE Access, 7*, 36380–36387.

Social Sensing Applications for Public Health

"Montaj": A Gaming System for Assessing Cognitive Skills in a Mobile Computing Platform

Saikat Basu, Sudipta Saha, Sourav Das, Rajlaksmi Guha, Jayanta Mukherjee, and Manjunatha Mahadevappa

Abstract Attention is an integral part of human beings. Attention deficit occurs mostly in young adult populations. We have developed a game-based software named 'Montaj' for the measurement of cognitive skills like attention, working memory, etc. The software has also a unique feature to add a new apk into the main module. Independent studies can be conducted using this software. In different studies, a set of suitable games for assessing cognitive skills, etc. are created under a defined framework that could be included. In these studies, diverse populations can be addressed. An active study can be suspended, reactivated, or permanently closed. In its base

S. Basu (✉) · M. Mahadevappa
School of Medical Science and Technology, Indian Institute of Technology Kharagpur,
Kharagpur 721302, West Bengal, India
e-mail: saikat.basu@smst.iitkgp.ac.in

M. Mahadevappa
e-mail: mmaha2@smst.iitkgp.ac.in

S. Basu
Department of Computer Science and Engineering, Maulana Abul Kalam Azad University
of Technology, Kolkata 700064, West Bengal, India
e-mail: saikat.basu@makautwb.ac.in

S. Saha
Department of Information Technology, Maulana Abul Kalam Azad University of Technology,
Kolkata 700064, West Bengal, India
e-mail: sudipta.30.saha@gmail.com

S. Das
Department of Industrial Engineering and Management, Maulana Abul Kalam Azad University
of Technology, Kolkata 700064, West Bengal, India
e-mail: sou.das123@gmail.com

R. Guha
Centre for Education Technology,Indian Institute of Technology Kharagpur, Kharagpur 721302,
West Bengal, India
e-mail: rajg@cet.iitkgp.ac.in

J. Mukherjee
Department of Computer Science and Engineering, Indian Institute of Technology Kharagpur,
Kharagpur 721302, West Bengal, India
e-mail: jay@cse.iitkgp.ac.in

feature, the system hosts four games that are internally added to measure attention. Another external game is considered to demonstrate the feature of the flexibility of supporting any new game designed and implemented under the given framework specified in the system. Its integration with this platform is also discussed. The main focus of the software is the young adult population. It is challenging to engage young adult populations in studies, so proper gamification is done to create interest among them. Android platform is used for development as Android is the most popular operating system in mobile platforms.

Keywords Attention · Working memory · Cognition · Gamification · Android games · Dynamic environment

1 Introduction

Cognitive control covers a wide range of cognitive processes that are necessary to achieve a chosen goal (Chan et al., 2008). Cognitive controls and executive functions include but not limited to cognitive processes such as attention control, cognitive inhibition, working memory capacity, planning ability, fluid intelligence, and cognitive flexibility (Chan et al., 2008; Diamond, 2013), etc. The meaning of attention control is paying attention to relevant things while overcoming distractions. Cognitive inhibition is an ability to control natural or habitual behaviors by overriding strong internal bias or external allure. Working Memory (WM) is responsible for holding easily accessible information required for guidance on the action. Fluid intelligence is required for reasoning and new problem-solving. Cognitive flexibility denotes the ability to switch between different concepts. These cognitive processes are responsible for the variation of general intellectual ability among humans (Baddeley and Hitch, 1974). Several already existing studies tried to find correlation between the efficiency of two or three cognitive processes at a time with academic success, and they found a positive correlation between them Lan et al. (2011); McClelland et al. (2007).

Authors in Szalma et al. (2018, 2014) measured sustained attention (the ability to monitor specific targets over a prolonged period) by a vigilance task, and in Grunebaum et al. (1974); Kupietz and Richardson (1978) by a Continuous Performance Task (CPT). Cancellation Task (CT) was used to measure visual neglect severity in Rorden and Karnath (2010). Authors use the Stroop task in De Giglio et al. (2015) for measuring sustained attention, response inhibition, ability to filter target information, and in Zhang and Goh (2018) for measuring sustained selective attention. Researchers in Nouchi et al. (2013) also used the Stroop task to measure executive functions like response inhibition and impulsivity. The operation span task uses a list of stimuli, where each stimulus contains a pair of mathematical operations and a subsequent unrelated word. Participants need to recall words in previous order on completion of the entire list of the stimulus. Authors of Unsworth et al. (2004); Hutchison (2007) varied length of the operation-word list from two to five or six items and the sum of recalled words of the correctly recalled sets were assigned as working memory span score of participants.

In this work, a system for assessing cognitive skills using computer games developed for testing the executive functions of young-adult students. Here, as a base feature, four games were developed that implement different tasks to test various cognitive controls. However, it has the flexibility of integrating new gaming modules for assessing different kinds of cognitive skills. It was motivated by the fact that Gamification can improve users' experience and engagement in non-game applications(Deterding et al., 2011b). Gamification is the usage of game design elements in non-game contexts, emphasizing rule-based and goal-oriented playing (Deterding et al., 2011a). A few examples of game design elements are point, badge, leaderboard, levels, progress bar (Deterding et al., 2011a). Gamification of tasks was done by current score displays, emojis, progress bars, music, transient green-correct marks, and red-wrong marks. Games consist of levels, but there is no concept minimum score requirement to the next higher level from a lower level. Time constraints on the representation of stimuli are present in some cases. Time constraints are absent for user response as it was required to measure and analyze users' reaction time. In the implementation, an Android platform was used to develop the games.

The name of the system developed is 'Montaj.' The name 'Montaj' is a conglomeration of two Bengali words, namely 'Mon' means mind, and 'Taja' means fresh. By playing the games, it was tried to measure different psychological parameters of mind. Names of five games are Test Your Brain (TYB) Game, Card Game, Chess Objects Game, Stroop Game, and NBack game. The system has the flexibility of supporting a new set of games adhering to the framework specified. The first four games were developed as internal parts of 'Montaj,' whereas the NBack game was developed as an external game application to demonstrate its flexibility to support integration with the base module.

In all games, skills related to attention and working memory are focused. Since the Stroop task is a well-recognized measure of cognitive control (Miyake et al., 2000), the Stroop task was implemented in the fourth game with the name Stroop Game to verify whether the experimentation with this task corroborates with existing facts about this test. Software testing was incorporated to remove the bugs. A new version of the software was built to make the platform robust. An additional purpose of these studies is to collect and analyze user feedback on different game characteristics for the sake of future improvement of the games. In the future, we will try to find a composite score of the participants with the help of the Analytic Hierarchy Process (AHP) and the Technique for Order of Preference by Similarity to Ideal Solution (TOPSIS).

This paper is organized in the following way: Sect. 2 presents the detailed design and development. Detailed internal games and the cognitive tasks implemented in these games are also discussed in this section. Section 3 highlights the testing and validation section briefly. Section 4 consists of some novel features of the system 'Montaj' and its four internal games. Section 5 includes usability analysis depending on feedbacks. Comprehensive concluding remarks are presented in Sect. 6.

2 Design and Development

A game-based software named 'Montaj' was developed for measuring cognitive skills. Figure 1 depicts the major modules of 'Montaj'. Brief descriptions of the main functionalities implemented by these modules are shown in Table 1.

2.1 Device Compatibility and System Installation

The software application has complied with compileSdkVersion = 25 (compiler uses API level 25). It uses Android SDK version 7.1, which uses API level 25, and whose code-name is Nougat. This software has minSdkVersion = 15, which means the software cannot be installed on a device with an API Level is lower than 15 or SDK version lower than 4.0.3 (Ice Cream Sandwich).

2.2 Life Cycle of a Study

Every action in 'Montaj' has to be conducted under a distinct/ independent study. Every study needs to be created by a set of games and a period of its conduction. 'Montaj' can be used for conducting multiple studies with the same or different group of participants; a list of participants may overlap in studies. The administrator

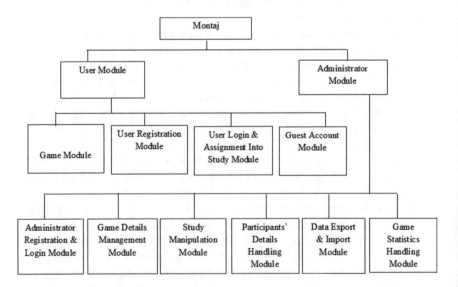

Fig. 1 Major modules of 'Montaj'

Table 1 Functionalities implemented in major modules of 'Montaj'

Modules	Functionalities
Game module	Contains core logic and scoring method of games
User registration module	Accepts personal details including email-id, password from user and save into database
User login and assignment into study module	i. Ask administrator to select an active study for assigning user ii. Ask user to provide registered email-id and password
Guest account module	Lists all the available games (internal as well as external games) for guest playing
Administrator registration and login module	Provide facility for new administrator registration and existing administrator login
Game details management module	Provide facilities for i. New game registration ii. Game details modification iii. Detailed listing existing games iv. Deleting selected games v. Deleting all games at once
Study manipulation module	Provide facilities for i. New study creation ii. Study end date extension iii. Incorporating games under studies iv. Altering list of included games into studies v. Changing study status vi. Deleting selected studies
Participants' details handling module	Listing participants' details and deleting selected participants
Data export and Import module	Providing facilities for i. Exporting complete database from a device ii. Importing total database into a device
Game statistics handling module	Provide different search options to administrator and to export the selected data into .csv format

needs to specify a name, a creation date, a start date, and a finish date at the time of study creation. During the study's creation, a study is associated with a list of 'Games' available in the system. Any registered user can join a study. A study can be in the state of 'active,' 'suspended,' or 'completed.' Participants can be assigned to a study only if the study is in an 'active' state. A study may be resumed from its 'suspended' state to 'active.' The administrator can change the status of an 'active' study to 'suspended,' or he forcefully makes the study 'completed' if necessary. Completed studies are not permitted to make them 'active' directly. A study automatically 'completed' if the current date exceeds the study finish date. The administrator can extend the study end date if necessary. Extension of finish date beyond the current date, make 'completed' study 'active' again. Any study deletion implicitly deletes all game performance data

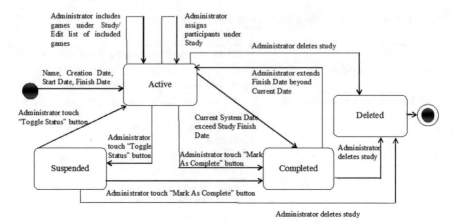

Fig. 2 Life cycle of a study

under that particular study. In Fig. 2, a state transition diagram depicts the life cycle of a study. 'Montaj' has a concept of the guest account, from which any user can play games available games of 'Montaj' any number of times. Registered users can play games at most once as a part of a single study.

2.3 Use Cases Diagram

Three types of actors of the software 'Montaj' are Guest, Registered User, and Administrator. A use case diagram of 'Montaj' is shown in Fig. 3. Table 2 lists important use cases, associated actors, and a brief description of functionalities provided by those use cases.

2.4 Data Flow Diagram (DFD)

Data Flow Diagram is a graphical tool. It represents a system in terms of the input, various processing, and the output generated by the system. Different levels of DFDs of software 'Montaj' are shown in the Figs. 4, 5 and 6. Figure 4 shows the context diagram of software 'Montaj'. While Fig. 5 represents level 1 DFD for Registered users and guests of software. Figure 6 depicts level 1 DFD for Administrator of this software. Here Yourdon approach is followed throughout the work.

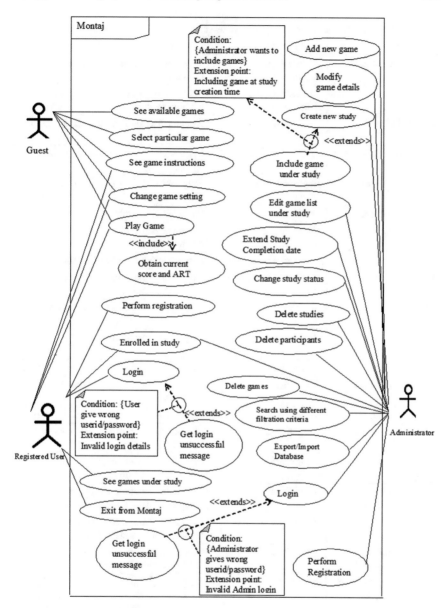

Fig. 3 Use case diagram of software 'Montaj'

Table 2 Brief descriptions brief descriptions of use cases and associated actors

Use case	Associated actors	Functionalities provided
Perform registration	Registered User, Administrator	Help new user or new administrator to get registered
Login	Registered User, Administrator	Verify login id and password of user or administrator
Enrolled in study	Registered User, Administrator	Assign a user into an active study selected by administrator
See games under study	Registered User	Display all games included in the study one by one
Exit from 'Montaj'	Registered User	Help user to exit from system on successful completion of all games included in study
See available games	Guest	Show list of available games to guests
Select particular game	Guest	Accept selection of one game form guest and load that game
See game instructions	Registered User, Guest	Show detailed level specific instructions
Change game setting	Registered User, Guest	Help user to manipulate sound setting and play session time
Play game	Registered User, Guest	Display stimulus and accept response from users
Obtain current score and ART	Registered User, Guest	Display updated score and ART
Add new game	Administrator	Help administrator to register new games
Modify game details	Administrator	Provide facilities for game details modification
Create new study	Administrator	Help administrator to create new studies
Include game under study	Administrator	Help administrator to include games under studies
Edit game list under study	Administrator	Provide facility to alter the list of included games under a study
Extend study completion date	Administrator	Give administrator option to extend study completion date if necessary
Change study status	Administrator	Help administrator to change study status between active and suspended
Delete studies/ participants/games	Administrator	Provide studies'/participants'/games' deletion facility to administrator
Search using different filtration criteria	Administrator	Help administrator to search data based on different criteria for display and help them to export selected data into .csv format
Export/import database	Administrator	Help administrator to export/import database from/to a device

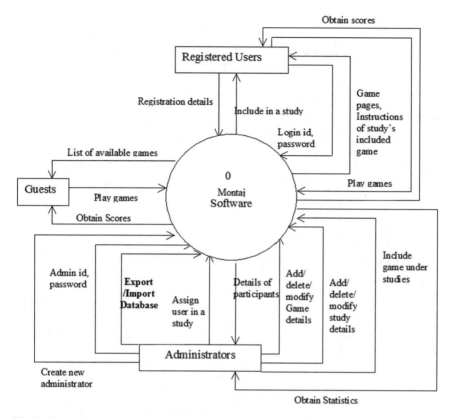

Fig. 4 Context diagram or zero level DFD of software 'Montaj'

2.5 Entity Relationship (ER) Diagram

The entity-relationship model is a conceptual data model. It assumes a real-world that consists of a collection of basic objects- called entities and relationships among these objects. Figure 7 represents Entity-Relationship diagram of 'Montaj'. ADMINISTRATORS schema contains administrators' login details. STUDIES table holds the name, start date, creation date, and end date of individual studies. Participants logging details, personal details, and their academic data are stored in PARTICIPANTS schema. GAMES schema contains unique game id, game name, description details of games, unique score saving table name, game location, etc. Every score table, like TYB SCORES, CARD SCORES, etc. hold the score and ART data of participants under different studies. pid, StudyName is the composite primary key for all score tables. For all scores table, GameComplete and LevelComplete fields exist to indicate playing status (not played, partially completed, completed) of particular game participants under a particular study. TYB HIGHEST field exists only for TYB Game to fetch the highest performance data of any specific level. PAR-

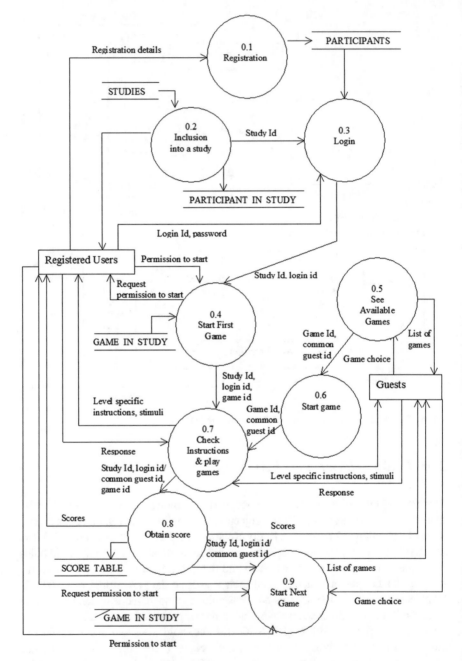

Fig. 5 Level 1 DFD for registered users and guests of software 'Montaj'

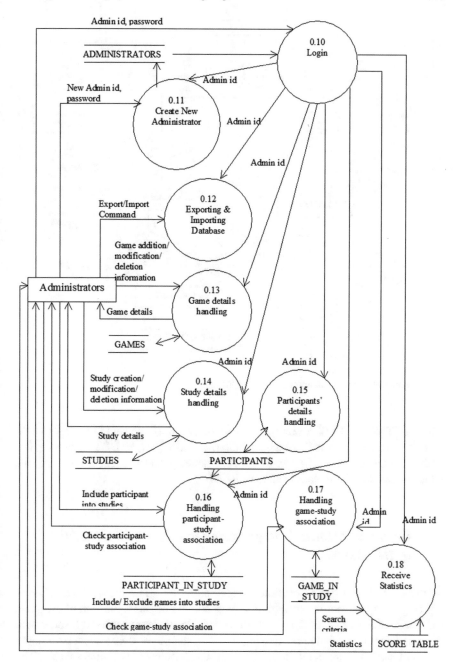

Fig. 6 Level 1 DFD for administrator of software 'Montaj'

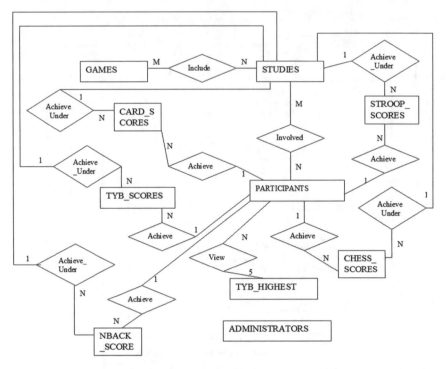

Fig. 7 Entity relationship diagram of software 'Montaj'

TICIPANT_IN_STUDY schema exists with pid, StudyName composite key to hold association of players with studies. Similarly, GAME_IN_STUDY schema exists with pid, gameid composite key to indicate games included under a study. All the tables in the 'Montaj' database achieve BCNF.

2.6 Games in 'Montaj': Registration and Removal-Flexibility of the System

At the time of new game insertion or registration, the game name, the number of levels, game type, scoring method, first-page address of game, location of the game (internal/external), and a unique name of score saving table are needed to be provided. A game becomes available for playing in this system only after a successful registration. Game is represented in the 'Montaj' database using GAMES schema. The Score saving table is automatically generated in the background with the administrator's provided name at the time of game registration. The administrator can modify the game type, scoring method, first-page address, location of a game. One or more games can be removed from the system at a time. Game deletion neither deletes actual game pages in case of internal games nor deletes any external games' .apk file. It only deletes particular game entries from the database. As a result, those specific games become unavailable to users. Any game deletion also implicitly deletes the corresponding score table from the database.

2.7 Games Made Available with the System

Score (in integer) and Average Response Time (ART) of participants are primarily the interest of measure in all games. For all games, every trial reflects updated score. Only the first game has a negative score for the wrong answer. Four games implemented in the system are briefly discussed below. Figure 8 depicts screen of available games with 'Montaj'.

2.7.1 Test Your Brain Game

This game has five levels. Each level of this game has different matching criteria. A participant has to touch "Green Tick Button" if the criteria match, and the participant has to touch "Red Cross Button" otherwise. TYB Game details are shown in Table 3. Dividing total playing time by the number of touches (i.e., no of correct/wrong responses), we calculate ART. Level 1 of the TYB Game implements a

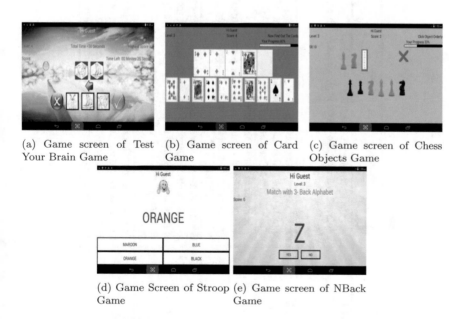

(a) Game screen of Test Your Brain Game

(b) Game screen of Card Game

(c) Game screen of Chess Objects Game

(d) Game Screen of Stroop Game

(e) Game screen of NBack Game

Fig. 8 Pictures of the platform

Table 3 TYB game details

Level	Level specified tasks	Cognitive task implemented	Time constraint	Scoring pattern
Level 1	Participants to touch "Green Tick", if 1 animal displayed in the middle screen is present out of three, else "Red Cross"	Cancellation task (CT)	Four available timing options 30, 60, 90 s or 120 s	+1 for correct response −1 for wrong response No upper or lower limits of scores
Level 2	Participants to touch "Green Tick", if both of two animals displayed in middle screen are present out of three else "Red Cross Button"	Unordered pair cancellation task		
Level 3	Participants to touch "Green Tick", if both of two animals displayed in middle screen are present out of three animals shown at the bottom screen at same order else "Red Cross"	Pair cancellation task		
Level 4	One has to touch "Green Tick Button", if both of two animals displayed in middle screen are present in set of three animals shown at the bottom of the screen at opposite order else "Red Cross Button" else "Red Cross"	Pair cancellation task		
Level 5	One has to touch "Green Tick Button", if both of two animals displayed in middle screen are present in set of three animals shown at the bottom screen at order directed by the violet arrow else "Red Cross Button"	Pair cancellation task		

cancellation task (CT), which is a strong predictor of visual neglect. Paper pencil form of CT requires marking only target items while ignoring nontargets from the randomly mixed items (Rorden and Karnath, 2010). Level 2 of TYB Game implements an unordered pair cancellation task while level 3 to level 5 of the TYB game implement Pair Cancellation task (McGrew et al., 2007). In pair Cancellation tasks, participants needed to mark out ordered ball-dog pairs from mixed pictures of dogs, balls, and cups (McGrew et al., 2007). Pair cancellation task measures the ability to control interference and processing speed in terms of attention and concentration (Schrank et al., 2016). Level 5 of TYB also implements divided attention tasks (Corbetta et al., 1991) as in level 5 of the TYB Game, as the participant needs to pay attention to requisite order along with identifying the correct pair of animals. TYB Game implements CPT also, as there are no options of leaving this game without completing up to 5th level and no options to jumping upper levels without completing low levels. For the entire duration, participants have to hold attention. The CPT examines human vigilance or sustained attention over continued periods of time (Corkum and Siegel, 1993; Klee and Garfinkel, 1983). Overall, TYB Game determines participants' visual neglect, sustained attention or vigilance, divided attention, impulsivity, concentration, and ability to control interference.

2.7.2 Card Game

This game has four levels. Five different cards with different numbers will be displayed for 10 s at the upper portion of the screen, and then they will disappear. An array of ten cards that must also contain five previously displayed cards will appear at the lower portion of the screen. A participant has to touch correct, i.e., previously shown five cards among ten cards in any order. A participant only gets five chances to select the cards correctly. By dividing the total time of five touches by five, we get ART. Details of Card Game are shown in the Table 4. Card Game implements a free recall task (Glanzer and Cunitz, 1966) as the order of recalling is unimportant. Since memory span depends on remembering only items without any order (Baddeley and Hitch, 1974), the free recall task measures memory span, and consequently, Card Game implements a span Task to measure memory span. Any span tasks have already proved reliable as well as valid measures of Working Memory Capacity (WMC) (Conway et al., 2005), and we expect WMC can be measured by Card Game. In simple span tasks, participants only need to remember previously displayed/heard items serially, and it can measure short term memory capacity (Unsworth and Engle, 2007). In complex span tasks, participants are assigned a memory task along with some processing activity, and it can measure WMC (Unsworth and Engle, 2007). An important characteristic of the processing component of WM span tasks is that it creates interference with rehearsal (Conway et al., 2005). Task difficulty of Card Game is increased with the increasing level number, as a participant has to remember card numbers along with increasing card type and card type interferes in the task rehearsal

Table 4 Card game details

Level	Level specified tasks	Cognitive task implemented	Time constraint	Scoring pattern
Level 1	Participants to remember 5 different cards of only one suit for later identification	Free recall task	• Initially 5 cards displayed for 10 s • No time constraints for later response	• +1 for correct identification of cards and 0 for wrong identification • Maximum score 5, minimum score 0
Level 2	Participants to remember 5 different cards of at most two suits for later identification			
Level 3	Participants to remember 5 different cards of at most three suits for later identification			
Level 4	Participants to remember 5 different cards of at most four suits for later identification			

of card number. We can say that Card Game actually turns from simple span task to complex span task with increasing game level. Overall, Card Game measures the free recall span of WM.

2.7.3   Chess Objects Game

This game has four levels. Six chess objects will be displayed in random order for 10 s at the upper portion of the screen, and then they will disappear. An array of the same six chess objects will appear again at the lower portion of the screen but in a different order. A participant has to touch the chess objects in the same or opposite order of the initial display. A participant only gets six chances to select chess objects in order. For a particular position, only one try is acceptable. After a wrong attempt for a particular position, participants should try for next position. Chess Objects Game details are shown in the Table 5. By dividing the total time of six touches by six, we get ART. Chess Objects Game implements serial-recall task (Thomas et al., 2003), as participants have to recall and touch chess objects in the same order or reverse order of initial presentation. In level 1 and level 3, chess objects implement forward recall task (Thomas et al., 2003) as chess objects need to be remembered and touched the

Table 5 Chess objects game details

Level	Level specified tasks	Cognitive task implemented	Time constraint	Scoring pattern
Level 1	Participants to remember order(same) of 6 different Chess objects of one colour	Forward Recall task	• Initially chess objects displayed for 10 s • No time constraints for later response	• +1 for correct in requisite order and 0 for wrong • Maximum score 6, minimum score 0
Level 2	Participants to remember opposite order of 6 different Chess objects of one colour	Backward recall task		
Level 3	Participants to remember order of 6 different Chess objects of mixed colour	Forward recall task		
Level 4	Participants to remember opposite order of 6 different Chess objects of mixed colour	Backward recall task		

same order of their initial presentation. While in level 2 and level 4, chess objects implement backward recall task (Thomas et al., 2003), as chess objects need to be remembered and touched opposite order of their initial presentation. So some form of processing, transformation, working memory update (Morris and Jones, 1990) is needed in level 2 and level 4 in addition to the required skill for level 1 and level 3 of the game. Since memory span depends on remembering items in order (Baddeley and Hitch, 1974), forward and backward recall task measure memory span. As a span task is a reliable measure of WMC (Conway et al., 2005), we expect Chess Objects Game can measure WMC. In Schofield and Ashman (1986), authors found that forward span task measures of sequential processing and backward-span tasks are closely related to planning and sequential processing. Level 1 and level 2 of Chess Objects Game implement simple span tasks as participants need to remember chess objects of only one color. Level 3 and level 4 of the game implement complex span tasks as chess objects of two colors are mixed, and color creates interference in chess objects' rehearsal task. With increasing level Chess Objects, Game actually turns from simple span task to complex span task. Overall, Chess Objects game measures forward and backward span of WM, planning ability, sequential processing ability, and ability to perform the cognitive transformation.

Table 6 Stroop game details

Level	Level specified tasks	Cognitive task implemented	Time constraint	Scoring pattern
Level 1	• Participants given a colour-word in either same/different colour • Participants to response with ink colour of colour-word • Participants to touch one button out of four buttons, labelled with four different colour names	Stroop task	No time constraints	• +1 for correct identification of ink colour and 0 for wrong identification • Maximum score 20, minimum score 0

2.7.4 Stroop Game

This game has only one level, consisting of 20 trials. Stroop Game details are shown in the Table 6. By dividing the total response time of twenty trials by twenty, we get ART. Our Stroop Game implements the Stroop task. Stroop task is one of the most commonly used measures of cognitive control (Miyake et al., 2000). Human has a natural habit of pronouncing a written word instead of saying ink colors of its printing. Still, the Stroop task expects from participants the name ink color of a word when the word itself is the name of another color (Stroop, 1935). This response is slower and more error-prone, and this is called the Stroop effect. Stroop task test inhibitory control (West and Alain, 2000) of a person by asking him/her to identify the color of a color-word by avoiding their natural habit to respond with the lexical meaning of the word (Prasad, 2014). In the Stroop task, a word stimulus creates interference in the task of responding with a color stimulus (Stroop, 1935). In our Stroop Game, we first four trials are congruent, and the last 16 trials are incongruent. In the congruent stimulus, the color-word, and its ink color are the same color; in an incongruent stimulus, the color-word and its ink color are different colors (van Maanen et al., 2009). Stroop task measures executive functions including impulsivity control and response inhibition (Nouchi et al., 2013), selective attention (Lamers et al., 2010) and divided attention (Lowe and Mitterer, 1982). Overall our Stroop Game measures interference resolution ability, selective attention, divided attention, response inhibition.

2.8 Built in Search Facilities of 'Montaj'

A number of search options to get the data about a group of participants are present in this system. Gender wise search, age range wise search, combined age range, and gender-wise search, selected game-wise search, and selected participants wise search facilities are some of the examples.

2.9   Provision for Importing New Games

2.9.1   Assumptions and Constraints of Adding a Game

The basic assumption of importing a new game in the 'Montaj' environment is that the game should be in .apk format. Two constraints of importing new games are listed below:

– New game should have a minimum of 1 level and a maximum of 10 levels
– For each level, only score and ART as players' performance can be saved into the database of 'Montaj.' If ART is irrelevant, then 0.0 can be saved for ART fields in all levels of the game.

2.9.2   Schema Used for Game Addition into 'Montaj'

The game registration process inserts a row in the GAMES schema, and from that moment, a new game becomes a part of 'Montaj' and available for inclusion to any study or from the guest account. For game registration, the administrator needs to provide game name, a short description of games, number of game levels, scoring method, fully qualified name of .apk file, game location, and a unique score saving table name. The system does not register a game and repeatedly asks the administrator to re-enter until the administrator gives the score saving table's unique name. A flowchart of the game insertion page is provided in Fig. 9.

2.9.3   Core Mechanism of Game Integration with 'Montaj'

1. When the Game runs from a registered user account, it should accept five arguments from Montaj. The same five arguments with unaltered values should return to 'Montaj.' These five arguments are the Game's unique id, user name, unique user's id, the unique study id, and 'GameSequence.' The Game also needs to return back scores and ARTs of participants for all game levels. If the new Game is running from the guest account, the Game needs not to return back anything.
2. If a user under a particular study had already played a complete game, then the Game should have a provision to block the user from replying. If a user, under a particular study, already played some levels of the Game. In that case, a Game should have a provision to block already played levels, play the rest of the levels, and send player's scores and ART of user for all levels of Game to 'Montaj.'
3. The system 'Montaj' has not any option of auto checking whether external games adhere or not protocols set by 'Montaj.' 'Montaj' can't function properly after returning control from those disregarding games.
4. Figure 10 represents the core mechanism of game integration with 'Montaj.'

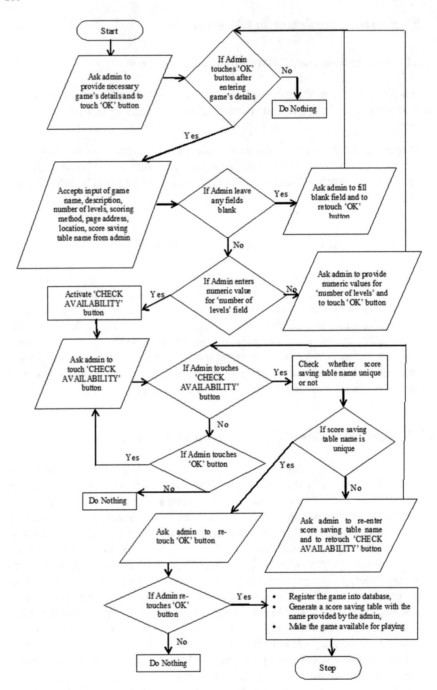

Fig. 9 A flowchart of game insertion page

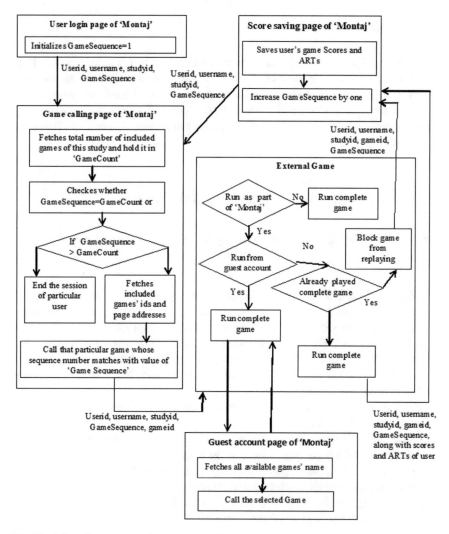

Fig. 10 A flow diagram to depict core mechanism of game integration with 'Montaj'

2.9.4 Example of Importing a New Game

The fifth game, i.e., NBack Game, was designed by completely adhering protocol listed in Sect. 2.9.3 to integrate it with 'Montaj.' The NBack Game implements the N-Back task (a psychological task). This game takes five arguments from 'Montaj'. These are unique user id, unique study id, user name, unique game id, unique sequence no of game among the game enlisted under the study. At the end of playing the game, the NBack Game returns scores and ARTs of all game levels of user with previous five received parameters value in unaltered state to software Montaj'.

3   Testing and Validation

In 'Montaj' software, testing has been performed, and in the latest version, bugs have been removed. Tests were conducted on user registration, administrator panel for creating games and studies, the administrator and user login and registration, hosting a study, importing and exporting psychological games for users to play, guest playability, and the uninterrupted execution of imported games and recording of the test results.

4   Novelty of System Implemented in the System

4.1   Capability of Accommodating Externally Implemented Games

1. 'Montaj' is capable of incorporate any external games developed by other programmers till they follow the protocols provided. This software provides same data manipulation facility for internal as well as external games.
2. A separate score table is automatically generated at the time of game registration, and it will automatically be deleted at the time of game deletion.
3. 'Montaj' automatically change the study status to 'completed' when the current date exceeds the study end date.
4. If a study entity is deleted, all performance tuples for this study from all the game score table will be deleted.
5. Automatic blocking of already played total game/ game levels in case of repeated participation of a participant as part of the same study.
6. 'Montaj' forbids the alteration of included game lists under a study if at least one participant has already taken part in this study.
7. It also forbids the alteration of number of levels of a game if at least one registered participant has already played this game.

4.2   Novelty of the Games Implemented in the System

The four internal games were designed by following previous works reported in the literature Rorden and Karnath (2010), Wojciulik et al. (2004), McGrew et al. (2007), Mussgay and Hertwig (1990), Rundus and Atkinson (1970), Masur et al. (1973), Roodenrys and Hinton (2002), Keeney et al. (1967), Hutchison (2007), etc. While the basic concepts were borrowed from these works, a number of improvements are also made.

In both Rorden and Karnath (2010), Wojciulik et al. (2004) cases, authors designed a letter cancellation task that needed to mark only the target alphabet distributed among other alphabets. Image cancellation is used in level 1 of the TYB game instead of letter cancellation, which is more attractive than letter cancellation. In McGrew et al. (2007), it is asked to mark out the ordered pair of the ball-dog from rows containing repeating pictures of dogs, balls, and cups as a pair cancellation task. The task of finding the same ball-dog pair repeatedly in McGrew et al. (2007) demands less attention and concentration than identifying new ordered pair of animals each time, which is implemented in level 3 to level 5 of the TYB game. In Klee and Garfinkel (1983), Oades (2000), and Overtoom et al. (1998) authors implemented CPT by pair cancellation task. In Klee and Garfinkel (1983), participants are asked to respond when S followed by the letter T (ordered pair TS), which was repeated a number of times in a total of 500 stimuli. CPT by pair cancellation is also implemented in Overtoom et al. (1998) and Oades (2000) with ordered pair AX. TYB Game uses different images in CPT rather repetitively using same letters like Klee and Garfinkel (1983), Oades (2000), and Overtoom et al. (1998). It demands more attention and concentration. The TYB Game implements a pure CPT task by removing the working memory component from CPT-AX or CPT-ST format task Klee and Garfinkel (1983), Oades (2000), Overtoom et al. (1998), which needs to remember the previous stimulus.

In Hertzog et al. (1998) and Rundus and Atkinson (1970) participants were asked to recall in any order from lists of English nouns words. In Tulving and Colotla (1970), examinees were needed to recall nouns in any order from unilingual, bilingual, and trilingual lists of words. Card game implements free recall tasks on images instead of noun words like Tulving and Colotla (1970), Rundus and Atkinson (1970), and Hertzog et al. (1998). It makes this game more attractive and gives participants a feeling of the game rather than a simple task. Card Game does not require knowing more than one language like Tulving and Colotla (1970), neither requires good card gaming skills; a preliminary knowledge about card suits is enough for scoring in this game. Participants in Masur et al. (1973) are needed to free recalling from lists of line drawings of 36 common objects like toys, animals, etc. Recall tasks on images of completely different objects like in Masur et al. (1973) are easy than recalling from a list of only card objects because all the items are cards, and one needs to remember card numbers and card suits.

Serial recall task is implemented by authors of Gupta (2003), Roodenrys and Hinton (2002), Keeney et al. (1967), Oyen and Bebko (1996), Turner and Engle (1989), Kane et al. (2004), Schofield and Ashman (1986), and Reynolds (1997) participants were needed to recall digits serially from lists of digits, and in Roodenrys and Hinton (2002) participants were asked to recall serially from lists composed of four consonant-vowel-consonant (CVC) non-words. Chess Objects Game implements serial recall tasks on images instead of letters or digits like in Gupta (2003) and Roodenrys and Hinton (2002), it makes this games more attractive and gives participants a feeling of a game rather than a simple task. In Keeney et al. (1967) and Oyen and Bebko (1996) subjects were needed to verify whether all previously displayed picture is still present or not in an array of 6 pictures of common objects and point the pictures in a previously displayed order. Remembering different object pictures is less demanding than remembering a set of only chess objects of mixed color. Backward recall task is absent in Gupta (2003), Roodenrys and Hinton (2002), Keeney et al. (1967), Oyen and Bebko (1996), what is present in level 2 and level 4 of Chess Objects Game. Participants were asked to read the operation aloud and verify its correctness orally and needed to read a word loudly following the equation in Turner and Engle (1989). After all items of the sequence ends, participants needed to remember the word for later recall. Turner and Engle (1989). In Kane et al. (2004), participants were required to remember isolated letters presented at the end of each sentence, along with verifying the sentence. It requires grammatical knowledge in English, but Chess Objects does not. Authors of Schofield and Ashman (1986) and Reynolds (1997) gave the ideas about the forward-and-backward digit span and forward-and-backward letter recalling tasks. Both Schofield and Ashman (1986) and Reynolds (1997) are less difficult than Chess objects Game as two colors chess objects are mixed in level 3 and level 4 of the game.

Hutchison (2007), and Durgin (2000) implement stroop task. In Hutchison (2007), stimuli consisted of four-color words red, green, blue, and yellow and four neutral words bad, deep, poor, and legal. Large numbers of congruent and incongruent stimuli were used in Hutchison (2007), so the experiment is time-consuming. In our Stroop game, nine colors are used; these are black, silver, red, blue, yellow, maroon, green, pink, and orange. Instead of using only four colors used in many pieces of literature like Hutchison (2007), Durgin (2000), etc. The labels (show color name) of four response buttons presented at the bottom screen of our Stroop Game is changed from trial to trial, so participants had to provide attention at the time of pressing the button. This is in contrast with the cases where four fixed color patches Durgin (2000) or color button were used as a medium of accepting a response.

5   Usability Analysis

We had conducted a study among young adult students from two institutions—Institution A and Institution B. Ethical clearance was taken from the corresponding Institutional Ethical Committees. After successful completion of all games by the students, feedback on games were collected in the printed feedback form. Participants were asked to evaluate games based on seven points. These are efficient use of screen layout, understand-ability of the user interface, necessity of games' levels, appropriateness of games' speed, understand-ability of games' instructions, appropriateness of games' durations, and integration of various games' elements. Participants were given seven assertions, and they were asked to answer whether they were completely agreed or partially agreed, or disagreed with these assertions. Table 7 shows feedbacks of institution A, Institution B, and overall feed-backs and percentages of complete agreement. Figure 11 depicts percentages of complete agreements, partial agreements, and disagreements by pie charts. Table 7 does not show complete statements; it shows only topics of assertions. From Table 7, it is observed that all assertions on games achieved complete agreement over 75% except the assertion on

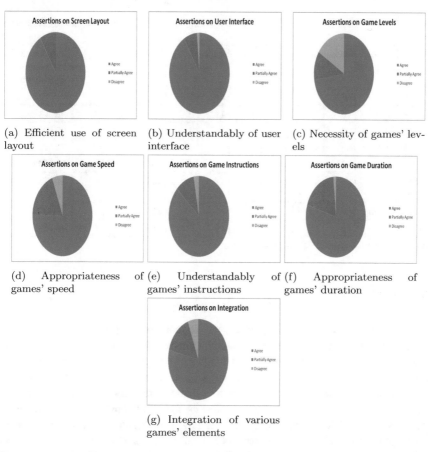

Fig. 11 Pie Charts depicting percentage of complete agreement, partial agreement and disagreement on seven assertions

Game Levels, which is "Playing any level of games is necessary to succeed next upper level". That means they were tried to say some game levels are redundant. The percentage of complete agreement with assertions is calculated as

$$\frac{\text{Number of completely agree}}{\text{Total number of students}} \times 100 \qquad (1)$$

Cronbach's alpha is calculated to determine the internal consistency of seven assertions, and it is found 0.47. Inter-class Correlation Coefficient (ICC) is also determined to determine the inter-judge reliability of 143 judges (participants of study). For the purpose of calculating ICC two-way random effects, absolute agreement, multiple raters/measurements Koo and Li (2016) model is used, and fair inter-judge reliability (ICC = 0.76) was found.

Table 7 Feedbacks of institution A, institution B, overall feedbacks, overall percentage of complete agreement

Assertions on	Institution A			Institution B			Overall			Percentage of complete agreement
	A	PA	D	A	PA	D	A	PA	D	
Screen layout	76	2	0	54	11	0	130	13	0	90.9090
User interface	78	0	0	52	11	2	130	11	2	90.9090
Game levels	60	8	10	43	9	13	103	21	19	72.0279
Game speed	60	12	6	48	15	2	108	27	8	75.5344
Game instructions	70	8	0	54	7	4	124	15	4	86.7132
Game duration	60	16	2	54	11	0	114	27	2	79.7202
Integration	56	14	8	56	9	0	112	23	8	78.3216

A—Agree, PA—Partially Agree, D—Disagree

6 Conclusion

The software 'Montaj' is mainly developed as an aid of research work on cognitive psychology. Cognitive psychology research generally uses different tasks to test the cognitive control of a human. One of the popular ways to test humans' cognitive control is embedding the tasks inside games and involving human beings to play games. The software 'Montaj' contains four games internally to test a large number of humans' cognitive controls and provides an extensible environment to integrate any new number of external games with it as long as those games will design adhering protocol fixed by 'Montaj.' The flexibility of software was verified by integrating the NBack game, which was developed independently of 'Montaj.' This software can be used in multiple studies with different sets of games with different participants. It is expected that the extensible feature of the software will greatly help future research workers by providing them a well-developed platform for integrating their games and using the data manipulation facility provided by the software. However, the software can not provide support if a game has more than 10 levels. Also, it can accept only the score and ART of players as results for each level of external games. By fixing all uncovered bugs earlier version was converted into the latest version.

References

Baddeley, A. D., & Hitch, G. (1974). Working memory. In *Psychology of learning and motivation* (Vol. 8, pp. 47–89). Elsevier.

Chan, R. C., Shum, D., Toulopoulou, T., & Chen, E. Y. (2008). Assessment of executive functions: Review of instruments and identification of critical issues. *Archives of Clinical Neuropsychology, 23*(2), 201–216.

Conway, A. R., Kane, M. J., Bunting, M. F., Hambrick, D. Z., Wilhelm, O., & Engle, R. W. (2005). Working memory span tasks: A methodological review and user's guide. *Psychonomic Bulletin and Review, 12*(5), 769–786.

Corbetta, M., Miezin, F. M., Dobmeyer, S., Shulman, G. L., & Petersen, S. E. (1991). Selective and divided attention during visual discriminations of shape, color, and speed: Functional anatomy by positron emission tomography. *Journal of Neuroscience, 11*(8), 2383–2402.

Corkum, P. V., & Siegel, L. S. (1993). Is the continuous performance task a valuable research tool for use with children with attention-deficit-hyperactivity disorder? *Journal of Child Psychology and Psychiatry, 34*(7), 1217–1239.

De Giglio, L., De Luca, F., Prosperini, L., Borriello, G., Bianchi, V., Pantano, P., & Pozzilli, C. (2015). A low-cost cognitive rehabilitation with a commercial video game improves sustained attention and executive functions in multiple sclerosis: a pilot study. *Neurorehabilitation and Neural Repair, 29*(5), 453–461.

Deterding, S., Dixon, D., Khaled, R., & Nacke, L. (2011a). From game design elements to game-fulness: Defining gamification. In *Proceedings of the 15th International Academic MindTrek Conference: Envisioning Future Media Environments* (pp. 9–15). ACM.

Deterding, S., Sicart, M., Nacke, L., O'Hara, K., & Dixon, D. (2011b). Gamification. Using game-design elements in non-gaming contexts. In *CHI'11 Extended Abstracts on Human Factors in Computing Systems* (pp. 2425–2428). ACM.

Diamond, A. (2013). Executive functions. *Annual Review of Psychology, 64*, 135–168.

Durgin, F. H. (2000). The reverse Stroop effect. *Psychonomic Bulletin and Review, 7*(1), 121–125.

Glanzer, M., & Cunitz, A. R. (1966). Two storage mechanisms in free recall. *Journal of Verbal Learning and Verbal Behavior, 5*(4), 351–360.

Grunebaum, H., Weiss, J. L., Gallant, D., & Cohler, B. J. (1974). Attention in young children of psychotic mothers. *American Journal of Psychiatry, 131*(8), 887–891.

Gupta, P. (2003). Examining the relationship between word learning, nonword repetition, and imme-diate serial recall in adults. *The Quarterly Journal of Experimental Psychology Section A, 56*(7), 1213–1236.

Hertzog, C., McGuire, C. L., & Lineweaver, T. T. (1998). Aging, attributions, perceived control, and strategy use in a free recall task. *Aging, Neuropsychology, and Cognition, 5*(2), 85–106.

Hutchison, K. A. (2007). Attentional control and the relatedness proportion effect in semantic priming. *Journal of Experimental Psychology: Learning, Memory, and Cognition, 33*(4), 645.

Kane, M. J., Hambrick, D. Z., Tuholski, S. W., Wilhelm, O., Payne, T. W., & Engle, R. W. (2004). The generality of working memory capacity: A latent-variable approach to verbal and visuospatial memory span and reasoning. *Journal of Experimental Psychology: General, 133*(2), 189.

Keeney, T. J., Cannizzo, S. R., & Flavell, J. H. (1967). Spontaneous and induced verbal rehearsal in a recall task. *Child Development*, 953–966.

Klee, S. H., & Garfinkel, B. D. (1983). The computerized continuous performance task: A new measure of inattention. *Journal of Abnormal Child Psychology, 11*(4), 487–495.

Koo, T. K., & Li, M. Y. (2016). A guideline of selecting and reporting intraclass correlation coeffi-cients for reliability research. *Journal of Chiropractic Medicine, 15*(2), 155–163.

Kupietz, S. S., & Richardson, E. (1978). Children's vigilance performance and inattentiveness in the classroom. *Journal of Child Psychology and Psychiatry, 19*(2), 145–154.

Lamers, M. J., Roelofs, A., & Rabeling-Keus, I. M. (2010). Selective attention and response set in the Stroop task. *Memory and Cognition, 38*(7), 893–904.

Lan, X., Legare, C. H., Ponitz, C. C., Li, S., & Morrison, F. J. (2011). Investigating the links between the subcomponents of executive function and academic achievement: A cross-cultural analysis of Chinese and American preschoolers. *Journal of Experimental Child Psychology, 108*(3), 677–692.

Lowe, D. G., & Mitterer, J. O. (1982). Selective and divided attention in a Stroop task. *Canadian Journal of Psychology/Revue Canadienne de Psychologie, 36*(4), 684.

Masur, E. F., McIntyre, C. W., & Flavell, J. H. (1973). Developmental changes in apportionment of study time among items in a multitrial free recall task. *Journal of Experimental Child Psychology, 15*(2), 237–246.

McClelland, M. M., Cameron, C. E., Connor, C. M., Farris, C. L., Jewkes, A. M., & Morrison, F. J. (2007). Links between behavioral regulation and preschoolers' literacy, vocabulary, and math skills. *Developmental Psychology, 43*(4), 947.

McGrew, K. S., Woodcock, R. W., & Schrank, K. A. (2007). *Woodcock-Johnson III normative update technical manual*. Riverside Pub.

Miyake, A., Friedman, N. P., Emerson, M. J., Witzki, A. H., Howerter, A., & Wager, T. D. (2000). The unity and diversity of executive functions and their contributions to complex "frontal lobeâĿž tasks: A latent variable analysis. *Cognitive Psychology, 41*(1), 49–100.

Morris, N., & Jones, D. M. (1990). Memory updating in working memory: The role of the central executive. *British Journal of Psychology, 81*(2), 111–121.

Mussgay, L., & Hertwig, R. (1990). Signal detection indices in schizophrenics on a visual, auditory, and bimodal continuous performance test. *Schizophrenia Research, 3*(5–6), 303–310.

Nouchi, R., Taki, Y., Takeuchi, H., Hashizume, H., Nozawa, T., Kambara, T., et al. (2013). Brain training game boosts executive functions, working memory and processing speed in the young adults: A randomized controlled trial. *PLoS One, 8*(2), e55518.

Oades, R. D. (2000). Differential measures of 'sustained attention' in children with attention-deficit/hyperactivity or tic disorders: Relations to monoamine metabolism. *Psychiatry Research, 93*(2), 165–178.

Overtoom, C. C., Verbaten, M. N., Kemner, C., Kenemans, J. L., van Engeland, H., Buitelaar, J. K., Camfferman, G., & Koelega, H. S. (1998). Associations between event-related potentials and measures of attention and inhibition in the continuous performance task in children with ADHD and normal controls. *Journal of the American Academy of Child and Adolescent Psychiatry, 37*(9), 977–985.

Oyen, A.-S., & Bebko, J. M. (1996). The effects of computer games and lesson contexts on children's mnemonic strategies. *Journal of Experimental Child Psychology, 62*(2), 173–189.

Prasad, J. (2014). *Connecting the dots between N-back, operation span, and Raven's progressive matrices*. Ph.D. Thesis, Wake Forest University.

Reynolds, C. R. (1997). Forward and backward memory span should not be combined for clinical analysis. *Archives of Clinical Neuropsychology, 12*(1), 29–40.

Roodenrys, S., & Hinton, M. (2002). Sublexical or lexical effects on serial recall of nonwords? *Journal of Experimental Psychology: Learning, Memory, and Cognition, 28*(1), 29.

Rorden, C., & Karnath, H.-O. (2010). A simple measure of neglect severity. *Neuropsychologia, 48*(9), 2758–2763.

Rundus, D., & Atkinson, R. C. (1970). Rehearsal processes in free recall: A procedure for direct observation. *Journal of Memory and Language, 9*(1), 99.

Schofield, N. J., & Ashman, A. F. (1986). The relationship between digit span and cognitive processing across ability groups. *Intelligence, 10*(1), 59–73.

Schrank, F. A., Decker, S. L., & Garruto, J. M. (2016). *Essentials of WJ IV cognitive abilities assessment*. Wiley.

Stroop, J. R. (1935). Studies of interference in serial verbal reactions. *Journal of Experimental Psychology, 18*(6), 643.

Szalma, J., Daly, T., Teo, G., Hancock, G., & Hancock, P. (2018). Training for vigilance on the move: A video game-based paradigm for sustained attention. *Ergonomics, 61*(4), 482–505.

Szalma, J. L., Schmidt, T., Teo, G., & Hancock, P. A. (2014). Vigilance on the move: Video game-based measurement of sustained attention. *Ergonomics, 57*(9), 1315–1336.

Thomas, J. G., Milner, H. R., & Haberlandt, K. F. (2003). Forward and backward recall: Different response time patterns, same retrieval order. *Psychological Science, 14*(2), 169–174.

Tulving, E., & Colotla, V. A. (1970). Free recall of trilingual lists. *Cognitive Psychology, 1*(1), 86–98.

Turner, M. L., & Engle, R. W. (1989). Is working memory capacity task dependent? *Journal of Memory and Language, 28*(2), 127–154.

Unsworth, N., & Engle, R. W. (2007). On the division of short-term and working memory: An examination of simple and complex span and their relation to higher order abilities. *Psychological Bulletin, 133*(6), 1038.

Unsworth, N., Schrock, J. C., & Engle, R. W. (2004). Working memory capacity and the antisaccade task: Individual differences in voluntary saccade control. *Journal of Experimental Psychology: Learning, Memory, and Cognition, 30*(6), 1302.

van Maanen, L., van Rijn, H., & Borst, J. P. (2009). Stroop and picture-word interference are two sides of the same coin. *Psychonomic Bulletin and Review, 16*(6), 987–999.

West, R., & Alain, C. (2000). Age-related decline in inhibitory control contributes to the increased Stroop effect observed in older adults. *Psychophysiology, 37*(2), 179–189.

Wojciulik, E., Rorden, C., Clarke, K., Husain, M., & Driver, J. (2004). Group study of an "undercoverâŁž test for visuospatial neglect: Invisible cancellation can reveal more neglect than standard cancellation. *Journal of Neurology, Neurosurgery and Psychiatry, 75*(9), 1356–1358.

Zhang, Y., & Goh, W. B. (2018). The influence of peer accountability on attention during gameplay. *Computers in Human Behavior, 84*, 18–28.

Social Data Analysis Techniques and Applications

Safikureshi Mondal◉, Zeenat Rehena◉, and Nandini Mukherjee◉

Abstract There is an ongoing trend towards delivery of quality healthcare services in public healthcare domain that can effectively incorporate the social network analysis according to human needs. Social data analysis allows us to make understanding the link between physical symptoms, mental health symptoms, and their expression in social interactions and behavior. The interdependent relationships between these, are not well understood, due to limitations of existing clinical diagnosis and public health tools, but play an important role in medical detection, treatment and management of conditions. There are so many research opportunities in public health domain like epidemiologic monitoring, situational awareness, risk assessment, diagnosis or prediction, disease control or outbreak, cancer prevention and control intervention, mental health, prediction brain function etc. These researches are need to be figured out as social data applications to continue more research on it. On the other hand, social network analysis (SNA) is a modern research approach which measures or discovers hidden relationships, connection or trends of complex healthcare systems and used for both methodological tool and theoretical paradigm that answer the important ecological questions in public health. This chapter concerns about the research to trace the history of social data analysis with providing different sources for different social data in public health with state of art of social data analysis and techniques. Also, when and how different SNA techniques are used in public health as SNA techniques, are discussed. It is also shown in this chapter that how the SNA techniques and measures are used in different public health applications.

Keywords IOT · Social sensing application · Social data · SNA · Public health

S. Mondal (✉)
Narula Institute of technology, Kolkata, India
e-mail: msafi.cse@gmail.com

Z. Rehena
Aliah University, Kolkata, India

N. Mukherjee
Jadavpur University, Kolkata, India
e-mail: nandini.mukhopadhay@jadavpuruniversity.in

1 Introduction

One of the important uses of Internet of Things (IoT) is social sensing applications in public health domain. In several surveys (Aggarwal and Abdelzaher, 2013; Abdelzaher, 2007), the idea and objective of social sensing applications are depicted. People-centric sensing (Aggarwal and Abdelzaher, 2011; Campbell et al., 2008; Miluzzo et al., 2008) and participatory sensing (Burke et al., 2006) are both considered as social sensing applications. The main aim of social sensing applications in public health is to collect or capture the runtime sensor's health data to monitor the patient's vital sign, tracking and feedback. Different types of sensors are used in public health for sensing the application. Medical sensors are used to predict or track the personal medical condition of individual. Some sensors such as, fitness and activity sensors, vital sign sensors, Blood Constituent Sensor and Ambient sensors etc. are used in social sensing applications in public health. These sensors are the active role player for the public health domain, There are many challenges which are faced by social sensing applications and these are common as healthcare applications due to used sensor in public health domain: such as (1) privacy of the sensor collected data (2) Energy efficiency challenges (3) processing large amount of sensor data (4) trust-worthiness of collected data (5) request-response challenges of large sensor data etc.

There are several research papers are published (Hou et al., 2020; Wang et al., 2014) to study the survey the data analysis and application on social media platform. Natural language processing, news analytics, opinion mining techniques, scraping, sentiment analysis, text analytics and SNA are the important techniques and these are also used as social data analysis techniques in public health. SNA is highlighted in this chapter.

SNA plays a significant role to share the vital information and transferring the knowledge among different actors, groups in various areas in social data analysis. The various actors in public health are shown Fig. 1. SNA concepts are built from various

Fig. 1 Actors in public health

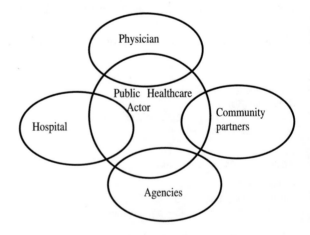

domains (Lewis et al., 2008; Krempel and Plumper, 2003; Klofstad et al., 2013; Rubinov and Sporns, 2010; Chen et al., 2007) such as: social science, economics, politics, epidemiology, neuroscience etc. SNA finds new objective as analysis and prediction to focus on the interconnectedness properties between different actors in a system. SNA is used on complex graph systems which must be represented as graph nodes interconnected though social relationships. The relationship may be friendship, collaboration, co-occurrence etc. SNA is used to create a model to map, characterize the system, and identify the complex relation and recognize the different role of a group of actors in SNA methodologies to analyze the complex graph data by both structural and dynamic analysis techniques and also helps to find the hidden relationship of nodes and trends of complex system etc. In public health domain particularly social sensing application with sensor data, modeling and analyzing are the important research problems due to dynamic complex behavior of actors which interact to each other. These important challenges in public health domain make the use of SNA techniques to overcome the challenges. The SNA techniques can be used as node level analysis, network level analysis, clustering, community detection and flow analysis to solve the current challenges of public health domain.

The remainders of this chapter are as follows: Sect. 2 will introduce social sensing applications in Public Health. After that, different variations of social data are figured out in public health in Sect. 3. A brief review of social data analysis techniques are described with emphasizes of different SNA methodologies or techniques in Sect. 4. Next a state of the art of social data analysis approaches are categorized and described in Sect. 5. After that a details review is carried out for the SNA analysis techniques as social data analysis in public health in Sect. 6. Finally, concluded the chapter by Sect. 7.

2 Social Sensing Application in Public Health

Sensors and social network are actively involved in social sensing applications. Public healthcare is one of the best examples of social sensing applications in where not only sensors are performed in these applications, but also human are acted as versatile sensor. Actors can be serve itself as information sources like patient's feedback in public health sensor operators like geo-tagging (track the location of patient) applications in public health, sensor conveyors such as smartphone equipped sensors in continuous monitoring and sensor data processor which are the best example of crowd sensing applications in public health.

A lot of opportunities of research are available in social sensing applications. There are lot of applications are treated as social sensing applications which are used as social data applications in public health domain. Social sensing application can be divided into three broad applications according to their function. Such as Data centric application, statistics or machine learning based application, model centric based application.

– Data centric application: In this type of social sensing applications, individual
  actors share the data which are used to make a decision. In public health domain,
  as individual actor's patient share the feedback, history or location (continuous
  monitoring) to make a decision of provider
– Statistics or machine learning based application: Statistical functions or machine
  learning based statistical function computed on sensor based data to convert appropriate format of data which is required data for consumer or provider. Such as for
  continuous monitoring in public health, statistical functions are computed the data
  from sensing based data.
– Model centric applications: In this type of social sensing application, models are
  learned from sensory data which is used later outside of that application. Such as
  sharing data which is to be collected as sensory data from fitness enthusiasts can
  lead to better life style which promotes better healthier behaviors.

There are several social sensing applications (Longstaff et al., 2010; Cook, 2011;
Ganti et al., 2010) are used in public health domain as different mentioned type
applications. Social data is one of the important places of research in social sensing
applications.

3   Social Data in Public Health

Social data can be recognized as data individual which is created by actors (human)
with the objective to share others for specific goal. Social media can be important
platforms for creating social data. But data generated from sensing applications can
be good example of social data. Thus, public healthcare data is the example of social
data as social sensing or monitoring application. In Fig. 2, variations of social data
are shown.

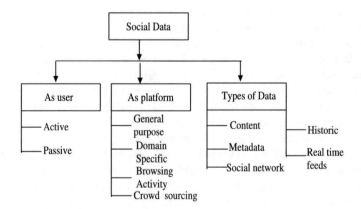

Fig. 2 Different corners of social data

Social data can be categorized as user, platform and contents or types of data. In user based social data tells us that the process of user participation in the generation of data such as actively or passively. As for example in social monitoring, active user based requires explicit participation from users and passive makes use of data already published by users without requiring user interaction. Heldman et al. discussed in the research paper (Ganti et al., 2010) that how public health agencies can use social media and Moorhead et al. and Thackeray et al. are shown in their research papers (Moorhead, 2013; Thackeray et al., 2008) that how medical profession can use social media to communicate with the population. Also, in Yazdavar et al. (2018) research papers authors has been work on mental health using social media analysis and Kuamri and Babu (2017), it is shown that how emotion can be detected using analysis of real time data.

Social data is published with different public health goals and purposes from different websites and online platforms. In general, the sources of social data are different blogs and microblogs. The popular examples of blogs are Tumblr, Blogger and Wordpress and Twitter is the example of microbloggers. Also Facebook and LinkedIn are the example of social network where users used to communicate other users and this is used in public health. Such as Morgan (2010) drug used captured videos which are shared in social network though YouTube.

As domain specific social data includes reviews websites, online reviews and patient communities. Social data is generated from this reviews and these are domain specific includes health of domain. Users are post their feedback of doctors through RateMDs.com websites and write medications review throughDrugs.com websites. In Harrison et al. (2012) research paper, researcher monitored food poising outbreaks through websites. Also patients can share their health condition, experiences with other through online communities, forums or creating thread etc. In PatientsLikeMe patient community, hundreds of patient shared their results and teat amyotrophic lateral sclerosis disease trial (Wicks, 2011). In research papers (Cook et al., 2013), author shown that approximately 10% twitter group chats on health. The Google Flu Trends system search engines is a good example where searching data is mostly used in public health. In Santillana et al. (2014a) obtained the search data from UptoDate disease database which is used by clinicians. There are lot of sources of public data in browsing activity such as Wikipedia, search engines etc.

Crowdsourcing can be defined as a process where feedback and assistance can be get from group of peoples through online services. Crowdsourcing can be used in public health. Such as users are asked to share their health status through FluNearYou application (Baltrusaitis, 2017; Crawley et al., 2014; Smolinski et al., 2015). Social data can be available in various forms, such as text, locations information's and social network information. Social data is published as form of text that came from web content. Other content come in the form of images such as Instragram. In a research paper (Garimella et al., 2016), it is found that extracted Instragram images can be useful for some health applications like detecting excessive drinking. Time, location of the data are the component of metadata and these are used as the patient information in public health domain. Social network data is another important source of social data. These are important for some type of public health surveillance such as predicting disease (Sadilek et al., 2012a,b).

A discussion is done about several social applications in previous section and their benefits in IoT based e-health care system. However, several challenges are there which need to be addressed. In this section, some of the current challenges are discussed that are hampering the extensive acceptance of e-health care.

4   Social Data Analysis Techniques in Public health

Generally, data or information can be analyzed with the help of machine learning, statistical functions and qualitative method. In Fig. 3, general data analysis methods are show in pipelines. First method is content analysis and filtering method which is filtered the data to the research relevant data. This filtering method may be rule based approaches, machine learning classification, unsupervised clustering etc. In several research papers (Wasserman, 1994; Chew and Eysenbach, 2010; Culotta, 2010), researcher finds the twitter based influenza surveillance to filter the "flu" or "fever" which are one of the social data application of public health by rule based social data analysis, approach. Also keyword and phase-based filtering are used for public health to filter the social data. In Lampos and Cristianini (2010), Aramaki et al. 2011 research papers, authors built a machine learning classifier to identify flu related tweets. Also, regression model, support vector machine and natural language processing techniques used as classifier in public health.

Clustering is a one type of unsupervised machine learning technique. Such as in research papers (Achrekar et al., 2012; Brody and Elhadad, 2010; Chen et al., 2015a; Ghosh and Guha, 2013) clustering method is applied for social data analysis. As filtering method, there are three techniques are used in public health: keyword filtering, topic modeling and classification. These approaches are used in their different data techniques and data properties itself. After filtering method relevant social data are used for prediction, validation etc. in analysis. In Paul and Dredze (2011), Chew and Eysenbach (2010) research papers, authors analyzed the trend to compute the volume of filtered data (flu tweets per week) to see the time, location and measure.

There are so many techniques are used in public health which are related to analyzing unstructured textual health data like natural language processing, news analytics, opinion mining techniques, scraping, sentiment analysis and text analytics. But, SNA technique is, one of the important techniques in Social data analysis. SNA technique is an interdisciplinary areas like social science, economics, politics,

Fig. 3 A general data analysis techniques

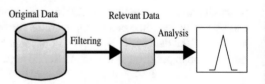

epidemiology, neuroscience etc. and these areas are represented as a complex network in which system actors and their relationship are represented as network nodes and edges. The social network analysis techniques (Lamb et al., 2013; Albert, 2002; Barabasi, 2002; Newman, 2003; Watts, 2004; Christakis, 2012) are broadly divided into two categories such as structural analysis and dynamic analysis. Structural data analysis is find the existing social interaction between users and their behavior which the help of graph theory method. But dynamic analysis finds the changes of topology of network nodes and due to the lack of structure and multi-modality of the data.Data can be different form like text, image, video and audio etc. The analysis is the biggest challenge for these techniques. Structural analysis techniques includes the network nodes, communities etc. and dynamic analysis measured by adding or removal of nodes, edges or link weight, examines the diffusion process etc.

In this section social data analysis techniques are discussed with concentration of SNA's techniques in public health domain with different measures which are depicted in the following.

4.1 Natural Language Processing

It is a field with Computer Science, AI and linguistics (human and computer language). It is the process to extract the meaningful health information from natural language input or output.

4.2 News Analytic

This analytic method is the measurement of qualitative and quantitative attributes of some health unstructured news stories data. Sentiment, relevance, novelty are attributes.

4.3 Opinion Mining

It is required to make a automatic system to determine human opinion from text written about healthcare.

4.4 Scraping

Collecting online data as social health data in the form of site scraping, web harvesting etc.

4.5   Sentiment Analysis

It is the process which is a application of natural language processing with computational linguistics to identify subjective information.

4.6   Text Analytics

This analysis involves the information retrieval, visualization and predictive analysis etc.

4.7   Social Network Analysis

Social network analysis is a new perception of analysis and prediction of large complex networks. It finds the interconnectedness between the system actors. The analysis is based on graph theories to represent the complex systems as a collection of nodes which are interconnected through social relationships. The main objective of SNA analysis is to find the network properties, identify patterns of relations and recognize the roles of actors of the system. SNA analysis can be done by some measures which are depicted in the following.

4.7.1   Structural Analysis

The objective of structural analysis is to study the network topology to find the properties of the network. There are two perspectives to find the properties of network. At first, it is used to focus on selected actors and find other neighbors. This is is called ego-centric view. In another perspective socioeconomic view, it is find the structural pattern of the interactions of nodes. A lot of measures or basic metrics are used for the structural based analysis which are used by graph theory algorithms.
Network Metrics

- Centrality: Centrality network metrics is used to find the structural importance of a node in a network. Centrality measure is mainly used to assess the important or influential node in a network. There are several measures are used for centrality.

  1. Degree centrality is used for the nodes which has more rank with more connections.
  2. Eigenvector centrality is used after generalization of degree centrality.
  3. PageRank can be evaluated by the number of outgoing link from the node.
  4. Between centrality measures the number of shortest path between two paths. Highest value can be treated as "bridge" of two subgraph.

5. Closeness centrality can be based on node average distance to all other nodes. If there are more central nodes then it is easier to reach other nodes. Means, the smaller the average shortest path length is, the centrality value of the node will be higher.
6. K-shells centrality is came from diffusion models. Network decomposes into many shells to identify influencing node who spread information.
7. Group centralities is similar like degree centrality, but it measures to a group of nodes.

- Transitivity and reciprocity: These are used to represent linking behavior in a network. Higher transitivity in a graph means denser graph which is closer to complete graph. Global clustering coefficient and local clustering coefficient are used for the network and nodes.
- Balance and status: Social balance and social status are used to determine the consistency in signed networks. Social balance theory says that friend/foe relationships are consistent when the transitivity between nodes can be propagated. A signed graph is a graph in which each edge has a positive or negative sign. This sign is used in Online Social Networks (OSN) to represent interpersonal relationships. This kind of graph is balanced if the product of edge signs around every cycle is positive.
- Assortatively or social similarity: In social networks connections between individuals are not random; a connection between two similar individuals is more likely than between two dissimilar ones. This similarity can be manifested as similar hobbies, language, behavior, or nationality among others. Therefore, measuring assortatively in OSN helps to better understand user interactions. Many forces creates assortatively in OSN, among them Homophily and Influence are the most common ones (Barabasi, 2016). Nevertheless, Homophily and Influence are two sides of the same coin, while the latter is the force that an individual (influencer) applies to other individuals so they became similar to him and the former is the force that makes two already similar individuals connect.
- Community detection: Community detection is defined to divide or partition the graph into clusters and nodes belonging to the same cluster are referred as strong interconnected. As random walks, spectral clustering, modularity maximization, or statistical approaches are used to find communities. A good community is one whose nodes are highly connected and it has few connections to the nodes of other communities.
  Node-centric community: Node-centric community finding methods: in this case, each node of the network must satisfy the properties of mutuality, reachability and degrees. Mutuality property relies on the concept of the clique, which is the maximal complete subgraph of three or more nodes in such a way that all of them are adjacent to each other. Reachability property considers that two nodes may belong to the same community if there is a path connecting them. This property assigns the nodes belonging to the same connected component to the same community. degree property establishes that the nodes of a group must be adjacent to a relatively large number of group members.

- Dynamic Analysis: Social network modeling deals with analysis of social network in terms of structural relationships that exists among various entities or nodes present in the network. The most important aspect in the social network analysis is its evolution with time and its dynamicity and dynamic social network analysis explicitly deals with this aspect effectively.

5 State of Art Social Data Applications

There are several origin of social data are discussed and how the social data analysis are measured by different metrics are discussed in previous section. What are the different social data applications are used in public health are discussed in this section.

In Fig. 4, a state of the art of different social data applications are shown. The Disease surveillance category includes infectious disease, non-infectious disease and influenza applications. There are many functions are done as influenza surveillance social data applications like track the trends of seasonal influenza, early detection of diseases, and the transmission pattern of diseases etc. Also as non-infectious diseases, the functions are track the spread diseases like dengue, West Nile and done the awareness of ebola, Zika virus etc. Tracking the geographic patterns in chronic illness, progress of the diseases and discover the correlates of diseases etc. are the function of the chronic diseases. In behavioral medicine social data applications are used like disease awareness, prevention, substance use and fitness. Dieting and fitness patterns are discovered among different populations and correlates the health outcome by discovering dietary correlates. Also substance measuring attitudes is done for different substances like tobacco and e-cigarettes, alcohol, and other drugs.

In environmental social data applications category, emergencies and disaster, Foodborn illness and vilolence are categorized. Social data is used at situational awareness during emergencies like disaster and also it is used for the understanding of population behavior during disaster. Foodborn illness can be identified through

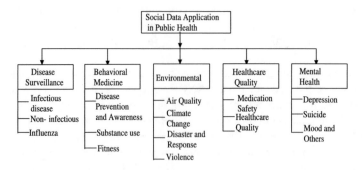

Fig. 4 Different social data applications

reports, feedback on social media. Air quality measuring requiring urban areas to measure the pollution for the people awareness and responses data are used for climate change.

Quality of healthcare of centre or hospital is estimated by measuring perceptions of social media reports, feedback or reviews of doctors and these are the important of function of healthcare quality. People are reported the drug and medication side affects through online for the medication safety.

There are several social data applications are used in mental health category as public health like depression, suicide and moods etc. Predicting the depressive episodes, finding the symptoms or indicators of depression are the category of depression and suicide. The risk factors of suicide, detecting the instances of suicidal mood, emotions of online users are the functions of mood and understanding patterns of mental illnesses.

6 SNA Techniques and Applications in Public Health

In this section, SNA techniques are concentrated as social data analysis techniques and rigorous reviews are done with different analysis techniques with appropriate SNA measures metrics in public health domain (Table 1).

7 Conclusion

Social data analysis is a new emerging research area in data analysis world which needs to be focused in public health for future research. It can be used to answer social scientific questions. Public health research is depends on data and social data describe the research on sharing of health information over the communication network. Through this chapter, it is trying to show the overall research test of enormous potential of social data analysis. The impact of social data analysis and techniques are shown in public health through this chapter. Review of different corners of source of social data, applications and social data analysis techniques are done rigorously. SNA analysis is the important category of social data analysis techniques which are used heavily in public health domain. In this chapter SNA techniques with appropriate measures are described in public health domain.

Table 1 Different types of SNA techniques and its applications

Reference of research work	Details SNA application	Analysis techniques	Metrics used	Public health
Yoshimitsu (2016)	A descriptive analysis of medical waste by studying duplicative prescription practices in Japan has been conducted	Structural analysis	Pearson correlation co-efficient and scatter plots are used for statistical analysis and bipartite net-work, density as SNA analysis measure	Medical waste
Bramhachari (2016)	SNA used to explore the genesis of social ties of the RMPs with diverse health system actors and identify the gaps within the network	Structural analysis	Qualitative ego-network is used as SNA analysis	Rural Health
Guo et al. (2015)	SNA is used to explore the patients' transferring data of medical insurance Bureau	Structural analysis	Spinglass, edge betweenness, label propagation, walktrap method are used for community detection and degree, closeness centrality, betweenness centrality, eigenvector, centrality as linear regression	Medical Insurance
Soulakis (2015)	Provider collaboration network is used to describe collaboration between patients and providers	Structural analysis	Heuristic community detection algorithm, kCliques algorithm are used	Patient-provider relation
Schoen (2014)	SNA techniques used on contact and collaboration networks building community capacity and enhancing collaboration	Structural analysis	Average degree, density, degree centrlization are used for SNA	Public health programmes
Dianis (2016)	SNA is used for assessment of federal funding on the network of all stake holders in an excellence program	Structural analysis	Density, average distance is used as SNA	Health system stakeholder
Kawonga (2015)	SNA is used to measure communication between disease programme and district managers using networks of GHS and DCP	Dynamics of the network	Density, degree, betweenness centrality and homophile (E-Index) is used	Rural Healthcare

(continued)

Table 1 (continued)

Reference of research work	Details SNA application	Analysis techniques	Metrics used	Public health
Khosla (2016)	SNA is used to measure quality of coordination among HIV agencies	Structural analysis	Density, degree, centralization, weighted degree centralization, closeness centrality,betweenness centrality are used	HIV agency
Wang et al. (2014)	SNA is used to understand the nature of collaboration among doctors treating hospital inpatients and explore the impact of collaboration on cost and quality of care	Structural analysis	Degree centrality, closeness centrality betweenness centrality, density, clustering coefficient are used	Hospital Management System
Wu (2014)	SNA is used on authors, institution and countries collaborating on psychiatric research	Structural analysis	Centrality, K-plex analysis, Core periphery hierarchical clustering	Psychiatry research
Wu (2014)	SNA is used to identify leaders and influencers in a research collaboration network	Dynamics of the networks	centrality,path length, clustering coefficient,centrality leaders are used	Healthcare

References

Abdelzaher, T. F. (2007). Mobiscopes for human spaces. *IEEE Pervasive Computing, 6*(2), 20–29.

Achrekar, H., Gandhe, A., Lazarus, R., Yu, S., & Liu, B. (2012). Twitter improves seasonal Influenza prediction. In *International Conference on Health Informatics*.

Aggarwal, C. C., & Abdelzaher, T. (2013). *Social sensing in managing and mining sensor data*. Kluwer Academic Publishers.

Aggarwal, C. C., & Abdelzaher, T. (2011). *Integrating sensors and social networks, social network data analytics*. Springer.

Albert, R. (2002). Statistical mechanics of complex networks. *Reviews of Modern Physics*, 741–747.

Aramaki, E., Maskawa, S., & Morita, M. (2011). Twitter catches the u: Detecting influenza epidemics using Twitter. In *Empirical Methods in Natural Language Processing (EMNLP)*, pp. 1568–1576.

Baltrusaitis, K. (2017). Determinants of participants' follow-up and characterization of representativeness in Flu Near You, a participatory disease surveillance system. *JMIR Public Health Surveillance, 3*(2), e18.

Barabasi, A. L. (2002). *Linked: The new science of networks*. Perseus Books Group.

Barabasi, A. (2016). *Network science*. Cambridge University Press.

Bian, J., Xie, M., Topaloglu, U., Hudson, T., & Hogan, W. (2013) Understanding biomedicai research collaborations through social network analysis: A case study. In *2013 IEEE International Conference on Bioinformatics and Biomedicine (BIBM)*, pp. 9–16.

Bramhachari, R. (2016). a social network analysis of rural medical practitioners in the Sundarbans, West Bengal. *BMJ Global Health, 1*, A41–A42.

Brody, S., & Elhadad, N. (2010) Detecting salient aspects in online reviews of health providers. In *AMIA Annual Symposium Proceedings*.

Burke, J., Estrin, D., Hansen, M., Parker, A., Ramanathan, N., Reddy, S., & Srivastava, M. B. (2006). Participatory sensing. In: *WWW Conference*.

Campbell, T., et al. (2008). The rise of people centric sensing. *IEEE Internet Computing, 12*(4).

Caniato, M. (2015). Understanding the perceptions, roles and interactions of stakeholder networks managing health-care waste: A case study of the Gaza Strip. *Waste Management, 35,* 255–64.

Chen, Y. D., Tseng, C., King, C. C., Wu, T. S. J., & Chen, H. (2007). Incorporating geographical contacts into social network analysis for contact tracing in epidemiology: A study on Taiwan SARS data. In: *Intelligence and Security Informatics: Biosurveillance* (pp. 23–36). Springer, Berlin, Heidelberg.

Chen, B., Zhang, J. M., Jiang, Z., Shao, J., Jiang, T., Wang, Z., et al. (2015). Media and public reactions toward vaccination during the hepatitis B vaccine crisis' in China. *Vaccine, 33*(15), 1780–1785.

Chew, C., & Eysenbach, G. (2010). Pandemics in the age of Twitter: Content analysis of tweets during the 2009 H1N1 outbreak. *PLoS ONE, 5*(11), e14118.

Christakis, N., & Fowler., J. (2011). *Connected: The surprising power of our social networks and how they shape our lives*. Back Bay Books (Scott, 2012)

Cook, J., Kenthapadi, K., & Mishra, N. (2013). Group chats on Twitter. In *International Conference on World Wide Web (WWW)* (pp. 225–236). New York, NY, USA: ACM.

Cook, D. J. (2011). Multisensor selection to support practical use of healthmonitoring smart environments. *Wiley Interdisciplinary Reviews: Data Mining and Knowledge Discovery 1*(4), 339–351. https://doi.org/10.1002/widm.20

Crawley, A. W., Wojcik, O. P., Olsen, J., Brownstein, J. S., & Smolinski, M. S. (2014). Flu near you: Comparing crowdsourced reports of influenza-like illness to the CDC outpatient influenza-like illness surveillance network, October 2012 to March 2014. In *Council of State and Territorial Epidemiologists Annual Conference*

Culotta, A. (2010). Towards detecting influenza epidemics by analyzing Twitter messages. In *ACM Workshop on Social Media Analytics*.

Dianis, N. L. (2016). The NHLBI-united health global health centers of excellence program: Assessment of impact of federal funding through a social network analysis. *Global Heart, 11,* 145–48.e1.

Ganti, R. K., Srinivasan, S., & Gacic, A. (2010). Multisensor fusion in smartphones for lifestyle monitoring. In *Proceedings of the 2010 International Conference on Body Sensor Networks*, ser. BSN '10 (pp. 36–43). Washington, DC, USA: IEEE Computer Society. https://doi.org/10.1109/BSN.2010.10.

Garimella, V. R. K., Alfayad, A., & Weber, I. (2016). Social media image analysis for public health. In *Conference on Human Factors in Computing Systems (CHI)* (pp. 5543–5547). New York, NY, USA: ACM

Ghosh, D. D., & Guha, R. (2013). What are we 'tweeting' about obesity? Mapping tweets with topic modeling and geographic information system. *Cartography and Geographic Information Science, 40*(2), 90–102.

Guo, H., Wei, F., Cheng, S., & Jiang F. (2015). Find referral social networks. In *International Symposium on Security and Privacy in Social Networks and Big Data* (pp. 58–63).

Harrison, C., Jorder, M., Stern, H., Stavinsky, F., Reddy, V., Hanson, H., Waechter, H., Lowe, L., Gravano, L., & Balter, S.: Using online reviews by restaurant patrons to identify unreported cases of foodborne illness|New York City, 2012–2013. *Morbidity and Mortality Weekly Report, 63*(20), 441–445.

Heldman, A. B., Schindelar, J., & Weaver, J. B. (2013). Social media engagement and public health communication: Implications for public health organizations being truly social. *Public Health Reviews, 35*(1), 13.

Hou, Q., Han, M., & Cai, Z. (2020). Survey on data analysis in social media: A practical application aspect. *Big Data Mining and Analytics, 3*(4), 259–279. https://doi.org/10.26599/BDMA.2020.9020006.

Kawonga, M. (2015). Exploring the use of social network analysis to measure communication between disease programme and district managers at sub-national level in South Africa. *Social Science and Medicine, 135,* 1–14.

Khosla, N. (2016). Analysing collaboration among HIV agencies through combining network theory and relational coordination. *Social Science and Medicine, 150,* 85–94.

Klofstad, C. A., Sokhey, A. E., & McClurg, S. D. (2013). Disagreeing about disagreement: How conflict in social networks affects political behavior. *American Journal of Political Science, 57*(1), 120–134.

Krempel, L., & Plumper, T. (2003). Exploring the dynamics of international trade by combining the comparative advantages of multivariate statistics and network visualizations. *Journal of social structure, 4*(1), 1–22.

Kuamri, S., & Babu, C. N. (2017). Real time analysis of social media data to understand people emotions towards national parties. In *8th International Conference on Computing, Communication and Networking Technologies (ICCCNT)* (pp. 1–6). Delhi, India. https://doi.org/10.1109/ICCCNT.2017.8204059.

Lamb, A., Paul, M. J., & Dredze, M. (2013). Separating fact from fear: Tracking u infections on Twitter. In *North American Chapter of the Association for Computational Linguistics (NAACL)* (pp. 789–795).

Lampos, V., & Cristianini, N. (2010). Tracking the u pandemic by monitoring the social web. In *2010 2nd International Workshop on Cognitive Information Processing, CIP2010* (pp. 411–416).

Lewis, K., Kaufman, J., Gonzalez, M., Wimmer, A., & Christakis, N. (2008). Tastes, ties, and time: A new social network dataset using Facebook.com. *Social Networks, 30*(4), 330–342.

Longstaff, B., Reddy, S., & Estrin, D. (2010). Improving activity classification for health applications on mobile devices using active and semi-supervised learning. In *4th International Conference on no permissions Pervasive Computing Technologies for Healthcare (PervasiveHealth)* (pp. 1–7). IEEE.

Miluzzo, E., Lane, N., Fodor, K., Peterson, R., Eisenman, S., Lu, H., Musolesi, M., Zheng, X., & Campbell, A. (2008). Sensing meets mobile social networks: The design, implementation and evaluation of the cenceme application. In *SenSys*.

Moorhead, S. A. (2013). A new dimension of health care: Systematic review of the uses, benefits, and limitations of social media for health communication. *Journal of Medical Internet Research, 15*(4), e85.

Morgan, E. M. (2010). Image and video disclosure of substance use on social media websites. *Computers in Human Behavior, 26*(6), 1405–1411. Online interactivity: Role of technology in behavior change (2010).

Newman, M. E. J. (2003). The structure and function of complex networks. *SIAM Review 45*(2), 167–256.

Paul, M. J., & Dredze, M. (2011). You are what you Tweet: Analyzing Twitter for public health. In *International Conference on Weblogs and Social Media (ICWSM)*

Rubinov, M., & Sporns, O. (2010). Complex network measures of brain connectivity: Uses and interpretations. *Neuroimage, 52*(3), 1059–1069.

Sadilek, A., Kautz, H., & Silenzio, V. (2012a). Modeling spread of disease from social interactions. In *International Conference on Weblogs and Social Media (ICWSM)* (pp. 322–329).

Sadilek, A., Kautz, H., & Silenzio, V. (2012b). Predicting disease transmission from geo-tagged micro-blog data. In *AAAI Conference on Artificial Intelligence (AAAI)*.

Santillana, M. (2014). Using clinicians' search query data to monitor influenza epidemics. *Clinical Infectious Diseases, 59*(10), 1446–1450.

Schoen, Martin W. (2014). Social network analysis of public health programs to measure partnership. *Social Science and Medicine, 123,* 90–95.

Smolinski, M. S., Crawley, A. W., Baltrusaitis, K., Chunara, R., Olsen, J. M., Wojick, O., Santillana, M., Nguyen, A.T., & Brownstein, J. S. (2015). Flu Near You: Crowdsourced symptom reporting spanning two influenza seasons. *American Journal of Public Health*.

Soulakis, Nicholas D. (2015). Visualizing collaborative electronic health record usage for hospitalized patients with heart failure. *Journal of the American Medical Informatics Association?: JAMIA, 22,* 299–311.

Thackeray, R., Neiger, B. L., Hanson, C. L., & McKenzie, J. F. (2008). Enhancing pro-motional strategies within social marketing programs: Use of web 2.0 social media. *Health Promotion Practice, 9*(4), 338–343.

Wang, Z., Joo, V., Tong, C., & Chan, D. (2014). Issues of social data analytics with a new method for sentiment analysis of social media data. In *2014 IEEE 6th International Conference on Cloud Computing Technology and Science, Singapore, 2014* (pp. 899–904). https://doi.org/10.1109/CloudCom.2014.40.

Wang, F., Srinivasan, U., Uddin, S., & Chawla, S. (2014). Application of network analysis on healthcare. In *Advances in Social Networks Analysis and Mining (ASONAM)* (pp. 596–603).

Wasserman, S. (1994). *Social network analysis: Methods and applications* (Vol. 8). Cambridge university press.

Watts, D. (2004). *Six degrees: The science of a connected age.* Norton

Wicks, P. (2011). Accelerated clinical discovery using self-reported patient data collected online and a patient-matching algorithm. *Nature Biotechnology, 29*(5), 411–414.

Wu, Y. (2014). Social network analysis of international scientific collaboration on psychiatry research. *International Journal of Mental Health Systems.*

Yazdavar, A. H., Mahdavinejad, M. S., Bajaj, G., Thirunarayan, K., Pathak, J., & Sheth, A. (2018). Mental health analysis via social media data. In *2018 IEEE International Conference on Healthcare Informatics (ICHI)* (pp. 459–460). New York, NY, USA. https://doi.org/10.1109/ICHI.2018.00102.

Yoshimitsu, T. (2016). Social network analysis of duplicative prescriptions: One-month analysis of medical facilities in Japan. *Health Policy, 120,* 334–341.

Challenges and Limitations of Social Data Analysis Approaches

Safikureshi Mondal◉ and **Zeenat Rehena**◉

Abstract Health data are not only generated from different healthcare environments. They are also obtained from society itself such as through sensor monitoring and Internet of Things (IoT). The social environment is the new source for health data that allows information to be obtained at all community levels in public health. Many academics and practitioners use social data in different areas of public health and warn against the native uses of social data. There are some limitations, however, such as biases or inaccuracies that occur at the source of the data and in processing, as well as challenges which need improvement for a better quality of life of the population. The challenges of social data analysis approaches, data management and processing, social sensors and IoT devices are significant for public health. Also, important concerns like methodological limitations, ethical concerns and unexpected consequences are often overlooked when social data is used in public health. Self-reported data, the size of data and the reliability of third-party social data are concerns resulting in technical or methodological limitations. Reliability, the utility of web intelligence and decision-making are the important issues for the use of social data in analysis approaches. Public health data and user interaction are the important issues that have to be taken into account in social data analysis approaches as they concern the ethical side of the use of such data. Other issues from data collection to social data analysis approaches are also reported. This survey addresses all the challenges and limitations faced by different researchers and practitioners in the use of social health data in public health.

Keywords Social data analysis · Challenges · Limitations · Ethics · Public health

S. Mondal (✉)
Narula Institute of Technology, Kolkata, India
e-mail: msafi.cse@gmail.com

Z. Rehena
Aliah University, Kolkata, India
e-mail: zeenatrehena@yahoo.co.in

1 Introduction

Social data are generated from different software like social media platform recom-mendation, Question–Answer sites and collaborative sites or search platforms. These social platforms are used for the purpose of keeping in touch with friends, such as via Twitter, Pinterest or Facebook (Lampe 2008). Information can also be obtained from search engines (White 2013; Tufekci 2014). There are so many applications where social data are used such as (Ehrlich and Shami 2010) food (Abbar et al. 2015), health (Counts et al. 2014) and relations (Rama et al. 2014). After the initial success of Google Flu Trends (Ginsberg et al. 2009), the use of social data analysis is increasing in public health. But, there is not enough research work being carried out for social data analysis (Babbie 2016).

An unbelievable revolution is occurring in the public health domain due to the growing availability and accessibility of health data resources and the tremendous growth of technological development. Health dataset analysis can help early outbreak detection, improve diagnosis and shorten the time to market the drugs. But, extracting the knowledge from health data is a very important challenge due to unstructured health data and the lack of contexts and privacy algorithms in public health. Society gets help through the collection and analysis of the information generated (social data) from the social environment, via, for example, social networks, forums, chatrooms, social sensors, the Internet of Things (IoT) devices, surveillance systems and virtual worlds. These generated social data can be analysed and applied to benefit public health, thus allowing improvement in the quality of life of the population as well as reducing economic costs. Policymakers, researchers, health professionals and managers from public health research are still attempting with limited success to acquire health information upon which to base their decisions.

The new opportunities for research come with limitations regarding the use of social data and process in the public health domain. There are two important basic challenges found in public health:

1. When computer scientists are trying to develop health applications and use them to handle social data in the public health domain, they are faced with a lot of unfamiliar health data practices and conversations.
2. Healthcare researchers have no confidence in existing practices and methods of social data analysis, even after working for a long time in public healthcare.

Except for these two, there are a lot of challenges categorized as general methodolog-ical or related to data sources, process and analysis and ethical issues. The chapter will discuss the challenges and limitations of social data in public health, as shown in Fig. 1. This survey is intended for researchers, practitioners and health researchers who want to work on social data analytics in public health.

The rest of the chapter is organized as follows. The general challenges and limita-tions of social data analysis approaches are discussed in Sect. 2. Other issues of social data analysis, including collection, are discussed in Sect. 3. There is a discussion on the practical implementation of social data in Sect. 4. The chapter is concluded in Sect. 5.

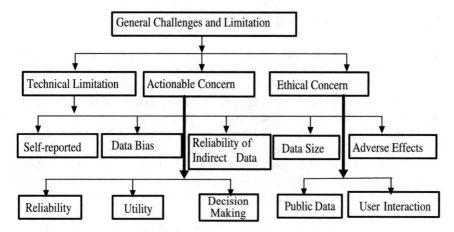

Fig. 1 General challenges and limitations

2 General Challenges

In this section, general challenges in social data analysis approaches in public health are discussed. The challenges can be categorized as the technical limitations of methodological challenges, actionable concerns and ethical concerns.

2.1 *Technical Limitations*

Social data are not perfect or not sufficiently complete that the data can be used in health research; the derivation of health data from these data is also imperfect. There is no reliability to make a decision from the creation to collection of data from public health application. These are very important concerns when using social data in public health. All the procedures of collection and creation of data without health applications are poorly biased, which are considered reliable for the patient and public health decisions. Since 2003, researchers have been investigating the use of web search engines in the health domain to obtain information (Eysenbach and Kohler 2004). There are lots of review works (Watts 2008; Ginsberg et al. 2009; Harford 2014; Broniatowski et al. 2013; Althouse et al. 2015) that address the challenges and limitations of social data in public healthcare. Some research has already been done on the common research limitations and challenges (Ruths and Pfefer 2014; Shah et al. 2015; Tufekci 2014; Mowery 2016) which are discussed only in social media research. In this section, the major technical challenges and limitations are discussed.

2.1.1 Self-Organizing or Self-Reported Data

Social data are generated from various social platforms and these are mainly self-reported or self-organizing data. Some problems arise when user's self-reports are passive rather than active, such as users who do not give information or do not respond in a timely way to a survey. Users may give misinformation on health conditions or health behaviour due to forgetfulness, self-diagnosis or complex medical terms.

In a research study (Mowery 2016), it was stated that approximately 40% of flu tweets on Twitter were diagnosed. Two other research papers corroborated this in Newell et al. (1999) and Saunders et al. (2011) show that there is no reliability in self-reported social data compared to intended dimensions and that self-diagnosis noise differs between groups and other factors. Also, users of social platforms are not always keen to report their health status. For example, for influenza, sexually transmitted diseases and mental health cases, users of social platforms are always less reported than unreported cases and these are the good examples of limitation of passive surveillance. There are positive and negative instances on Twitter.

Mohan et al. (2013) and Rubin (1976) show that Twitter users always speak the truth if they have flu. This is called data missing not at random (MNAR). In (Rubin 1976), it has been shown that there will always be a bias in a set of people in a group who wish to share information. Such as it is shown that for the privacy differ by age group. Another issue found with self-reported social data concerns medical terminology. Users do not always use the same medical terminology for reporting their health information. Flu and influenza are the same health condition but are different medical terminology. In (Nie et al. 2014a, b; Pimpalkhute et al. 2014), formal and informal terms to highlight this gap between medical professionals and Twitter users have been researched. In this research (Pimpalkhute et al. 2014), users were found to use phonetic spelling to solve the difficulty of drug names. In another research (Gesualdo et al. 2013; Velardi et al. 2014), Twitter-based influenza surveillance was used to focus on symptoms rather specific illness in reports.

2.1.2 Data Bias

Data quality is an important issue which varies with the analytic task and it is bound by the type of questions that can be answered with a dataset, whether it is valid or not. Social data suffers from noise, representativeness and bias. The noise of social data is referred to as the content of the data which is not reliable, or is credible and incomplete, or has typo graphical errors and so on. Data bias is an important challenge which is defined as systematic distortion in the data.

A lot of bias can affect the representation of social data (Ruths and Pfefer 2014). Social data and analysis bias issues can affect analysis research. This should be addressed and the bias removed. Some of the common sources of bias are studied here. First, there are several user-dependent factors that can influence the social data due to its direct origin in the user. Due to reduced knowledge, reports and discussions cannot be trusted on social platforms, especially if there is an uncommon disease with uncommon users. The nature of a discussion can affect the nature of the topic. Some conditions can be under-represented like a cold or sexually transmitted diseases due to privacy issues. Also external factors can increase topics which are induced in the data. Researchers must understand the factors that influence heath topics. Collected data can be influenced by user demographics (Gesualdo et al. 2013). Social platforms cannot represent the interests of the population appropriately (Velardi et al. 2014). Thus, there is a lack of demographic representation in social data representation.

Social data is not direct health information or data which is given by a user. Rather it is passive, which means that social data can be collected by searches for particular health information like medication or different diseases. The analytical results may be influenced by the data collection method. Platforms can allow both the unbiased and biased collection of data. For example, in Twitter, all messages can be omitted to find a keyword in all tweets. Also Facebook allows the collection of public messages even though most of the messages are private. Some studies have been done of common biases in social media as described in Paul et al. (2015b). Analytic methods like machine learning, statistical analysis and natural language processing can introduce bias. Discussion of these biases and comparison to other data types place these concerns in perspective. Consider telephone surveys, the bedrock of modern public health research. While results from telephone surveys comprise the primary data source for numerous public health topics, they also suffer from numerous biases (Mac Kim et al. 2016; Lazer et al. 2014b; Clark et al. 2016). Thus, data biases and other data quality issues arise regarding data collection, processing and data creation. The data biases can be categorized from the perspective of the cause of distortion without knowing the origin. The data biases include population bias, behavioural bias, linking bias and temporal variations.

2.1.3 Reliability of Third-Party Data

There are several drawbacks that can be seen regarding the data which are owned by third parties like Google and Twitter. Third-party data collection is an important concern for scientific reproducibility. It happens sometimes that the generated raw query from query logs is proprietary and that cannot be shared with other owners. It may be available for a certain time for study but not later. As, for example, tweet data can be available for a while but not so after deletion. Also, there is no control over third-party data which is a drawback. Changes of user behaviour can affect the process of the interpretation of data. Also updating platforms can alter the type of social data which was user created. In Belkin et al. (2003), user faced an issue that length of queries can be affected while choice a design of a search interfaces. Another issue arises concerning the variations across platforms which are used in different ways and with different populations. Thus, one built model cannot be applied to another.

Thus, the selection of data and how to build the research for these data sources should be kept in mind.

2.1.4   Data Size

The combination of unstructured and semi-structured data as heterogeneous data are generated from web applications and these data are called big data. But unfortunately only a small percentage of data is health-related data, and even that only concerns a single health issue. Thus, for a small percentage of health data or a single health issue, it is difficult to study the health issue in a population. In (Gesualdo et al. 2013), it has been found that there are much more tweets in USA but less in a city.

Another issue concerns the size of the samples of health data. For example, only 1% of data is available for all the sampled data on Twitter and Facebook. This percentage of data can available by not only random or statistical model basis. Instead data filtered for specific keywords can introduce further bias in the results in social data analysis approaches.

Also, data collection from social platforms can influence social data approaches. In a research paper, Velardi et al. (2014) performed a comparison among many Twitter data collection techniques to show the biasness to demographic interference. It is to be concluded from all these cases that concern must be taken with data collection procedures, sources of data and influencing methods that affect the result.

2.1.5   Adverse Concerns or Effects

The quality of data sources depends upon coordinated efforts by the group who have taken part in interaction on a social platform (Lazer et al. 2014b). In a research paper, (Clark et al. 2016) author showed that 70–80% of tweets mentioning e-cigarettes were posted by automated accounts which creates problems in under-standing the public regarding e-cigarettes. The presence of those accounts compli-cates the analysis of the resulting data. In (Nie et al. 2014a), a search filter to retrieve the e-cigarette-related tweets by keyword search has been developed. In (Allem and Ferrara 2016), it has been found that failure to exclude tweets from automated accounts distorts insights derived from the data. For Google Flu Trends (GFT), any-one can increase the flu estimates by creating many flu queries from multiple user accounts. This phenomenon can be found in a marketing campaign for influenza-related medical products. This type of fake concern can be addressed, by not sharing the list of search terms that are used in the GFT model.

2.2   Actionability Concern

There are some action-ability concerns and questions that must be addressed in public health. Such as how social media platforms are used by public health authorities and practitioners, how trustworthy social media platforms are and what happens if these systems fail.

2.2.1 Reliability of Web Intelligence

The action-ability of public health based on social data is limited reliability of the system prediction and quality of the data. Data reliability is important for disease surveillance. Negative results come from poor predictions of epidemics. Early diagnosis of disease outburst is very important for mitigating its spread and effect.

Much research has proved that digital systems fail to detect crises in public health. For example, a swine flu outbreak in North America in 2009 and an ebola outbreak in West Africa in 2014 (Allem and Ferrara 2016; Ruths and Pfefer 2014).

Not only the failure to detect an outbreak, but also unnecessary action taken in an epidemic has negative consequences. For example, mass immunization increases costs (http://foreignpolicy.com 2020) and immunization campaigns can erode public health trust (Krause 2006). All these limitations and concerns relate to traditional surveillance but in the case of digital surveillance, which involves the same actions, care and more research are needed to ensure the reliability of these systems. Another limitation is the validation of social data. In (Doshi 2009), authors show that informal data from social media data creates problems of validation. Many researchers concluded that social data analysis techniques can be done with both traditional and digital techniques.

2.2.2 Utility of Web Intelligence

Another concern of social data analysis is that the amount of utility that social data offers beyond traditional data.

In (Blouin-Genest and Miller 2017), it has been pointed out that the surveillance of influenza must be improved little bit so as to use reliable social data, though traditional data is perfectly accurate for the same purpose.

In (Lazer et al. 2014b; Dugas et al. 2012), the authors aimed to show that forecast accuracy can be improved so as to use either type of data alone. In so many papers, it is shown that there is much more utility for locations that do not conduct formal surveillance (Olson et al. 2013; Paul et al. 2015a). Also, other authors argue that social data is used in behavioural medicine more than disease surveillance, such as the example of the prevalence of behaviour in smoking surveys.

2.2.3 Decision-Making and Intervention

There is always a challenge with social data as to how to proceed with social media information, even when the social platform delivers important and reliable data. Always it should be noted that policy-makers and health officials need to find the web-based data sources to incorporate into decision models. Another decision involves pursuing intervention with individuals. Suppose an algorithm found that a person has poor mental health and something can be done for the support of this person and simple, non-arguable interventions are in place. How and when to perform such interventions are the difficult questions that will need to be addressed.

2.3 Ethical Considerations

There are so many ethical challenges in using social data (Broniatowski et al. 2015; Benton et al. 2017; boyd and Crawford 2012; Conway 2014; McKee 2013; Mikal et al. 2016). There are two important ethical issues which arise in public health, which are mentioned below:

1. Users' data.
2. Health data, particularly sensitive information.

Data are made public for particular reasons. Users share their public data under the terms of service agreed when first using social media platforms. The Institutional Review Board (IRB) guidelines govern research ethics in the USA for the use of social data publicly; after that there is no interaction between the user and this public data. Ethics research needs to be developed in the fields of medicine and the public health domain. A study and summary of community's current behaviour towards the ethics of social media platforms are shown in Vayena et al. (2015). In the following some ethical issues of social data analysis research are discussed.

2.3.1 Public Data

One of the important and difficult ethical research issues is related to public data (Golder et al. 2017). The current research of public data does not require informed consent according to IRB guidelines. This means that the owner of social public data may not be aware that their data is public or they cannot be want to create it public. Many social platforms, especially Facebook, have been criticized for having unclear privacy management systems. A lot of directions are unclear to differentiate the boundaries between public and private data research in public health.

1. First, users may not be aware that their data is fully public and accessible. Many users want privacy within their discussions and forums and other communities.
2. Second, if a user does not want privacy, they may not wish their data to be used for all possible purposes. Liu et al. (2011) show that users of online communities react negatively if the data is used for research. Hudson and Bruckman (2004) conducted a survey with Twitter users for diagnosed histories of depression and found that they had alternatively a positive view.
3. Another issue arises when public data is used for the research of private health information. Statistical and machine learning approaches can be used to conclude that a user has an illness based on public data, even when the user was not

willing to share their information publicly. There are so many papers demonstrating that analysis of social data from users can be used to detect mental health conditions (Coppersmith et al. 2014b; De Choudhury et al. 2013b).

Therefore, strong reasons are required for treating public data as private data. Thus, it is necessary to offer policies that are not too restrictive and allow for research work using social data to balance privacy concerns as well ethics.

2.3.2 User Interaction

For the interactions of researchers and social media users, ethical considerations and research protocols are required, like the full IRB review (Prieto et al. 2014). The direct recruitment of social media users needs to be studied, and there is no clear ethical answers for conducting studies. Thus, the uses of social data in public health pose complex ethical questions on data use, and the answers remain significantly debatable.

3 Other Issues for Social Data Analysis

There are many issues to be dealt with regarding social data in public health, from health data collection to the analyses of data, as shown in Fig. 2. There are four processes shown in this figure: data collection, data processing, analysing and assessment or results. In this section all the issues are discussed in general which are in the public health domain.

3.1 Issues of Social Data Collection

The selection of data sources or procedures to collect the data acquired and prepared is introduced as one of the limitations of social data analysis approaches. This happens when a certain data source affects the observations or datasets are affected by their source for platform reasons.

3.1.1 Data Acquisition

At the time of data acquisition, errors can be occurring and this must be accounted for at the collection time. Many social media platforms can't collect the data by third parties. Also, in some programs, social data can be accessed from a platform only with limitations. An Application Programmer Interface (API) can access the data with setting some quantity of data that can be collected. The platform can't capture

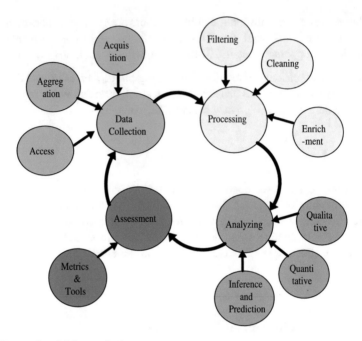

Fig. 2 Issues of social data analysis

all the relevant social data or user actions. Sometimes platforms may not provide access to all the data they capture.

3.1.2 Data Access

Access to social data can be made through API which defines the criteria for selecting, ranking and getting the data. These criteria constitute a filter in the form of a query with different APIs expressing this query. APIs have limited expressiveness regarding the data needed from queries.

3.1.3 Data Filtering

Data filtering is used for the removal of irrelevant portions of data. Removing outliers is one of the filtering steps which is used to remove inactive or unnaturally active accounts from a dataset and for the inactive user or accounts does not mean that they ignoring such users which lead to misguide the conclusion. For text filtering, words with pronouns, articles or prepositions can be there and these words may embed useful contain and filtering these text nay be big issue.

3.1.4 Data Aggregation

Data aggregation can be done by structure, organize and transform data which are either hide or prominence to distinct, even divergent, patterns of social data. These factors can be an issue for social data analysis approaches.

3.2 Issues for Processing Data

Data processing operations can be considered as cleaning, enrichment and data aggregations; building a data processing framework can affect data organization and distort datasets by altering the content and structure.

3.2.1 Data Cleaning

Data cleaning refers to relevant data representation by correction or substitution or incomplete or missing values. For this, results can be misleading or contain incorrect data patterns due to embedding important data. It involves mapping items from different sources to a common representation. This mapping affects the analysis result.

3.2.2 Data Enrichment

Data enrichment is done by adding annotations to data items of automatic classifications or human annotations which are both liable to error. Human annotations can be affected by certain factors which are given below:

– Unreliable annotators.
– Poor annotation guidelines.
– Poor category design.

Automatic annotation can be done by statistical and machine learning methods to enrich data. Natural language processing helps to process text and it can be complex. Machine learning or natural language processing are not 100%.

3.3 Issues Analysing Data

Analysing refers to pre- and post-analysing might be pitched the results. Deselecting an appropriate method is often characterized by different strengths and weaknesses. Due to the variations of data analysis methodologies and measurements, distinct approaches can be characterized by different strengths and weaknesses. Thus, it is always important to choose the right analysing method at the right time and the right place.

3.3.1 Qualitative and Quantitative Analysis

Qualitative analysis is used to analyse and extract trends from the data or support predictive modelling. But quantitative analysis can be done for the processing of large volumes of data. The basic goal of qualitative analysis is to understand the content by analysing social media data and providing more in-depth understanding of the data than quantitative methods that provide only aggregate trends. Nagar et al. (2014) and Heaivilin et al. (2011) show that for understanding Twitter-based influenza research, content-based analysis of tweets messages is performed during influenza epidemics. The combined method of qualitative and quantitative analysis is called a mixed-method. An example of qualitative analysis for social data analysis is pain related which is identifying medical mistakes in Twitter (Nakhasi et al. 2012; Agapie et al. 2013).

3.3.2 Descriptive Statistics

Descriptive statistics analysis is the foundation of studies where social data are quantitatively depicted with summaries of quantities such as the average number of messages for user demographics and geographical distribution of messages. This type of analysis method measures the distribution and correlations among variables of interest. The main goal is to summarize the datasets though they may harbour the important details that may mislead the user into a wrong conclusion. Social data research often relies on counting entities and a simple count can mislead for unlearning what is counted and why it is counted. Failing the distinction of volume based trends or uses language, may lead to bias and affect the validity of the study. Count based and correlation analyses are sensitive to bias and co-founders and issues with construct validity.

3.3.3 Inference and Prediction

There are so many limiting factors as inference and prediction like uncontrolled co-founders, bias in testing datasets and dealing with ambiguous cases. Performances can be varied across and within social datasets. Also the data samples of the composition of test and training datasets impact the results. In data analysis, the distinct target variables, class labels or representation of data may lead to different results. There are other issues where the inference task can be misguided regarding choosing an objective function.

3.3.4 Metrics and Tools

Social data analysis approach challenges exist for the evaluation and interpretation of findings. Metrics and tools can be used to quantify performance though they can suffer from reliability and validity issues. There are many issues related with metrics used for the analysis of social data. Another issue is that domain-specific performance indicators are not used much.

3.3.5 Assessment and Interpretation

There are some issues around result assessment and interpretation after social data analysis. The assumption of online social traces reflects in several ways real-world facts; this assumption can be a challenge due to the issues of construct validity and stability. The meaning of a social trace may change with context. The analysis should not be confined in a single dataset or method and should go beyond social data analysis studies.

4 Social Data in Real-World Applications

For the development of social data analysis, many real-world applications are built, such as Disease Spread Indicator (Sun et al. 2020), Crowdsensing-based Disease Tracking (Haddawy et al. 2015) and UAV-based Health Surveillance and Alerting (Minaeian et al. 2015). Disease Spread Indicator is used to analyse the COVID-19 disease from social media posts. In this application, a real-time data crawler collects people's opinions about disease tweets from Twitter. After that, these tweets are filtered and classified into some discrete categories. The categorized topics include the regions where people are most affected, when people realized the first symptom, the age at which the disease affected them most, the speed of the authorities, response and whether people were communicating to each other regarding the recovery of patients. After that the categorized or labelled Twitter data are analysed and trained on a server. This server constructs reliable information from the large, complex, unstructured data which is analysed by AI algorithms like Long-Term Memory networks or Gated Recurrent Units (GRU) (Ma et al. 2016). Finally, a smartphone app or website will give the alert or warnings to end users regarding disease spreading.

5 Conclusion

Social data analysis is a new emerging research area and has been started to be used for public health monitoring. It has seen growing interest regarding practitioners and researchers on social data analysis in public health for the last 3 years. Thus, a concrete survey is required on the challenges and limitations to focusing social data research on public health for future work. In this chapter, general challenges have been discussed, focusing on the social data analysis research in public health; all the issues have been reported while social data is used from social data collection to analysis in public healthcare.

References

Abbar, S., Mejova, Y., & Weber, Y. (2015). You Tweet what you eat: Studying food consumption through Twitter. In *Proceedings of CHI*.

Agapie, E., Golovchinsky, G., & Qvarfordt, P. (2013). Leading people to longer queries. In *Conference on human factors in computing systems (CHI)*.

Allem, J. -P., & Ferrara, E. (2016). The importance of debiasing social media data to better understand e-cigarette-related attitudes and behaviors. *Journal of Medical Internet Research, 18*(8).

Althouse, B. M., Scarpino, S. V., Meyers, L. A., Ayers, J. W., Bargsten, M., Baumbach, J., et al. (2015). Enhancing disease surveillance with novel data treams: Challenges and opportunities. *EPJ Data Science, 4*(1), 17.

Babbie, R. (2016). *The practice of social research*. Wadsworth Publishing Company, 14th edn.

Baltrusaitis, K., Santillana, M., Crawley, W. A., Chunara, R., Smolinski, M., & Brownstein, S. J. (2017). Determinants of participant' follow-up and characterization of representativeness in Flu Near You, a participatory disease surveillance system. *JMIR Public Health Surveillance, 3*(2), e18.

Belkin, N. J., Kelly, D., Kim, G., Kim, J.-Y., Lee, H. -J., Muresan, G., Tang, M. -C., Yuan, X. -J., & Cool, C. (2003). Query length in interactive information retrieval. In *Conference on research and development in information retrieval (SIGIR)*.

Benton, A., Coppersmith, G., & Dredze, M. (2017). Ethical research protocols for social media health research. In *EACL workshop on ethics in natural language processing*.

Benton, A., Coppersmith, G., & Dredze, M. (2017). Ethical research protocols for social media health research. In *EACL workshop on ethics in natural language processing*.

Blouin-Genest, G., & Miller, A. (2017). The politics of participatory epidemiology: Technologies, social media and inuenza surveillance in the US. *Health Policy and Technology, 6*(2), 192–197.

Blumberg, S. J., & Luke, J. V. (2007). Coverage bias in traditional telephone surveys of low-income and young adults. *Public Opinion Quarterly, 71*(5), 734–749.

Boyd, D., & Crawford, K. (2012). Critical questions for big data. *Information, Communication & Society, 15*(5).

Broniatowski, D. A., Paul, M. J., & Dredze, M. (2013). National and local inuenza surveillance through Twitter: An analysis of the 2012–2013 inuenza epidemic. *PLoS ONE, 8*(12).

Broniatowski, D. A., Dredze, M., Paul, J. M., & Dugas, A. (2015). Using social media to perform local inuenza surveillance in an inner-city hospital: A retrospective observational study. *JMIR Public Health Surveillance, 1*(1), e5.

Chew, C., & Eysenbach, G. (2010). Pandemics in the age of Twitter: Content analysis of tweets during the 2009 H1N1 outbreak. *PLoS ONE, 5*(11), e14118.

Clark, E. M., Jones, C. A., Williams, J. R., Kurti, A. N., Norotsky, M. C., Danforth, C. M., & Dodds, P. S. (2016). Vaporous marketing: Uncovering pervasive electronic cigarette advertisements on Twitter. *PLoS ONE, 11*(7), e0157304.

Conway, M. (2014). Ethical issues in using Twitter for public health surveillance and research: Developing a taxonomy of ethical concepts from the research literature. *Journal of Medical Internet Research, 16*(12).

Cook, S., Conrad, C., Fowlkes, A. L., and Mohebbi, M. H. (2011).: Assessing Google Flu Trends performance in the United States during the. (2009). Inuenza virus A (H1N1) pandemic. *PLoS ONE, 6*(8), e23610.

Coppersmith, G., Dredze, M., & Harman, C. (2014b). Quantifying mental health signals in Twitter. In *ACL Workshop on Computational Linguistics and Clinical Psychology (CLPsych)*.

Counts, S., Choudhury, M. D., Diesner, J., Gilbert, E., Gonzalez, M., Keegan, B., Naaman, M., & Wallach, H. (2014). *Computational social science: CSCW in the social media era.* In *Proceedings of CSCW Companion.*

De Choudhury, M., Counts, S., & Horvitz, E. (2013). Predicting postpartum changes in emotion and behavior via social media. *Conference on Human Factors in Compu-ting Systems (CHI)* (pp. 3267–3276). New York: NY, USA.

Doshi, P. (2009). Calibrated response to emerging infections. *BMJ, 339,* b3471.

Dugas, A. F., Hsieh, Y. H., Levin, S. R., Pines, J. M., Mareiniss, D. P., Mohareb, A., et al. (2012). Google Flu trends: Correlation with emergency department inuenza rates and crowding metrics. *Clinical Infectious Diseases, 54*(4), 463–469.

Ehrlich, K., & Shami, S. N. (2010). Microblogging inside and outside the workplace. In *Proceedings of ICWSM.*

Eysenbach, G., & Kohler, C. (2004). Health-related searches on the internet. *JAMA,291*(24), 2946–2946.

Gesualdo, F., Stilo, G., Agricola, E., & Gonantini, M. V., Pandol, E., Velardi, P., & Tozzi, A. E. (2013). Inuenza like illness surveillance on Twitter through automated learning of native language. *PLoS ONE,8*(12), e82489.

Ginsberg, J., Mohebbi, M. H., Patel, R. S, Brammer, L., Smolinski, M. S., & Brilliant, L. (2009). Detecting influenza epidemics using search engine query data. *Nature, 457,* 7232 (2009).

Ginsberg, J., Mohebbi, M. H., Patel, R. S., Brammer, L., Smolinski, M. S., & Brilliant, L. (2009). Detecting inuenza epidemics using search engine query data. *Nature, 457*(7232), 1012–1014.

Goel, S., Hofman, J. M., & Sirer, M. I. (2012). Who does what on the web: A large-scale study of browsing behavior. In *International conference on weblogs and social media (ICWSM).*

Golder, S., Ahmed, S., Norman, G., & Booth, A. (2017). Attitudes toward the ethics of research using social media: A systematic review. *Journal of Medical Internet Research, 19*(6), e195.

Haddawy, P., Frommberger, L., Kauppinen, T., De Felice, G., Charkratpahu, P., Saengpao, S., & Kanchanakitsakul, P. (2015). Situation awareness in crowdsensing for disease surveillance in crisis situations. In *Proceedings of the seventh international conference on information and communication technologies and development.*

Harford, T. (2014). Big data: A big mistake? *Significance, 11*(5), 14–19.

Heaivilin, N., Gerbert, B., Page, J. E., & Gibbs, J. L. (2011). Public health surveillance of dental pain via Twitter. *Journal of Dental Research, 90*(9), 1047–1051.

Hudson, J. M., & Bruckman, A. (2004). Go away: Participant objections to being studied and the ethics of chatroom research. *The Information Society, 20*(2), 127–139.

Iannacchione, V. G. (2011). The changing role of address-based sampling in survey research. *Public Opinion Quarterly, 75*(3), 556–575.

Kempf, A. M. and Remington, P. L. (2007). New challenges for telephone survey research in the twenty-first century. *Annual Review of Public Health, 28,* 113–126.

Krause, R. (2006). The swine u episode and the fog of epidemics. *Emerging Infectious Diseases, 12*(1), 40–43.

Lampe, C., Ellison, B. E., & Steinfield, C. (2008). Changes in use and perception of Facebook. In *Proceedings of CSCW.*

Lazer, D., Kennedy, R., King, G., & Vespignani, A. (2014a). Google Flu trends still appears sick: An evaluation of the 2013–2014 u season. https://gking.harvard.edu/files/gking/files/ssrn-id2408560_2.pdf.

Lazer, D., Kennedy, R., King, G., & Vespignani, A. (2014). The parable of Google Flu: Traps in big data analysis. *Science, 343*(6167), 1203–1205.

Leetaru, K. (2014). Why big data missed the early warning signs of ebola.

Liu, Y., Gummadi, K. P., Krishnamurthy, B., & Mislove, A. (2011). Analyzing Facebook privacy settings: User expectations vs. reality. In *ACM SIGCOMM conference on internet measurement conference* (pp. 61–70).

Ma, J., Gao, W., Mitra, P., Kwon, S., Jansen, B. J., Wong, K. F., & Cha, M. (2016). Detecting rumors from microblogs with recurrent neural networks. In *Proceedings of the 25th international joint conference on artificial intelligence (IJCAI 2016)*.

Mac Kim, S., Wan, S., Paris, C., Jin, B., & Robinson, B. (2016). The effects of data collection methods in Twitter. In *Workshops on natural language processing and computational social science (NLP+CSS)* (p. 86).

McKee, R. (2013). Ethical issues in using social media for health and health care research. *Health Policy, 110*(2–3), 298–301.

Mikal, J., Hurst, S., & Conway, M. (2016). Ethical issues in using Twitter for population-level depression monitoring: A qualitative study. *BMC Medical Ethics, 17*(1), 1.

Minaeian, S., Liu, J., Son, Y.J.: Vision-based target detection and localization via a team of cooperative UAV and UGVs. *IEEE Transactions on systems, man, and cybernetics: systems 46*(7) (2015)

Mislove, A., Lehmann, S., Ahn, Y. -Y., Onnela, J. -P., & Rosenquist, J. N. (2011). Understanding the demographics of Twitter users. In *International Conference on weblogs and social media (ICWSM)* (pp. 554–557).

Mohan, K., Pearl, J., & Tian, J. (2013). Graphical models for inference with missing data. In *Advances in Neural Information Processing Systems (NIPS)*, (pp. 1277–1285).

Mowery, J. (2016). Twitter inuenza surveillance: Quantifying seasonal misdiagnosis patterns and their impact on surveillance estimates. *Online Journal of Public Health Informatics, 8*(3), e198.

Nagar, R., Yuan, Q., Freifeld, C. C., Santillana, M., Nojima, A., Chunara, R., & Brownstein, J. S. (2014). A case study of the New York City 2012–2013 inuenza season with daily geocoded Twitter data from temporal and spatiotemporal pers-pectives. *Journal of Medical Internet Research, 16*(10), e236.

Nakhasi, A., Passarella, R. J., Bell, S. G., Paul, M. J., Dredze, M., & Pronovost, P. J. (2012). Malpractice and malcontent: Analyzing medical complaints in Twitter. In *AAAI fall symposium on information retrieval and knowledge discovery in biomedical text*.

Newell, S. A., Girgis, A., Sanson-Fisher, R. W., & Savolainen, N. J. (1999). The accuracy of self-reported health behaviors and risk factors relating to cancer and cardiovascular disease in the general population: A critical review. *American Journal of Preventive Medicine, 17*(3), 211–229.

Nie, L., Akbari, M., Li, T., & Chua, T. -S. (2014b). A joint local-global approach for medical terminology assignment. In *SIGIR workshop on medical information retrieval* (pp. 24–27).

Nie, L., Zhao, Y. -L., Akbari, M., Shen, J., & Chua, T. -S. (2014a). Bridging the vocabulary gap between health seekers and healthcare knowledge. *IEEE Transactions on Knowledge and Data Engineering*.

Olson, D. R., Konty, K. J., Paladini, M., Viboud, C., & Simonsen, L. (2013). Reassessing Google Flu Trends data for detection of seasonal and pandemic inuenza: A comparative epidemiological study at three geographic scales. *PLoS Computational Biology, 9*(10).

Paine, C., Reips, U.-D., Stieger, S., Joinson, A., & Buchanan, T. (2007). Internet users' perceptions of 'privacy concerns' and 'privacy actions'. *International Journal of Human-Computer Studies, 65*(6), 526–536.

Paul, M., Dredze, M., Broniatowski, D., & Generous, N. (2015a). Worldwide inuenza surveillance through Twitter. In *AAAI workshop on the world wide web and public health intelligence*.

Paul, M. J., White, R. W., & Horvitz, E. (2015b). Diagnoses, decisions, and outcomes: Web search as decision support for cancer. In *International conference on World Wide Web (WWW)*.

Pimpalkhute, P., Patki, A., Nikfarjam, A., & Gonzalez, G. (2014). Phonetic spelling filter for keyword selection in drug mention mining from social media. In *AMIA summits on translational science*.

Prieto, V. M., Matos, S., Alvarez, M., Cacheda, F., & Oliveira, J. L. (2014). Twitter: A good place to detect health conditions. *PLoS ONE, 9*(1), e86191.

Rama, V., Garimella, K., & Dai, S. (2014). From "I love you babe" to "leave me alone" romantic relationship breakups on Twitter. In *Social informatics*: Springer.

Retrieved December 15, 2020, from http://foreignpolicy.com/2014/09/26/why-big-data-missed-the-early-warning-signs-of-ebola/.

Rubin, D. B. (1976). Inference and missing data. *Biometrika, 63,* 581–592.

Ruths, D., & Pfefer, J. (2014). Social media for large studies of behavior. *Science, 346*(6213), 1063–1064.

Ruths, D., & Pfefer, J. (2014). Social media for large studies of behavior. *Science, 346*(6213), 1063–1064.

Saunders, T. J., Prince, S. A., & Tremblay, M. S. (2011). Clustering of children's activity behaviour: The use of self-report versus direct measures. *International Journal of Behavioral Nutrition and Physical Activity, 8,* 48.

Shah, D. V., Cappella, J. N., & Neuman, W. R. (2015). Big data, digital media, and computational social science: Possibilities and perils. *The ANNALS of the American Academy of Political and Social Science, 659*(1), 6–13.

Sun, K., Chen, J., & Viboud, C. (2020). Early epidemiological analysis of the coronavirus disease 2019 outbreak based on crowdsourced data: A population-level observational study. The Lancet Digital Health.

Tufekci, Z. (2014). Big questions for social media big data: Representativeness, validity and other methodological pitfalls. In *International Conference on Weblogs and Social Media (ICWSM)*.

Tufekci, Z. (2014). Big questions for social media big data: Representativeness, validity and other methodological pitfalls. In *Proceedings of ICWSM*.

Vayena, E., Salathfe, M., Madof, L. C., & Brownstein, J. S. (2015). Ethical challenges of big data in public health. *PLoS Computational Biology, 11*(2), e1003904.

Velardi, P., Stilo, G., Tozzi, A. E., & Gesualdo, F. (2014). Twitter mining for fine-grained syndromic surveillance. *Artificial Intelligence in Medicine, 61*(3), 153–163.

Watts, G. (2008). Google watches over u. *BMJ: British Medical Journal, 337.*

White, R. (2013). Beliefs and biases in web search. In *Proceedings of SIGIR*.

Reliability, Security and Privacy of Health Data

IoT-Based Secure Health Care: Challenges, Requirements and Case Study

Sohail Saif, Pratik Bhattacharjee, Koushik Karmakar, Ramesh Saha, and Suparna Biswas

Abstract Delivering health care to people has become revolutionizing due to the technological advancement of embedded systems and medical devices. Integration of different health sensors, handheld devices and the Internet can be a great potential for significant improvement of the quality of remote health care. Physiological sensor devices used for monitoring vital signs are gaining popularity. This network of sensor and coordinator devices has led to the growth of Body Sensor Network (BSN). Since patient health information is transmitted through this Body Sensor Network and stored in medical servers, these data are vulnerable to security threats. Security attacks on communication channels or malware in the sensor devices can lead to incorrect data collection by devices which can result in wrong diagnosis and treatment. So the security of health data is of utmost concern which needs to be handled carefully. This chapter intends to discuss recent advancements in security mechanisms to secure health data. This chapter can help the readers to get an overview of secure health care by discussing the traditional architecture, various security attacks on healthcare data, security requirements, available solutions and case studies. Open research issues in this field are also discussed which can motivate the researchers in this field.

Keywords MBSN · IoT · Security · Health care · IDS

S. Saif (✉) · S. Biswas
Department of Computer Science and Engineering, Maulana Abul Kalam Azad University of Technology, Kolkata, West Bengal, India
e-mail: sohailsaif7@gmail.com

P. Bhattacharjee
Department of Computational Science, Brainware University, Kolkata, West Bengal, India

K. Karmakar
Department of Computer Science and Engineering, Narula Institute of Technology, Kolkata, West Bengal, India

R. Saha
Department of Information Technology, Gauhati University, GUIST, Guwahati, Assam, India

© The Author(s), under exclusive license to Springer Nature Singapore Pte Ltd. 2022 327
S. Biswas et al. (eds.), *Internet of Things Based Smart Healthcare*, Smart Computing and Intelligence, https://doi.org/10.1007/978-981-19-1408-9_15

1   Introduction

Majority people of our country live in villages. But unfortunately in maximum villages, medical facility is inadequate. Neither it has well-equipped hospitals/health centres nor has it has qualified doctors. Village people are therefore the worst sufferers and in need of medical attention. Though lagging in medical facilities, some progress is taking place in villages in terms of the setup of better telecom infrastructure and electricity connections. Internet access is now possible even from remote villages of our country. These rapidly growing telecom infrastructure and Internet access may help the village people to overcome the inconvenience caused due to the shortage of adequate medical facilities.

IoT-based cloud-assisted healthcare systems are popular nowadays because of the timely and remote health data monitoring. It is a network of various wearable sensors in the body also known as Mobile Body Sensor Network (MBSN) (Saha et al., 2019). Biological sensors attached to the human body are used to collect various physiological changes in order to monitor the patient's health status and that information is transmitted to a Sink device. This device is used to instantly transmit the health data to a cloud-based medical server for storage and processing. Doctors and other medical facilities can access this cloud-based medical server to see the health parameters of the patient in real time.

Since this health information is transmitted through an insecure channel, data suffers from a lack of security and privacy. An adversary can apply different security attacks like Man-in-the-middle, replay attack, impersonation attack, modification attack (Movassaghi et al., 2014; Mucchi et al., 2019; Roy et al., 2020; Saif et al., 2018a), etc. to gather private information of the patient or can alter the information during the transmission. Also, insider attacks can take place on the cloud-based medical server to compromise the information stored there. Hence, corrective measures are needed to secure the data in transmission as well in storage. Proper use of security requirements such as Confidentiality, Integrity and Authentication (Hasan et al., 2019) is very much important. Also, Intrusion Detection System (IDS) (Newaz et al., 2020; Kore & Patil, 2020; Yuce, 2010) can help to fight insider attacks. Motivated by the recent literature, this chapter intends to discuss recent advancements in security mechanisms to secure health data during the collection, transmission and storage phase.

The rest of the chapter has been organized as follows: Sect. 2 shows the traditional and modern architecture of IoT-based health care, Sect. 3 discusses the possible security attacks on healthcare data, Sect. 4 presents security and privacy requirements. Sect. 5 discusses the available security solutions and Sect. 6 discusses a detail case study on intrusion detection systems for health care. In Sect. 6.4, several research issues have been explored, and finally Sect. 7 concludes the chapter.

2 Traditional Versus Modern Architecture

An end-to-end IoT-based healthcare monitoring system is divided into three layers as shown in Fig. 1; detailed working of each layer has been described in this section.

Tier-I: It is the first layer of MBSN communication where data transmission is done within the human body. Sensor nodes are used for sensing which directly touch the body. These small sensor devices can detect various physiological parameters from the patients' body such as body temperature, ECG, pulse rate, EEG and transmit them wired/wirelessly to the local coordinator device which is a special sensor node. Such sensor node is called 'Sink'.

Tier-II: It is the middle layer of MBSN where communication is done between 'Sink' and the 'Access Points (AP)'. AP is a gateway device outside the patient's body. Communication between the Sink and AP takes place through the Internet or other such networks. Such networks can be infrastructure-based or can communicate using ad-hoc networks.

Tier-III: This is the last part of MBSN communication where all information is transmitted to a cloud-based medical server routed through the AP. Only authorized people can access this server. Data kept in the server is periodically checked to monitor the health condition of the patients. If needed, automatic notifications are sent to the relatives of the patients. The patient party and doctors are open to communicate using video conferencing and Internet.

Now with the rapid advancement of machine learning/deep learning techniques, health care has become smart in terms of decision-making. Health vitals collected through the sensor devices can be analysed to extract meaningful information in the cloud platform. Here, machine learning-based algorithms are deployed to perform various tasks such as disease prevention and risk monitoring, diagnosis and treatment

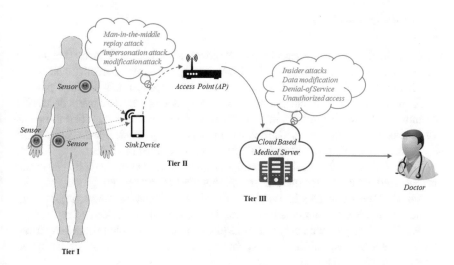

Fig. 1 Traditional architecture of IoT-based health care

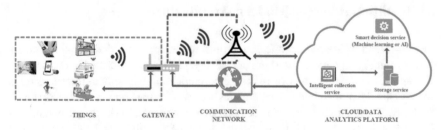

THINGS   GATEWAY   COMMUNICATION   CLOUD/DATA
                                      NETWORK   ANALYTICS PLATFORM

Fig. 2 Modern architecture of IoT-based smart health care (Alam et al., 2018)

and health management. Modern architecture of IoT-based smart health care has been presented in Fig. 2.

The above architecture has been divided into four parts such as things, gateways, communication network and cloud platform. Gateways are also referred to as Fog nodes. Fog nodes are introduced to perform some rapid analysis based on the sensor data, for example, if the blood pressure of a patient crosses the threshold limit, then alert/corrective measures should be taken immediately. Since the latency for blood pressure data transmission from the patient to the cloud platform for processing and analysis might cause havoc in patient's life, therefore, analysing data in edge nodes can be beneficial for patient health diagnosis. Cloud infrastructure can be used to store the high volume of health data since it is constituted of a set of servers and storage which are interconnected. In such infrastructures, machine learning or deep learning-based models are deployed to analyse the sensor data to extract useful information for decision-making.

3   Security Threats

IoT-based health care is vulnerable to a considerable number of security threats and attacks. Security issues can be divided into two types: system security and information security. Also, they can be divided into two types in another way: passive attack and active attack. Security attacks can take place in different layers of MBSN communication architecture. In the following sections, we have classified the security attacks in different layers. The details of each security attack (Hasan et al., 2019; Roy et al., 2020) in different layers of MBSN are described in Table 1.

Tier-I: It deals with intra-body communication. Possible attacks in this layer are unauthorized attack, impersonation attack, repudiation and replaying.

Tier-II: Security attacks in Tier-II involve data modification, network jamming, eavesdropping, impersonation attack, repudiation, Denial of service and replaying.

Tier-III: Different attacks that can take place in this layer include data tampering, fake packet injection, sniffing attack, routing attack, jamming attack, Distributed Denial of Service (DDos) attack, etc.

Table 1 Layer-wise security threats in MBSN

Threats type	MBSN layer where it occurs	Description
Data modification	Tier-II, Tier-III	While transmitting data from source to destination, if some unauthorized entity inserts some new information or modifies or deletes some vital information, then it can be fatal for the patient's life. It is an attack on the integrity of the data. If some vital health information is modified in the middle, doctor will get wrong information about the patient. This can result in a great disaster
Unauthorized attack	Tier-I	It may occur when an attacker gets control of the sensor and other nodes of the health monitoring system and thus subsequently takes control of the entire system. As a result, the hacker can have unauthorized access to the sensitive and vital information about the patient
Interruption/Network jamming	Tier-II, Tier-III	It results in the destruction of a component of a remote terminal of the health monitoring system. As a result, normal communication is disrupted and in case of a patient's emergency, it may pose threat to patient's life
Eavesdropping	Tier-II, Tier-III	An attacker can easily steal information from the open communication system between the sensor nodes. Stolen information may be used for malicious activity
Impersonation attack	Tier-I, Tier-II, Tier-III	If any attacker gets information on the identity of a sensor node, the same can be used to cheat other nodes

(continued)

Table 1 (continued)

Threats type	MBSN layer where it occurs	Description
Repudiation	Tier-I, Tier-II, Tier-III	It occurs when a sender or receiver denies the fact that they have actually sent or received the information. This threat must be removed for a safe healthcare monitoring system
Denial of Service (DoS)	Tier-II, Tier-III	It occurs when the targeted system is overflowing with data beyond its normal capacity and is related to the effect caused by the compromised system. DoS attack may affect the physical, data link, network and transport layers of the Open System Interconnection (OSI) model
Replaying	Tier-I, Tier-II, Tier-III	An attacker can eavesdrop valid information and can resend them later to the same destination. It will hamper the 'data freshness' requirement of the sensor-based health monitoring system

In the last few years, the healthcare industry has been heavily targeted by attackers. Year-wise attacks on healthcare data have been shown in Fig. 3. In 1989, Becker's Hospital suffered the first Ransomeware attack, resulting in 20,000 floppy disc data being lost. Later on, in 2017 another WannaCry Ransomware attack occurred in the healthcare and military sector. Due to this ransomware attack, crucial data of 1,60,000 persons was lost. Healthnet data theft attack happened in 2009 which stole 5,31,400 patients' records. In 2010, Lincoln Medical and Mental Health Center in New York suffered an AVIMEdInc attack and as a result 1,80,111 patient data was stolen. In 2011, 49,01,432 patients' medical data of Tricare was hacked. In 2012, attackers hacked the sensitive health data of 7,80,000 users at US Medicaid. In 2013, Advocate Medical Group was targeted by hackers and the sensitive information of 40,00,000 users was compromised. In 2014, cyber-attack on Community Health Systems affected 45,00,000 users' data. In 2015, CareFirst BlueCross, Maryland, faced cyber-attack and about 1,00,000 data records were stolen. In 2016, 21st Century Oncology records were compromised by attackers resulting in 22,00,000 users' crucial data being stolen. In 2017, Grozio Chirurgija was compromised due to the WannaCry Ransomeware attack and healthcare data of 6,700 users was encrypted by the attackers. In 2018 and 2019 due to cyber-attacks on health database 75,000 and 8,08,000 users were affected, respectively.

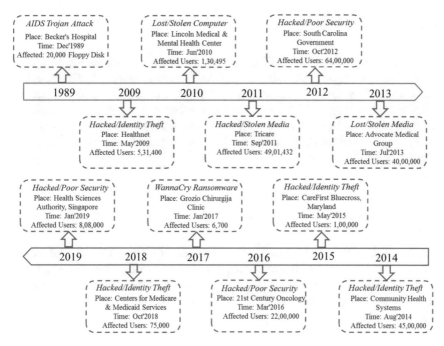

Fig. 3 Year-wise cyber-attacks on healthcare industry

4 Importance of Privacy and Security

The privacy and security requirements for IoT-based health care is a challenging task which includes authentication, confidentiality, user anonymity, key agreement, etc. These are the important factors to ensure the privacy and security of health data.

4.1 Mutual-Authentication

Kerberos authentication protocol is one of the widely used mutual authentication protocols. In traditional communication, secure socket layer (SSL)/transport layer security (TLS) is used to ensure the flow of communication but lacks the ability to verify the user or device; here, mutual-authentication is used (He & Zeadally, 2015). It allows only the authorized user to access the information stored on the server (Mutlag et al., 2019).

4.2 Confidentiality

To ensure the confidentiality of health data, symmetric cryptographic algorithms such as AES, DES, 3-DES and Blowfish, CAST can be used (Saif & Biswas, 2020). These algorithms ensure confidentiality by encrypting the data at the sink node using the shared secret key and the encrypted data are sent and stored in a cloud medical database. Doctors or users can access those data if they have the secret key only. Using the key, they can decrypt the data. But key sharing is another challenging task which needs to be explored.

4.3 Anonymity

Privacy of the patient can be in danger if an attacker compromises the identity of the user. Thus, anonymity is another important security requirement in health care to ensure the privacy of the users. User authentication must be present to prove the doctors' and patients' identities. Identity can be encrypted using symmetric encryption algorithms.

4.4 Data Freshness

Destination node should always receive fresh data, i.e. data received in proper order and time. Attackers may capture data during transmission and send them later to confuse the receiver, which can mislead the diagnosis of the diseases.

4.5 Data Integrity

An attacker can alter the health data during transmission from sink node to the cloud server; this can be fatal for the patient. Since the doctor makes his/her decision based on these data, health data should be intact and not manipulated in any way. Here, hashing algorithms such as MD5 and SHA are widely used.

4.6 Data Availability

Uninterrupted connectivity is an important feature of a healthcare monitoring system. Vital information about the patient must reach the doctor in time. Presence of an unwanted node in between is a threat. It may result in loss of data and ultimately prove to be life-threatening for the patient. As such, the communication must be secured and uninterrupted connectivity must be maintained.

5 Taxonomy of Privacy and Security in Health Care

Several security techniques are adopted in IoT-based health care till now. Based on the security requirements, it can be classified into different categories such as Access control-based schemes, authentication-based schemes and Encryption-based schemes. Taxonomy of secure healthcare solutions is presented in Fig. 4.

5.1 Access Control Schemes

Cloud-oriented Electronic Healthcare System has several stakeholders such as patients, healthcare professionals, hospitals, pharmacist and government agencies. Most health data collected through wearable sensors are stored in the cloud-based storage server where healthcare users share their data. But cloud-based storage servers suffer various security attacks such as Masquerade attacks, Denial of Service (DoS), Flooding attack and Insider attack (Zeadally et al., 2016). Sensitive nature and Openness of the healthcare applications lead to several vulnerabilities and trust issues among the stakeholders. Here, trust has an important role to control the access of users based on the degree of trust.

In (Singh & Chatterjee, 2019a), the authors proposed a Trust-Based Access Control model for healthcare systems which ensures trusted and authorized users access the data and resources. In the first step, user is connected to the cloud server and to access data user needs to submit a request query to the authentication server; if the user is authenticated then the request query is sent to the trust assessment module to calculate the trust value of that user. The trust value is sent to the access control module to generate an access token depending on the access control rules and request query. Finally, the access decision checker determines whether the access is to be accepted or rejected. Performance of the scheme has been evaluated using standard parameters such as MAE. SMAPE and MAPE.

Another study presents the use of the dynamic Access Control Model (ACM) to secure the Electronic Healthcare System (EHS) (Singh & Chatterjee, 2019b). The authors have proposed a set of new rules to dynamically control the access. Beta distribution technique has been considered in the proposed model to evaluate the degree of trust; also, a multi-criteria decision-making technique called Analytic Hierarchy Process (AHP) has been considered to assign the weight of each trust parameter. Experimental result shows that the proposed model error (MAE) is 0.068 and 0.055 after 500 and 1000 interactions, respectively.

Fig. 4 Solution taxonomy of privacy and security in IoT-based health care

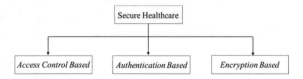

In (Bhattasali et al., 2018), the authors presented an adaptive workflow-based Access Control Model (ACM) to maintain the quality of trust and context between the stakeholders. This model has been considered for the kiosk-operated rural healthcare medical system. To avoid the bottleneck problem, workflow phases have been executed either online or in offline mode. To evaluate the performance of the model, several scenarios for kiosk-based rural healthcare medical system have been presented and analysed using the Workflow Petri Net Designer (WoPeD) tool. Experimental result shows that the proposed model performs better than the state of the art.

In (Banyal et al., 2014), the authors proposed an Access Control Model (ACM) based on trust and multi-factor authentication. Trust value is calculated by the model to provide the access permission. Depending on the trust value, decision is made whether the user request is granted or denied.

5.2 Authentication Schemes

In a remote healthcare environment, patient and doctor communicate with each other using a cloud server, where patient transfers his/her manifestations and doctors can view and upload the diagnosis report of the patient. Furthermore, the communication is done via a public channel, which is prone to several security attacks. Since the patient medical records are extremely critical in nature, they should not be revealed widely. Hence, it must be ensured that only authenticated users can access the records, and to do that various authentication schemes are available. Biometric features of the human body such as thumb, palm, iris and ecg can be used for authentication.

In Kumar et al., (2018) a mutual authentication protocol has been proposed for Telecare Medicine Information Systems (TMIS). This protocol consists of five phases such as Healthcare centre upload phase (HUP), where the patient registers himself/herself and the healthcare centre assigns OTP and a dynamic pseudo random identity to the patient using a mobile device. Next, the healthcare centre forms mutual authentication with the cloud server to upload the patient medical report. Another phase is patient data upload phase (PUP); in this phase, patients' health information is collected through body sensors and the information is sent to cloud server using patient identity and OTP. The third phase is Treatment phase (TP) where doctor and cloud server communicate with each other in an authenticated manner. The fourth phase is Checkup phase (CP) where patient receives the diagnosis report from the doctor in an encrypted format. Another phase is called Emergency phase (EP) which can be used in case of an emergency; here, patient needs to input his/her identity, sequence number and the request is forwarded to the cloud, and after verification the doctor sends necessary advice. This proposed five-phase scheme is compared with other models; also, it is found that the framework is resilient to several security attacks.

In (Khan & Kumari, 2013), a mutual authentication scheme has been proposed for secure exchange of patient medical information through the Internet. The proposed scheme consists of four phases such as initial phase, registration phase, login-authentication phase and password change phase. In the first phase, healthcare server generates two large prime numbers and using the prime numbers a master secret key is formed as well as a one-way hash function. In the registration phase, patient registers himself/herself in order to be a valid user; registration contains several steps. In the third phase, patient needs to login to the healthcare server using a login request. Healthcare server needs to verify the request if it is coming from a valid user or not; upon verification, request is either accepted or denied. The proposed scheme supports forward secrecy method, and also the scheme is secure from offline password guessing attack, denial of service attack, insider attack, replay attack, impersonation attack and stolen verifier attack.

In another recent study (Zhang et al., 2018), the authors presented the use of ECG features for authentication purposes; their proposed scheme is called PEA: Parallel Electrocardiogram-based Authentication. There are three types of Biometric features such as Behavioural Biometrics, Multimodal Biometrics and Physiological Biometrics which includes electrocardiograms (ECGs) and electroencephalograms (EEGs). The authors have used a hybrid feature extraction technique by combining fiducial- and non-fiducial-based features. These features are employed to build a parallel ECG pattern recognition framework. ECG features are used to retrieve patient medical information in case of an emergency. MIT-BH ECG dataset has been used for the experiments which contains 100 samples of ECG, each sample containing 200 ECG signal files, hence a total 20,000 ECG signals are used for the experiments.

In (Saif et al., 2018b), biosignals (thumb impression data) of patients and doctors have been used for authentication. Thumb impression of the patient and doctor is first registered, then the doctor makes a request to the patient device to get patient health information; this device is equipped with various body sensors. During the request, the doctor's thumb impression is matched; if a match is found then the request is accepted. Similarly, to authenticate the patient, the patient thumb impression is sent to the doctor's device and that is matched with the thumb data stored in the cloud server; once matched, the patient identity is verified and the requested patient data is available to the doctor for necessary advice. Another study shows the use of Palm impression data for identification and authentication of doctor and patients (Karmakar et al., 2018).

5.3 Encryption Schemes

Data confidentiality is one of the security principles to secure any kind of data; here in case of health data, it must be secured by applying cryptographic algorithms. Encryption of health data at the sensor node and transmitting that encrypted data will prevent several security attacks. Encrypted data is stored at the cloud server, and healthcare users can access those data if they have a decryption key.

In (Gupta et al., 2020), the authors have considered simple XOR and cryptographic hash functions to ensure the confidentiality and integrity of health data.

Security attacks such as intermediate node capture attack, sensor node imperson-ation attack and Hub node impersonation attack are considered as a threat model. The proposed scheme has four phases such as initialization, registration, authentication and dynamic node update phase. The system administrator starts the initialization process by selecting a master key for the hub node and that key is stored in the hub node's memory. In the registration phase, intermediate node and sensor nodes are registered by the system administrator. Registration consists of a few steps. The proposed scheme has been validated using the BAN-Logic, Real-Or-Random (ROR) model.

In (Saif & Biswas, 2019), a secure data transmission framework between tier 2 and tier 3 of MBSN has been proposed. The proposed framework uses AES and Triple DES to encrypt the health data; fingerprint information is used to generate the secret key; SHA-3 has been used to generate the hash of the health data. All this information is stored in the cloud medical server; whenever a doctor wishes to access the health data of the patient, first the encrypted health data is decrypted using a shared secret key and hash of the plain text is generated and matched with the hash stored in the cloud database. If matching is done successfully, then the health data is intact and free from attack such as man-in-middle attack. Experimental results satisfy the delay constraints for healthcare applications such as real-time health condition monitoring.

In (Jabeen et al., 2020), the authors have presented a genetic-based lightweight encryption scheme to encrypt the health data collected through the body sensors. MQTT protocol has been used in this study where health data collected through the sensors are sent to the MQTT broker to request for publishing. MQTT broker responds with a subscribe message which includes a data topic. Once subscribed, encrypted data is transmitted to the cloud server. 8-bit encryption key is generated using a simple mathematical operation; this key is used in the genetic encryption algorithm. To generate the secret key, a random integer is chosen and converted to binary, next 1's compliment is applied. Then, 2 bit is shift operation to the right is performed to obtain the 8 bit secret key. To encrypt the health data, first the plain text is converted into binary and divided into 8-bit blocks. Next, mutation and cross-over areapplied on the key and binary plain text in order to get the ciphertext. Ciphertext is stored on the cloud server; to decrypt the ciphertext into plain text, reverse steps are followed. Since the scheme is lightweight and simple, it can be used for healthcare applications.

In Table 2, a brief survey of the state-of-the-art work on MBSN security is described. All the techniques mentioned in the survey are for medical application. This survey mentions the nature of the work considered, like security and authentica-tion, and the methods adopted in the work like cryptography, biological methods like ECG reading, etc. It also discusses how the experiments were done, like simulation or analytical comparison. Also, the survey describes the scope of the work, whether the current work is energy-efficient or not, specifies its computational complexity and how accurate the current work is.

Table 2 Summary of the recent research findings on security issue of MBSN

Authors, year	Security parameters considered	Key generation (biological/non-biological)	Experiment done	Security attack considered	Energy-efficient?	Computational complexity	Accuracy
Almuhaideb & Alqudaihi (2020)	Anonymity, un-traceability, integrity	Non-biological key: based on randomly generated number	Scheme is validated using BAN logic	Sensor node replay attack, impersonation attack, brute force attack, replay attack, collision attack	Reduced system overhead increased energy efficiency	Less compared to Kompara et al., (2019)	Security analysis proves the system to be secure enough
Konan & Wang (2019)	Authentication, privacy, integrity	Non-Biological: public key cryptography	Performance Analysis conducted using Dual Core CPU consisting of 4 GB RAM	Eavesdrop, Impersonation attack	Data aggregation and batch authentication improve energy efficiency	Reduced computational cost	Comparison with other schemes makes the proposed scheme to be more accurate
Oberoi et al., (2016)	Authentication	Non-biological key: Based on data collection by the motion sensor and key generation based on that value which is used for further processing	Device with accelerometers attached to a person	No specific attack was addressed	Nothing specifically mentioned	Nothing specifically mentioned	More secure as more numbers of unpredictable keys are generated
Shen et al., (2015)	Confidentiality, integrity	Non-biological key: ECC and Hash chain key management using shared symmetric key	Analytical proof	Passive and active adversaries, malicious intruder	Better compared to Li et al.'s protocol (Li et al., 2010)	Better compared to Li et al.'s protocol (Li et al., 2010)	Better in many respects compared to Li et al.'s protocol (Li et al., 2010)

(continued)

Table 2 (continued)

Authors, year	Security parameters considered	Key generation (biological/non-biological)	Experiment done	Security attack considered	Energy-efficient?	Computational complexity	Accuracy
Li et al., (2013)	Security and authentication	Non-biological key: Based on symmetric key cryptography	Prototype sensor network platform with 10 devices having a central controller	Eavesdropping, impersonation attack	Energy-efficient than Scheme I (Li et al., 2013)	No discussion found	Accurate results given than some other related previous methods (Li et al., 2013)
Shi et al., (2013)	Confidentiality, authenticity	Non-biological key: Based on distinct RSS channels among body channels	Crossbow's Telos B notes (TPR2400)	Impersonation attack	NA	NA	More efficient even when a number of strategic attackers are present
Hu et al., (2013)	Security and elasticity	Non-biological key: Cryptography using fuzzy attribute-based signcryption (FABSC) scheme	Chipcon CC1000 radio chip used	Active and passive attacks	Efficient compared to some other previous methods (Shi et al., 2013)	Lower compared to some other previous methods (Shi et al., 2013)	Better results than some previous methods (Shi et al., 2013)
Hu et al., (2013)	Security, authentication	Non-biological key: Based on symmetric cryptography key exchange method	Chipcon CC1000 radio chip used	Brute force attack	Lower compared to PSKA (Hu et al., 2013)	Lower compared to PSKA (Hu et al., 2013)	Accurate results than PSKA (Hu et al., 2013)

(continued)

Table 2 (continued)

Authors, year	Security parameters considered	Key generation (biological/non-biological)	Experiment done	Security attack considered	Energy-efficient?	Computational complexity	Accuracy
Liang et al., (2012)	Source and data authentication during data routing	Non-biological key: Based on symmetric key encryption scheme	Simulation-based performance evaluation	Exhaustive source authentication attacks, data replay attacks	NA	NA	NA
Chang et al., (2013)	Confidentiality, Integrity	Biological key: Based on a communication channel in the body	Experiment done on a dead mouse	Eavesdropping	Yes	Lower	NA
Mana et al., (2011)	Security, privacy, integrity, authentication, confidentiality	Biological key: ECG-generated key	Analytically proved	Node capture attacks	Yes, compared to SSSL, SKERBEROS (Cheng et al., 2013)	NA	Efficient and energy-saving compared to SSSL, SKERBEROS (Chang et al., 2013)
Selimis, et al., (2011)	Integrity and authentication	Non-biological key: symmetric key-based cryptographic technique	Micro-controller (MSP430)-based test bed used	Eavesdropping	Yes, compared to Kaps & Sunar, (2006)	Lower compared to other works (Kaps & Sunar, 2006; Suarez et al., 2009)	Better performance compared to other works (Kaps & Sunar, 2006; Suarez et al., 2009)

6 Case Study on Intrusion Detection System for Health Care

Electronic Healthcare Data (EHD) is both private and sensitive in nature. As information systems in healthcare industries are rapidly advancing and evolving, so does the intimidation for such systems. In the present medical scenario, Patient Health Information (PHI) is very easy to access. The simplicity of access benefits medical service providers to be further effective and offer improved healthcare services. However, this ease of access also poses dangers which have to be taken care of to confirm that the data is secured. Further, the Health Insurance Portability and Accountability Act (HIPAA) has alreadily made it obligatory for all healthcare service providers (Ness, 2007). Protecting resources such as EHD in a healthcare facility is a very difficult task. The threats to health data arise in various forms and from numerous sources. One may think that viruses and external invaders are the only possible threats which need to be addressed, but that is not the actual case and in fact, it is far from the truth. Several threats often originate from insiders such as a user modifying files or elevating access levels (Thamilarasu, 2016).

In the effort of protecting the health data and the structures on which they are stored, Intrusion Detection Systems (IDS) may come as an important tool. By using IDS, one may recognize an attack and alert appropriate staff instantly so that the risk is minimized. IDS may be a handy tool in documenting forensic evidence which may be necessary for lawful proceedings when the offender of a breach needs to be prosecuted. It should be remembered that IDS does not shield resources by itself; it can only alert people of the threat and allow for suitable measures to be taken. Intrusion Detection Systems are characterized by their installation locations and the way they recognize threats. The category of IDS is identified by the installed location (on a host or the network). The diverse IDS models are identified by the method the system identifies an invasion. The target is to detect threat behaviour with a minimum false alarm. It is difficult to tag any one system better than the others as each one has its advantages. The establishment requirements and resources can fix the appropriate system.

6.1 Models

Intrusion Detection Systems also differ in their nature in determining attacks and threats. The most predominant models are based on rules-based detection (Mitchell & Chen, 2012, 2015), statistical anomaly detection (Begli et al., 2019) and a hybrid of the two (Thamilarasu et al., 2020).

Each model has its advantages and disadvantages similar to the type of IDS. The idea is to choose the model which is most suitable for the environment of the organization.

Statistical-anomaly model searches for statistical abnormalities (Begli et al., 2019; Thamilarasu et al., 2020). This model assumes that any abnormal behaviour is an indication of a threat. This model uses log files, file/folder properties, audits and traffic patterns to detect abnormal system behaviour. The principle of the statistical-anomaly model is how a normal behaviour is classified. It is required to specify the amount of deviation required from the normal profile, to be classified as an 'attack'. These types of IDS models rely on the deviation from normal readings.

Rule- or Signature-based model is another popular model. Most attacks are categorized by a series of events that helps in creating signature definitions of these threats (Mitchell & Chen, 2012). The Signature-based system inspects its data source for a possible match with the predefined signatures or activities. The system generates an alert of the attack if any matching signature is identified in the data. Such a model is less complicated and easier to maintain compared to the anomaly model. However, it is possible to detect attacks only for those, which it has signatures for. This signature requirement may fail to detect new threats or 'Zero Day' attacks. On the other hand, such a system has very precise events to search, so it has a very low failure (false positive) rate for known threats compared to Anomaly-based IDS.

The basic idea with healthcare data is that a greater level of care may be provided with the increase in accessibility of the patient information. This is evident from the rapid application of VPNs to connect Picture Archiving Computer Systems (PACS) to remote offices for accessing patient data. However, with the implementation of these novel technologies and systems, new vulnerabilities are exposed which can be potentially exploited by the attacker (He et al., 2019). Careful security planning using the IDS can be the sole method for a healthcare organization to counter these vulnerabilities.

6.2 Desired Features of Healthcare IDS and IPS

Ideally, an Intrusion Detection System (IDS) or Intrusion Protection System (IPS) should possess the following functionalities and satisfy HIPAA regulations (Annas, 2003).

Pattern Matching: The IDS and IPS must have updated threat signature definitions to compare network traffic with them and an option to keep the system updated with the utmost fresh threat patterns.

SSL Inspection (Inbound and Outbound): The IDS will decrypt and examine encrypted traffic and monitor onboard capability versus off-load to a secondary appliance.

Heuristics and Behaviour-Based Analysis: Associating the behaviour and nature of the network flow to the norm and desired output.

Granular Application Service Control: The facility to administer and implement policy regulations.

Network Visibility of User and Application: Generate local analytics and report about network bandwidth consumption of individual users and applications.

Web Category-Based Network Access Policy: The ability to create and impose the organization's policies to prohibit the access of workers to legitimate sites that are considered to be inappropriate (such as social media sites).

Access Policy Built on URL/IP Reputation and Location: Facility to create blacklist and whitelist of known Ips that are already classified as bad or good.

Amalgamation with Other Protection Solutions: Facility to provide a web service API to deploy commercial/open standard web services of various external components that are additionally required for virtual security.

Protection Against Data Leakage: Create and enforce a policy to detect and block sensitive distinguishable personal information like social security numbers or credit card numbers, whenever such information appears in the network. This facility is particularly beneficial for the auditors performing HIPAA and PCI assessments.

Forensics: Need to provide a packet capturing mechanism for the organization's forensics team with necessary evidence for an attack investigation.

Embedded Bypass Mechanism: Guarantees that network traffic flow will remain unaffected in the event of appliance failures.

6.3   Commercial IDS and IPS

The following are the major IDS in health care offered by commercial vendors.

Cisco Systems

As soon as Cisco's IDS and IPS (Santos et al., 2016) detects a threat that may compromise a medical device, Cisco's Identity Services Engine and Cisco TrustSec are informed of an immediate updation of the network segmentation policy, and the origin of the threat is immediately quarantined. This restricts the threat from reaching the device.

Features: Firepower NGIPS (Next-Generation IPS) and NGFW (Next-Generation Firewall) appliances use a software subscription model for URL Filtering, Threat (IPS) and Advanced Malware Protection (AMP).

Availability: The system is available separately or in combinations for one-, three- and five-year terms. Additionally, Cisco also has maintenance and support contracts for the appliances.

Fortinet Systems

Fortinet system (Ruoslahti, 2020) uses its own chipsets which offer a targeted level of performance in contrast with an IDS and IPS commodity chipset. The system provides higher capacity and lower latency by off-loading computational aspects onto its chipsets. A dedicated healthcare team is present to provide a greater level of understanding of the key healthcare challenges.

Features: Fortinet's security appliance provides multi-threat protection across all sites using FortiGate-60CX and a Cluster FortiGatge-200B. It integrates VPN, antivirus, SSL, anti-spam, firewall, intrusion prevention, web filtering and IPSec into a single device. Both the internal traffic and perimeter are scanned by Fortinet IDS and IPS components to protect not only the medical devices but the data centre as well.

Availability: A single subscription per appliance covers all required functionalities.

IBM Security Systems

The Next-Generation Intrusion Prevention System (NG-IPS) (Chakrabarty et al., 2020) of the big blue is a component of its original Security Network Protection (SNP) system also known as XGS. It uses both hardware and software to protect the virtual network environment. The Protocol Analysis Module (PAM) relies on heuristic data for threat identification and control.

Features: IBM QRadar acts as a backbone of XGS and analyses the network data from XGS. Any ongoing attack if identified, it immediately triggers an alert resulting in quarantine and isolation of the misbehaving node.

Availability: The subscription is based on dynamic pricing depending on the amount of protection needed. A Flexible Performance License permits subscribers to procure a performance level for present requirements and upgrade through a software license to new levels as and when needed.

Juniper Network Systems

Juniper (Adeleke, 2020) looks at a document whether it's from the outside or inside and uses static and dynamic check-ups to manipulate the file to see if it identifies itself as malware. Even without a known malware signature by putting the file in a place where it can be manipulated, it makes the file expose itself before it does its damage. Singling out just the IDS and IPS portion of the solution Juniper offers the ability to create a signature-based attack object. This attack object is used to block any user trying to download files using an executable passing through an File Transfer Protocol (FTP).

Features: With the advent of EMRs kept in multiple locations and the cloud as well, data processing power is key. It needs to decrypt SSL traffic at wire speeds, recognize valid and invalid application traffic and use advanced AI-type heuristics and signature mapping, aka dynamic inspection, which goes beyond merely identifying a known signature.

Availability: IDS is embedded into the firewall. Pricing is set for hardware plus software with licenses for different features. A basic and a premium service are offered. Basic service includes free static inspection. Premium uses dynamic inspection.

Damballa Failsafe System

Dynamic signature identification is a key feature at Damballa (Finding Advanced Threats Before They Strike, 2021). With the use of machine learning, it creates generic signatures and inspects each packet looking for 'patterns of activity' to determine which devices a file is communicating with and what looks suspicious. Compromised systems exhibit identifiable behaviours and Damballa's solution models how these systems communicate. It can determine within hours whether the network or a device on the network has been attacked.

Features: The solution includes a Failsafe Dashboard that employs what Damballa calls a Threat Discovery Center. Damballa sensors observe traffic and send it on to its behavioural analysis tool. If the risk assessment tool identifies the traffic as a true positive threat, the Breach Response team is alerted. The Center has been collecting data since 2006 and using machine learning; it identifies unusual behaviour that might indicate an attack.

Availability: Subscription-based on the number of devices in the system.

Symantec Endpoint Protection System

Symantec Endpoint Protection (Dhanda et al., 2020) shields endpoints while Symantec Data Center Security offers built-in IPS. Data Center Security uses a combination of host-based intrusion detection (HIDS), intrusion prevention (HIPS) (Hussain et al., 2021) and least privilege access control. Using HIPS, system administrators can restrict application and OS behaviour, allowing only the behaviour that's known to be safe across data centres and endpoints. It accomplishes this feat by tracking over 1400 actions a program can take. It then correlates the behaviour and if it figures out that the behaviour is suspicious, the file is blocked.

Features: Symantec uses reputation-based technology which tracks a file's reputation so it can identify suspicious files. The system leverages the data from a worldwide civilian threat intelligence network.

Availability: Endpoint Protect and Data Centre Security solutions are offered as perpetual licenses.

6.4   Open Research Issues

In this chapter, we have discussed IoT-based Mobile Body Sensor Network (MBSN). This emerging technology faces several challenges such as security, routing, energy efficiency and Quality of Service (QoS) which are trending research areas, and proper research can handle these issues. Security requirement confidentiality can be ensured only if the patient health information is not disclosed to the adversaries during transmission and storage. To do this, cryptographic measures are needed, but the sensor nodes are mostly resource-constrained and cannot adopt complex cryptographic algorithms. Hence, research should be made to design a secure and simple cryptographic algorithm which can encrypt the health data at the sensor node or in the sink device. Another important issue is key generation and sharing; this is the most important phase of cryptographic algorithms. The secret key should be generated in an efficient manner and must be shared in a secure way with the communication parties such as patient and doctor. Routing is another important issue, since the improper routing of sensor data will affect the network which may decrease the network lifetime, introduce several security attacks such as black hole and sink hole attacks. Several routing schemes are present in the literature such as posture-based, temperature-based and cluster-based (Maitra & Roy, 2017; Roy et al., 2017). But there is an inadequacy of secure routing schemes. Another important challenge is the need for Quality of Service (QoS); the design of MBSN should be done in a way so that QoS is ensured. QoS includes delay, throughput, packet delivery ratio, etc.; hence, to design a secure MBSN QoS parameters must be considered.

These are a few research issues pointed out in this chapter which should be addressed by researchers to make an end-to-end secure IoT-based remote health care, which can secure the health information starting from collection to delivery to the doctor.

7 Conclusion

Remote healthcare monitoring systems is the recent advancement in the healthcare sector where multiple stakeholders are involved related to sharing of patient health information. IoT and sensor network play a key role in this remote healthcare system which delivers the patient's physiological information to the doctor. But this advanced health monitoring system faces several challenges such as Security and privacy of patient data. Patient's Health data collected through the body sensors are transmitted to Doctor's device mostly through the Internet, which is an insecure channel for communication. Disclosure of health data to any adversaries will breach the patient's privacy, and also alternation of those data during transmission can be dangerous. This even can lead to death of the patient due to wrong diagnosis based on altered data. Thus, to make a successful health monitoring system, end-to-end security mechanism must be ensured. This chapter discusses all relevant security attacks on healthcare industries, security requirements and various secure solutions available. This chapter also presents a case study on an Intrusion detection system for healthcare applications.

Acknowledgements This work has been carried out with a grant received from WBDST sanctioned research project on secure remote health care with project sanction no. 230(Sanc)/ST/P/S&T/6G-14/2018.

References

Adeleke, O. (2020). Intrusion detection: Issues, problems and solutions. In: *2020 3rd International Conference on Information and Computer Technologies (ICICT)*. IEEE, pp. 397–402.

Alam, M. M., Malik, H., Khan, M. I., Pardy, T., Kuusik, A., & Le Moullec, Y. (2018). A Survey on the roles of communication technologies in IoT-based personalized healthcare applications. *IEEE Access, 6*, 36611–36631.

Almuhaideb, A. M., & Alqudaihi, K. S. (2020). A lightweight and secure anonymity preserving protocol for WBAN. *IEEE Access, 8*, 178183–178194.

Annas, G. J. (2003). HIPAA regulations—a new era of medical-record privacy? *New England Journal of Medicine, Massachusetts Medical Society, 348*, 1486–1490.

Banyal, R. K, Jain, V. K, & Jain, P. (2014). Dynamic trust based access control framework for securingmulti-cloud environment. In: *Proceedings of the 2014 international conference on information andcommunication technology for competitive strategies, ICTCS 14*. ACM, New York, pp 29:1–29:8.

Begli, M., Derakhshan, F., & Karimipour, H. (2019). A layered intrusion detection system for critical infrastructure using machine learning. In: *2019 IEEE 7th International Conference on Smart Energy Grid Engineering (SEGE)*. Oshawa, ON, Canada, pp. 120–124.

Bhattasali, T., Chaki, R., Chaki, N., & Saeed, K. (2018). An adaptation of context and trust aware workfloworiented access control for remote healthcare. *International Journal of Software Engineering and Knowledge Engineering, 28*(06), 781–810.

Chakrabarty, B., Kothekar, A., Mujumdar, P., Raut, S., Patil, S., & Ukirde, D. (2020). Securing data on threat detection using IBM spectrum scale and IBM QRadar.

Chang, S. Y., Hu, Y. C., Anderson, H., Fu, T., & Huang, E. Y. L. (2012). Body area network security: Robust key establishment using human body channel. In: *Proceedings of the USENIX Conference on Health Security and Privacy*, pp. 5–5.

Dhanda, S. S., Singh, B., & Jindal, P. (2020). IoT security: A comprehensive view. In: *Principles of Internet of Things (IoT) Ecosystem: Insight Paradigm*. Springer, Cham, pp. 467–494.

Finding Advanced Threats Before They Strike: A Review of Damballa Failsafe Advanced Threat Protection and Containment. (2021). http://www.sans.org/readingroom/whitepapers/analyst/finding-advanced-threatsstrike-review-damballa-failsafe-advanced-threatprotecti-34705. (Accessed 7 March 2021).

Gupta, A., Tripathi, M., & Sharma, A. (2020). A provably secure and efficient anonymous mutual authentication and key agreement protocol for wearable devices in WBAN. *Computer Communications, 160*, 311–325.

Hasan, K., Biswas, K., Ahmed, K., Nafi, N. S., & Islam, M. S. (2019). A comprehensive review of wireless body area network. *Journal of Network and Computer Applications, 143*, 178–198.

He, D., & Zeadally, S. (2015). Authentication protocol for an ambient assisted living system. *IEEE Communications Magazine, 53*(1), 71–77.

He, D., Qiao, Q., Gao, Y., Zheng, J., Chan, S., Li, J., & Guizani, N. (2019). Intrusion detection based on stacked autoencoder for connected healthcare systems. *IEEE Network, 33*(6), 64–69.

Hu, C., Zhang, N., Li, H., Cheng, X., & Liao, X. (2013). Body area network security: A fuzzy attribute-based signcryption scheme. *IEEE Journal on Selected Areas in Communication, 31*(9), 37–46.

Hu, C., Cheng, X., Zhang, F., Wu, D., Liao, X., & Chen, D. (2013). OPFKA: Secure and efficient ordered-physiological-feature-based key agreement for wireless body area network. In: *2013 Proceedings of IEEE Infocom*, pp. 2274–2282.

Hussain, S., Ahmad, M. B., & Ghouri, S. S. U. (2021). Advance persistent threat—a systematic review of literature and meta-analysis of threat vectors. *Advances in Computer, Communication and Computational Sciences*, 161–178.

Jabeen, T., Ashraf, H., Khatoon, A., Band, S. S., & Mosavi, A. (2020). A lightweight genetic based algorithm for data security in wireless body area networks. *IEEE Access, 8*, 183460–183469.

Kaps, J. -P., & Sunar, B. (2006). Energy comparison of AES and SHA-1forUbiquitous computing. In: *Proceedings of Emerging Directions Inembedded and Ubiquitous Computing (EUC 2006 Workshops)*, pp. 372–381.

Karmakar, K., Saif, S., Biswas, S., & Neogy, S. (2018). WBAN Security: study and implementation of a biological key based framework. In: *Fifth International Conference on Emerging Applications of Information Technology (EAIT)*, Kolkata, pp. 1–6.

Khan, M. K., & Kumari, S. (2013). An authentication scheme for secure access to healthcare services. *Journal of Medical Systems, 37*, 9954.

Kompara, M., Islam, S. H., & Hölbl, M. (2019). A robust and efficient mutual authentication and key agreement scheme with untraceability for WBANs. *Computer Networks, 148*, 196–213.

Konan, M., & Wang, W. (2019). A secure mutual batch authentication scheme for patient data privacy preserving in WBAN. *Sensors, 19*, 1608.

Kore, A., & Patil, S. (2020). IC-MADS: IoT enabled cross layer man-in-middle attack detection system for smart healthcare application. *Wireless Personal Communications, 113*, 727–746.

Kumar, V., Jangirala, S., & Ahmad, M. (2018). An efficient mutual authentication framework for healthcare system in cloud computing. *Journal of Medical Systems, 42*, 142.

Li, M., Yu, S., Lou, W., & Ren K. (2010). Group device pairing based secure sensor association andkey management for body area networks. In: *Proceedings of IEEE INFOCOM*, pp. 1–9.

Li, M., Yu, S., Guttm, J. D., Lou, W., & Ren, K. (2013). Secure ad-hoc trust initialization and key management in wireless body area networks. *ACM Transactions on Sensor Networks, 9*(2).

Liang, X., Li, X., Shen, Q., Lu, R., Lin, X., Shen, X., & Zhuang, W. (2012). Exploring prediction to enable secure and reliable routing in wireless body area network. In: *2012 Proceedings IEEE Infocom*, pp. 388–396.

Maitra, T., & Roy, S. (2017). SecPMS: An efficient and secure communication protocol for continuous patient monitoring system using body sensors. In: *Proceedings of the 9th International Conference on Communication Systems and Networks (COMSNETS)*, Bangalore, India, pp. 322–329.

Mana, M., Feham, M., & Bensaber, B. A. (2011). Trust key management scheme for wireless body area network. *International Journal of Network Security, 12*(2), 75–83.

Mitchell, R., & Chen, I. (2015). Behavior rule specification-based intrusion detection for safety critical medical cyber physical systems. *IEEE Transactions on Dependable and Secure Computing, 12*(1), 16–30.

Mitchell, R., & Chen, I. (2012). Behavior rule based intrusion detection for supporting secure medical cyber physical systems. In: *2012 21st International Conference on Computer Communications and Networks (ICCCN)*. Munich, pp. 1–7.

Movassaghi, S., Abolhasan, M., Lipman, J., Smith, D., & Jamalipour, A. (2014). Wireless body area networks: a survey. *IEEE Communications Surveys & Tutorials, 16*(3), 1658–1686.

Mucchi, L., Jayousi, S., Martinelli, A., Caputo, S., & Marcocci, P. (2019). An overview of security threats, solutions and challenges in WBANs for healthcare. In: *13th International Symposium on Medical Information and Communication Technology (ISMICT)*. Oslo, Norway, pp. 1–6.

Mutlag, A. A., Ghani, M. K. A., Arunkumar, N., Mohammed, M. A., & Mohd, O. (2019). Enabling technologies for fog computing in healthcare IoT systems, future gener. *Computing Systems, 90*, 62–78.

Ness, R. B. (2007). Influence of the HIPAA privacy rule on health research. *JAMA, American Medical Association (AMA), 298*, 2164.

Newaz, A. I., Sikder, A. K., Babun, L., & Uluagac, A. S. (2020) HEKA: A novel intrusion detection system for attacks to personal medical devices. In: *IEEE Conference on Communications and Network Security (CNS)*. Avignon, France, pp. 1–9.

Oberoi, D., Sou, W. Y., Lui, Y, Y., Fisher, R., Dinca, L., & Hancke, G. P. (2016). Wearable security: Key derivation for body area sensor networks based on host movement. In: *Industrial Electronics (ISIE), 2016 IEEE 25th International Symposium on 8–10 June*. IEEE.

Roy, M., Chowdhury, C., & Aslam, N. (2020). Security and privacy issues in wireless sensor and body area networks, In: *Handbook of Computer Networks and Cyber Security: Principles and Paradigms*. Springer, ISBN: 978–3–030–22276–5. https://doi.org/10.1007/978-3-030-22277-2.

Roy, M., Chowdhury, C., Kundu, A., & Aslam, N. (2017). Secure lightweight routing (SLR) strategy for wireless body area networks. *IEEE Ants, 2017*, 1–4.

Ruoslahti, H. (2020). Business continuity for critical infrastructure operators. *Annals of Disaster Risk Sciences: ADRS, 3*(1).

Saif, S., & Biswas, S. (2019). Secure data transmission beyond tier 1 of medical body sensor network. In: M. Chakraborty, S. Chakrabarti, V. Balas, & J. Mandal (Eds.), *Proceedings of International Ethical Hacking Conference 2018. Advances in Intelligent Systems and Computing*, Vol. 811. Springer.

Saha, R., Naskar, S., Biswas, S., et al. (2019). Performance evaluation of energy efficient routing with or without relay in medical body sensor network. *Health Technology, 9*, 805–815.

Saif, S., & Biswas, S. (2020) On the implementation and performance evaluation of security algorithms for healthcare. In: S. Kundu, U. Acharya, C. De, & S. Mukherjee (Eds.), *Proceedings of the 2nd International Conference on Communication, Devices and Computing*. Lecture Notes in Electrical Engineering, Vol. 602, pp. 629–640.

Saif, S., Gupta, R., & Biswas, S. (2018a) Implementation of cloud-assisted secure data transmission in WBAN for healthcare monitoring. In: S. Bhattacharyya, N. Chaki, D. Konar, U. Chakraborty, & C. Singh (Eds.), *Advanced Computational and Communication Paradigms. Advances in Intelligent Systems and Computing*, Vol. 706. Springer.

Saif S., Gupta, R., & Biswas, S. (2018b). Implementation of cloud-assisted secure data transmission in wban for healthcare monitoring. In: S. Bhattacharyya, N. Chaki, D. Konar, U. Chakraborty, & C. Singh (Eds.), *Advanced Computational and Communication Paradigms. Advances in Intelligent Systems and Computing*, Vol. 706. Springer.

Santos, O., Kampanakis, P., & Woland, A. (2016). Cisco next-generation security solutions: All-in-one cisco ASA firepower services, NGIPS, and AMP. Cisco Press.

Seimis, G., Huang, L., Masse, F., Tsekoura, I., Ashouei, M., Catthoor, F., Huisken, J., Stuyt, J., Dolmans, G., Penders, J., & Groot, H. D. (2011). A lightweight security scheme for wireless body area networks: Design, energy evaluation and proposed microprocessor design. *Journal of Medical System, 35*(5), 1289–1298. Springer.

Shen, J., Tan, H., Moh, S., Chubg, I., Kiu, Q., & Sun, X. (2015). Enhanced secure sensor association and key management in WBAN. *Journals of Communications and Networks, 17*(5).

Shi, L., Li, M., Yu, S., & Yuan, J. (2013). BANA: Body area network authentication exploiting channel characteristics. *IEEE Journals on Selected Areas in Communication, 31*(9), 1803–1816.

Singh, A., & Chatterjee, K. (2019a). Trust based access control model for securing electronic healthcare system. *Journal of Ambient Intelligence and Humanized Computing, 10*, 4547–4565.

Singh, A., & Chatterjee, K. (2019b). ITrust: Identity and trust based access control model for healthcare system security. *Multimedia Tools and Applications, 78*, 28309–28330.

Suarez, N., Callico, G. M., Sarmiento, R., Santana, O., & Abbo, A. A. (2009). *Processor Customization for Software Implementation of the AES Algorithm for Wireless Sensor Networks*. Patmos, pp. 326–335.

Thamilarasu, G., Odesile, A., & Hoang, A. (2020). An intrusion detection system for internet of things. *IEEE Access, 8*, 181560–181576.

Thamilarasu, G. (2016). iDetect: An intelligent intrusion detection system for wireless body area networks. *International Journal of Security and Networks, 11*(82). Inderscience Publishers.

Yuce, M. R. (2010). Implementation of wireless body area networks for healthcare systems. *Sensors and Actuators A: Physical, 162*(1), 116–129.

Zeadally, S., Isaac, J. T., & Baig, Z. (2016). Security attacks and solutions in electronic health (e-health) systems. *Journal of Medical Systems, 40*(12), 263.

Zhang, Y., Gravina, R., Lu, H., Villari, & M., Fortino, G. (2018). PEA: Parallel electrocardiogram-based authentication for smart healthcare systems. *Journal of Network and Computer Applications, 117*, 10–16.

Applications of IoT and Blockchain Technologies in Healthcare: Detection of Cervical Cancer Using Machine Learning Approaches

S. Jaya and M. Latha

Abstract The Internet of Things is an emerging subject of specialized, social, and efficient inference. Such as User products, long-lasting goods, cars and trucks, business enterprise and utility elements, sensors, and many other devices which are connected with internet. Big Data, the term refers about the large amount of data will be stored for the purpose of data sharing, data mining, data storing in various fields and applications like Health care, Finance and Transportation. Blockchain technology is like a public ledger of patients medical records where maintained by the hospital with secret genetic technology. The blocks should not modify in the middle of the chain due to inbuilt mechanism. Machine learning is the one of the fast-growing methods in all kind of fields, especially in medical fields, it is used to detect the disease state of the patient at early stage. Thus, the paper refers about how the advanced technologies are IoT, Big Data, and Blockchain methodologies are helpful to diagnosis the Cervical cancer at earlier in medical fields. The dataset of Cervical cancer has been taken from MDE Laboratory with the amount of 150 records.

Keywords Internet of Things · Big Data · Blockchain · Cervical Cancer · Machine Learning

1 Introduction

1.1 IoT (Internet of Things)

IoT the term stands for 'Internet of Things', founded by Kevin Ashtonv in the year of 1999. The word 'Things' is mentioning any kind of electron device, sensors that has ability to collect and exchanging data over internet. The main goal of IoT is to

S. Jaya (✉)
Department of Computer Science, Sri Sarada College for Women (Autonomous), Salem-16, India
e-mail: jaisundar11@gmail.com

M. Latha
Department of Computer Science, Sri Sarada College for Women (Autonomous), Salem-16, India

run along to internet connectivity from any type of standard devices like computer, mobile, and tablet. The importance of IoT is connecting all the devices and intercommunicate with each other through the internet. IoT is a huge network of connected devices all of which aggregate and transfer data by controlling and manipulating device without human intervention. In order to protect the seclusion and safety for patients in the healthcare situation based on IoT, a regular mechanism is needed (Baker et al., 2017). The example for IOT device like smart appliances is remote door locks, smart phones, smart watches, electronic washing machine stoves, refrigerators, hair washers and dryers, coffee maker machines, temperature checker, and slow cookers. IoT applies unambiguously specifiable smart devices and objects for the formation of cyber-physical smart ubiquitous systems which are also capable to connect with the already existing internet structure (Hakim, 2018). For example, refrigerator's sensor will be collecting the data based on the outside temperature and consequently adjust the refrigerator's temperature itself. These are the electronic device adjust their temperature automatically which helps the user to communicate with IoT Platform.

1.2 Big Data

Big Data is tons of information obtainable that can be stored at a primary location. Big Data may be derived with a collection of Distributed System, Storage, Statistics, Artificial Intelligence, Data Mining, Sciences, and Parallel Processing. The main process of big data is capturing data, data storage, data analysis, data sharing and transfer, visualizing data, and updating data. Big data give the power to guess new business models or to attain an important competitive advantage on the business organization. The size and complexity of the data need suitable technology in order to obtain value from it. The use of Big Data is becoming frequent these days by the enterprise to exceed their peers. Big Data is the backbone for many organizations to explore new opportunities and entirely new categories of companies that can be used to analyze the data in industry. The Big Data is a new word related with the vast amounts of stored as well as acquired data due to the radical early in different technologies (Kalipe & Behera, 2019). This big data is massively used in various fields such as Banking, Financing, Industry, Health care, Routine human life, Planet, and Satellite. Big Data is very helpful in various applications and fields which is used to develop the growth of the fields by applying machine learning algorithms. A tiny processing portion called as cloudlet which is for storing and processing and also helps to assume patients medical data. By storing data in cloudlet, it can be manipulating the data anytime for data analytics (Tawalbeh et al., 2016). Big Data analytics is one of the moving forward technology followed by many organizations. Big data generally consists of volume, velocity, value, veracity, and variety. It may have a characteristic of Petabyte volumes, Real-time velocity, and multi-structured varieties. The goodness of cloud technologies for big data management is providing limitless storage space, many helpful services, and connects relationship between patients and doctors (Mudholkar, 2020). The 'Apache Hadoop' is one of the open-source package library structure where allow the distributed processing of vast data sets transverse clusters of devices using easy scheduling models. It is built from one-on-one servers to one thousands of computer machines, providing local problem solving, and depository.

1.3 Blockchain Technology

Bloch chain technology was inaugurated by Satoshi Nakamoto in the year of 2008. The meaning of blockchain technology is a form of digital information that can be distributed, and it is like a backbone of new kind of internet. Execution of artificial intelligence (AI) algorithms and new merger algorithms would be essential to make sense from this ample magnitude of data (Failed, 2020). For example, Digital currency and Bitcoin blockchain are process of online distributed transaction. Blockchain is in simply derived as 'Huge number of data can be linked with each other managed by the multiple computers. Each and every block will be secured and bound to each other and is called as Cryptographic (single block). One of the important characteristics of blockchain is healthcare field is decentralization (Martín et al., 2018). Bitcoin and other virtual currency supported by blockchain technology helps the businesses to work out funding-related problems (Kumar & Mallick, 2018). Blockchain is a ledger that can be visible to anyone and if any data is modified in a block, that will be shared to all other blocks. It is a simple way of transforming information from A to B with full sage manner. For example, we can say buying railway tickets through App or Internet. There are two parties in the transaction one is Passengers and another person is a Railway company. Credit card agent is acquiring charge for transaction process. Here, the ticket is considered as a block which is to be added to a ticket blockchain separately. Blockchain is growing rapidly in Healthcare area where the patient encrypted data will be transmitted in secured manner.

1.4 Cervical Cancer Summary

Cervical cancer is extraordinary unsafe cancer which ruins the women cervix. Nearly 2,88,000 women are reach the death rate worldwide. It may raise due to abnormal growth of the cell in the cervix. A single woman is suggested to go for screening test at least once in a year. This type of cervical cancer mostly affects the women under the age of 26 to 62. It rarely affects the women below the age of 21. The sample cell tissue will be taken by the doctor that will send to the pathologist laboratory using microscopic. The pathologist will decide the disease state based on the shape, structure of the Nucleus, and Cytoplasm. Cervical cancer may have normal and abnormal cell types. Normal cell has three stages as well as abnormal cell have four stages such as, Superficial squamous, Intermediate squamous, Columnar epithelial, and Mild dysplastic, Moderate dysplastic, Severe dysplastic, and Carcinoma in situ. There are various technologies available to detect the disease automatically like CAD Tool. In this chapter, used the role of IoT, Big data, and Blockchain technology how these technologies are applied in health care fields. Taken sample dataset of cervical cancer in this entire chapter with the experiment analysis. The main purpose of this chapter is analyzing various technologies and machine learning algorithms to detect the Cervical cancer disease at earlier.

2   Literature Review

Shah Nazir et al. described about a review of functionality of IoT health care system using mobile computing. Shown various article referred in Literature Review on m-health care system and advantages of IoT technology in medical field (Nazir et al., 2019). The author Abdulaziz displayed importance of IoT in healthcare area such as diagnostic applications, therapy and counselling application, medical education application, drug reference application, and clinical field (Albesher, 2019). Amine Rghioui et al. gave brief notes on sensors and actuators like home appliances and smart mobile phones using IoT technologies like Radio Frequency Identification (RFID), Near Field Communication (NFC), Machine-to-Machine Communication (M2M), and Wireless sensor networks (WSN) (Rghioui & Oumnad, 2018). Sathya et al. referred about IoT device based on healthcare monitoring system. As well explained the system architecture of IoT, starting from data collection and transmission, cloudlet processing and analytics and prediction (Sathya et al., 2018). Stephanie et al. show IoT technologies, challenges facing toward medical field and opportunities. The scope of internet of things are wearable sensor and central nodes, short-long range communications, role of machine learning were used in the article (Sathya et al., 2018). Sabyasachi Dash et al. developed a role of Big Data in Healthcare. Healthcare data requires big data repository, and it is a digitization. The management of medical records is securely digitized using Big Data. The tool Hadoop and Apache also clearly mentioned by the author (Baker et al., 2017). Karim et al. explained the importance of big data, how the data can be secured from the hackers and what are the advanced and latest technologies are available, that is also displayed (Dash, 2019). Cornelius et al. gave a systematical review on the Blockchain Technology toward Healthcare system. Mentioned overview of the blockchain technology and difference between the ledgers of centralized and decentralized (Abouelmehdi, 2018). Seyednima et al. referred Blockchain technology in healthcare fields using Electronic Medical Records (EMR). Blockchain supply management are Billing management and quality management which are very essential task in medical fields (Agbo et al., 2019). Min Xu et al. published a review article on latest technology of Blockchain (Seyednima Khezr et al., 2019).

3   Research Methodology

3.1   *Role of Iot*

IoT is playing important role in day-to-day life. It is a trending advanced technology wireless networks and sensors that can be handle and manage by the people in a smart way. IoT is basically a platform which is connected to the internet over embedded device. By doing so, it can collect and transfer data with each other. It enables devices to communicate, cooperate, and acquire from each other's experiences just as humans do. Traffic camera is one of the best examples for IoT. The camera can able to monitor the streets from traffic crowding, accidents, weather conditions, and communicate this data to a common gateway. This single gateway will receive the data from other cameras and process that information further to a city-wide traffic monitoring system.

3.1.1   IoT Applications

IoT applications assure to bring huge value into our regular lives. With new found wireless networks, powerful sensors, and radical computing capacity, the Internet of Things could be the next subject field. IoT playing a vital role in every electronic device where by using technology and algorithm that can be ability to grow faster and faster.

Figure 1 shows the flowchart of applications of IoT platform.

Smart Home Automation

Now a days, people are searching for 'smart home' in Google. Because of the trendy technology applied on the appliances in a smart way without human access. IoT based Smart Home is the first place in recent technologies where everyone preferring such

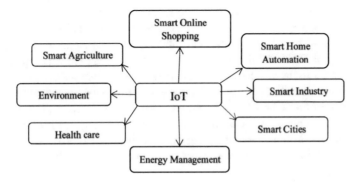

Fig. 1 IoT applications

a fashionable way. For example, Air Conditioner (AC), Refrigerator, Smart lights, Smart door, Smart car, Smart phones, Smart stove, Smart washing machine etc., there are many smart electronic devices applicable comes under home automation. These are the smart devices can be connected to the internet where the people can access and manipulate the device with their own convenient. Smart homes will be become as common as smart phones soon. The cost of owning a house is the difficult thing to middle class people but still these products are very useful to save time and energy. The smart home companies are Nest, Ring, and Ecobee, and many other companies. These companies are planned to deliver an unexpected products what we never expect.

(1) Switch on air conditioning before reaching home.
(2) Switch off lights after left from the home.
(3) Lock and Unlock door when you are at home or not.
(4) Stove off even forget to switch off after left from home.
(5) Car door lock is a function of IoT everyone knows.
(6) Smart Industry

IoT is a vast smart system used in the Industry which is called as 'Industrial Internet of Things' as well as Industry 4.0. This IIOT works on devices and machinery equipment used in business environment. The IIOT system consists of sensor devices, machinery, tools, software platforms, cloud server networks, and applications. These smart sensor networks frequently send data to the IoT gateway which act as a hub between IoT devices and cloud system. It receives the data and transfer to the cloud network server for analyzing the data. Ample amount of data is handling with the use of refined application programs with secured manner in smart phone application. The main advantage of this Industry IoT is comfortable workplace function, making employer safety, efficient and smart way work process, flexible environment like friendly system.

Smart Cities

IoT works on making the city in smart manner to become a healthier environment, traffic clearance for public safety smart city and providing best street lighting. For example, Road traffic—automatically clears the congestion vehicle by managing GPS on driver's car, speed of the car, vehicle number, and location of the vehicle. Smart Parking—The parking locations are noticed and make a real-time parking map with the help of GPS. The driver can easily get the paring map which place if free to park their car in faster. These facilities are only applicable with IoT Technology. Smart lighting—This technology works in a smart way that automatically adjust the enhancement of the light settings based on, while pedestrian cross the road, while bus entry into the bus stop, based on the climate such as rainy or sunny, movements of the people. Environment—monitoring water quality in an area based on the sensor measures the PH level as well as sensors checks the air quality by measuring CO, nitrogen, and sulfur oxides.

Energy Management

IoT is such an impact application for power consumption by the way of managing lightening, temperature, and vibration. These real time data are compared using sensor with program then only it can able to adjust the power energy automatically. Philips Hue and Ecobee 4 are lighting, it provides 85% less energy. WebNMS is an outstanding illustration of the Internet of Things energy management system for business enterprise and commercial spaces. Using the data point coming from a network of sensors and meters on-site, the solution supplying saving measures to analyze the utilization of energy and increase productivity. IoT application in the field of Energy management,

(1) Smart grid
(2) Power house
(3) Power supply controller for telecommunication, computer
(4) Photovoltaic installation

Health Care

The main problem for the patient is that interaction with doctor will be a difficult one in case of emergency. But after IoT, it made easy that the doctor can monitor the patient health continuously and it became easier to interact with doctor by enabled devices remote monitoring. The devices may in the form of wearable devices which are very helpful to check blood pressure, heart beat rate counting, if any abnormal cell growth identified, calorie count, and more. The primary advantage of IoT in health care is that it can avoid unnecessary visit to doctor, reduce length of days staying at hospital, helpful to diagnosis a disease earlier by doing regular monitoring by the doctor, and improving health care operations with the help of sensor devices.
   IoT technologies in Healthcare 2020,

(1) Telemedicine
(2) Internet of medical Things
(3) Cloud technology in healthcare
(4) AR(Augmented Reality) and VR(Virtual Reality) facility in healthcare sector
(5) Chatbots trends
(6) Predictive analytics

Environment

Environmental phenomena have a leading issue on our regular lives. The environment changes may affect the root of our lives such as water and air pollution which cause to degrade the purity. The word 'smart environment' is referred that the technology provides more facilities and resolution for few essential application issues based on water purity, air pollution, weather condition, radiation monitoring, waste product management, natural, and unnatural earth tragedy. 'Internet of Things' technology can ability to provide an innovative system tracking, remote sensing, and monitoring objects of the environment. The world can achieve a green world as soon as possible because of IoT. The process of IoT in environmental is that the sensor connected to the smart phones over Bluetooth or Wi-Fi for the purpose of sending tremendous data. By measuring degree of PH will determine the quality of water which can be an efficient water monitoring system. IoT is very helpful to protect the city from natural disaster like floods, volcano, earthquakes, cyclone, wildfires, snowstorm, and many more. Waste management also handled with the help of IoT technology by sensor solutions and cameras.

Smart Agriculture

IoT is being utilized in Agriculture field to help the farmers. Far more advanced sensors are being utilized. The sensors can be connected to the cloud through smart mobile and satellite network which may aid to know the real-time data from the sensors to making make the decision effective. The advanced IoT technology assists to monitor the water tank levels, decreasing cost expenses by increasing yields, rainfall prediction, and climate condition. Sensors are located in two places: inside and outside of the agriculture fields. It used to collect data from the situation which is helps to choose the right crops. Various IoT devices available to detect the crops in many ways based on the farmer requirements. By doing so, ability to increase the production and farmer can attain more benefits. Precision agriculture is used to control the water supply to the crop yields by maintaining reports in the sensors.

IoT 2020 latest technologies used to grow the smart agriculture by,

(1) Plant sensors
(2) Animal monitor and cattle monitor
(3) Smart drones
(4) Form the future using 5G
(5) Livestock track and Geo-fence
(6) Smart green house
(7) Predictive analytics for smart farming in agriculture

Smart Online Shopping

Automated checkout system is very beneficial to the shop manager as well as to the customer because of the crowd, and it is difficult for the manger to monitor the employers at busier time. The great IoT device helps to read the tag on each product while the customer leaving the shop. This checkout system assists to tally the items automatically deduct that price from the customers mobile payment app. Beacons is a small Bluetooth device that used to send alerts to smart phones based on location locality. The customers can get discounts, new arrival products, and any reminders when they are near to the store due to downloaded the store's app.

Retail business works using IoT 2020 technologies,

(1) Automated checkouts
(2) Personalized discounts
(3) Beacons

(4) Smart shelves
(5) Layout optimization
(6) Robot workers

3.1.2 Architecture of IoT

The concept of IoT Architecture is the system of unlimited features such as sensors, detectors, protocols, cloud networks, and distinct layers. And more over IoT Architecture layers are distinguished in order to measure the consistency of the system and also it considers a plan to improve the productivity of the organization's existing infrastructure and systems. IoT architecture is complicated when it is implemented in to reality. Need to check certain number of devices and sensor conditions. Generally, there are three basic IoT architecture layers:

(1) The customer side (IoT Device)
(2) Server side operator (Getaway)
(3) Connecting customer and server together (Platform)
(4) There are several types of architecture has been exposed by the researcher. The general form of IoT architecture is given below,

Figure 2 representing the basic structure of IoT with consists of four layers.

(a) **Application Layer**

Application layer is the top most first layer in the IoT Platform. This application layer extends to provide essential services to the user based on their requirements. The main duty of this layer is to link the leading gap between the users and the applications. This IoT layer is also contributing services to various fields to attain some solutions such as the fields are Online retail shopping, smart home appliances, healthcare monitor, agriculture water supply monitor, traffic checker, satellite sensors, etc.

Fig. 2 Architecture of IoT
(4 layers)

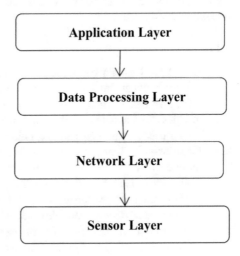

(b)   **Data Processing Layer**

Data processing layer otherwise called as 'Middleware Layer'. The primary task of this layer is storing, analyzing, and accessing the large amount of data where comes from transport layer. It has the ability to monitor and provide a different set of services to the lowest layers. It utilizes from many technologies like database system, analytics, cloud computing, and big data analytics modules. This layer makes decisions automatically based on the outputs where such data store in the database.

(c)   **Network Layer**

Network layer is also called as 'transmission layer'. The main work of this layer is transmitting data from sensor devices to the information processing system in a secured manner. This network layer can be divided into two layers such as routing layer and encapsulation layer. Routing layer defines about the data handles between the source and destination. Encapsulation layer is about to forming the data packets.

(d)   **Sensor Layer**

IoT sensors describe about that sensor can able to analyze the conditions close to the IoT device, for example, in agriculture application, sensor process is to check environmental conditions. There are various types of sensors available to apply on distinct fields to make more efficient. Sensors are used to collect the huge data to become a smarter such as temperature sensor, proximity sensor, pressure sensor, and chemical sensor.

3.1.3   Types of IoT Wireless Technology

The Internet of Things (IoT) begins with network connectivity as well as IoT is a wide diverse and multifarious domain and cannot able to find a one-size-fits-all communication method. Every solution has some advantage and disadvantage in several network criteria.

There are six types of IoT wireless technologies 2020 available. They are given below

(1)   **LPWANs (Low Power Wide Area Networks)**—It is a trendy wireless technology between machine to machine and IoT devices. This technology is recommended in many business cases and the term itself tells the characteristics of wide connectivity with low power consumption. For example, this sensor used in smart agriculture, building application and smart cities.

(2)   **Cellular**—Cellular networks like 3G,4G,5G. connection between the smart mobile phones. For example, car parking meters, smart house, hospital database connectivity, camera maintenance for public safety.

(3)   **Zigbee and mesh protocols**—Zigbee is a wireless technology which consumes low power and openly available in global standards. It has the facility of wireless network connectivity range of 70 m indoors and 400 m outdoors. It easily works on light monitoring and utilized in medical fields to find patients presence.

(4) **Bluetooth**—It may call as short range communication network as well as personal area network. This applicable in mobile to mobile connectivity or multi device connectivity with any wearable devices for transmitting purpose.
(5) **Wi-Fi**—Wi-Fi is widely used in many applications such as IT Industry, Study Organization, Hospitals, On board diagnostics.

3.2 Introduction to Big Data

Big data, the term talks about large amount of data maintained by some organization with huge quantity. For example, the Hervlet hospital maintains the Cervical cancer dataset of each and every patients that where stored in a huge database for future references. There are various algorithms and approaches available for representing the data. The four main characteristics of big data are Volume, Variety, Velocity, and Variability. The other example is Walmart manages 1 million customer transactions every one hour also social media Facebook. The use of big data is wanted in all industries to outperform their peers. Many companies are gathering data and storing it in a secured database for further analysis to improve their business. The main use of big data is 'decision taking', by the company as well as can improve the customer requirements. Big data is important in such a case,

(1) Cost savings—Hadoop is one of tool used in big data for storing the bulk data to analyzing depth by enterprise.
(2) Less time consumption—Many big data analytics tools are helpful to recover the data from database quickly and which may help to take decision fast.
(3) Update market conditions—By knowing big data strategies the company might know their future scope of the business based on the customer behavior/satisfaction.
(4) Knowing company reputations of the company by using big data analytics or knowing through online.

3.2.1 Application of Big Data

Big data, the term refers about the large size of unprocessed data. The main goal of big data analytics is to aid companies make business decisions by data analytics models, predictive models, and other analytics strategy toward handle the huge data. Big data technology is an influential tool in various applications to make them easy. Big data is used in several applications and fields. Some important fields are given below, education.

(1) Bank industry and securities
(2) Insurance protection
(3) Transportation
(4) Educational Activity
(5) Enterprises and manufacturing companies

Table 1 Employers table in company database

Customer acc. num	Customer name	Address	Contact number	Balance amount
2365 343	Kalpana rahena	India	435645645	650,000
3398 356	Pradeep joshi	India	565756756	650,000
7465 098	Roy renalut	India	565645656	500,000
7500 767	Shuba shree bhat	India	323987555	500,000

(6)   Energy services
(7)   Health care—Hospitality
(8)   Media and Entertainment
(9)   Agriculture

3.2.2   Types of Big Data

The use of Big data is increasing every year in IT field. The types of big data shall be derived into three types. Which are mentioned below,

(1)   Structured data
(2)   Unstructured
(3)   Semi-structured

(1)   **Structured data**—The large amount of data is in a structured way which is like an ordered manner. It is easy way of understanding the data which is representing in table form. For example, in Industry or Banking sector, they are used to maintain a record of employers and customer details in a database in form of table like employer name, employer id, salary details, address, contact number, etc., such as in Bank, customer name, account number, saving account, current account, and personal details.

Table 1 explains the employee's details that are maintained by a company.

(2)   **Unstructured data**—It is just opposite to the structured data where does not have clear format in storage. The best example for unstructured data is social media like Facebook and Instagram. Every second people are posting their photos and videos as well as chatting history. These are all stored as it is in the cloud data storage.

(3)   **Semi-structured data**—Semi-structured data will be in form of structured manner but that is not defined in the database. For example, semi-structured data will be represented in XML File format and.csv file.

3.2.3   Advantages and Disadvantages of Big Data Processing

Advantages

(1) In customer point of view, before buying any product people used to refer the feedback in social media about their rate of the product. This may be helpful to choose the product by the customer as well as the company can get to know their business state among the people. Based on the feedback the company can satisfy the customer requirements.

(2) Using big data can increase efficiency in term of Google map is used to reach the exact location without delay. It saves time and reduce travel expense. Use of business intelligence tool to estimate finance strategy that can project a clearer state of the business of where it stands.

(3) Big data is playing vital contribution in healthcare field. Many advanced technologies are developing by various researchers which helps to detect the disease of the person. For example, Cervical cancer is a dangerous kind of cancer which affects the women cervix. Various advanced tools are there to diagnosis the cancer state whether it is normal or abnormal. CAD tool is increased in medical area which helps to find the cancerous cell. More technologies and machine learning algorithms are used in classification phase.

(4) The industry can create product and services based on the customer needs and satisfaction by knowing trends of the customer requirements through big data analytics.

Disadvantages

(1) The capacity of storing big data is very large, and storage cost is high. Majority of the data will be in unstructured form. This is difficult to handle by the company. Big data tools are essential to resolve this problem due to need expert scientist.

(2) Data should be accurate if not prediction of the industry will be wrong.

The company maintain all data in a database where secured data may hack by Hack attackers.

3.2.4   Tools and Techniques of Big Data

Big data tools are very essential to implement the company strategy and can be able to know prediction analysis of the company based on the previous data. There are various tools available to access and manipulate the data. They are given below,

(1) **Apache Hadoop**—Apache Hadoop is a cluster-based file system which is used to handle the big data. It is an open source tool and frequently used by technologist and scholars. The data types can access like image, video, XML, and text file. This tool is mainly used in Research and Development sector.

(2) **CDH (Cloudera Distribution of Hadoop)**—It is open source software platform which controls Apache Hadoop and Apache spark etc. It is easy to handle the data implementation and it maintains the data in secured manner.

(3) **Cassandra**—It is free of cost tool consists of SQL and DBMS. Many companies are using this tool Accenture, Facebook, Yahoo, and Honeywell. It has ability to handle huge data very quickly, and it maintains data log structured storage.

(4) **Knime**—The term full form 'Konstanz Information Miner', which is an open source software, used for company data mining, data analytics, text mining, and business intelligence. The supporting operating systems are Linux, OS X, and Windows.

(5) **Datawrapper**—It is an open source tool for the purpose of visual representation to get quick chart results. It works well in laptop, tablet, and smart phones. It does not need any programming code.

(6) **MongoDB**—It is document-oriented database like C, C + + , and Javascript. It is open source software and supports multiple operating systems such as OS X, Linux, Solaris, and FreeBSD. The main advantage is reliable with low cost.

(7) **Lumify**—This tool is completely open source used for big data integration, data analytics, and visualization. It has facilities like 2D, 3D visualization, graphical design system, special, and multimedia analysis.

(8) **Rapidminer**—It is a cross platform tool used for machine learning, data prediction, and analytics. Rapidminer is used by Hitachi, BMW, Samsung, Airbus, and many more.

3.3 Blockchain Technology

All the transaction collected and stored in blocks where those data should be recorded. The term Blockchain is referred about the digital information recorded in a public database. It is peer to peer network connected with all network nodes. It is very difficult to change or modify the data in a block. The blockchain is used to build based upon the date and time to save the data. For example, consider land sale. Owner of the land property has been sale to other third party with all approved evidence. Those proofs will be stored in a computer database along with land documents. This is the final stage of the land sale because of the land should not sell to another person again. In blockchain the date of the property sale and who is the owner of the land, these details will be in the technology called 'Blockchain'.

(1) Blockchain is a ledger to maintain a financial transaction. It is a common book because everyone can monitor the transaction.

(2) Hash value is a function that converts the input values into encrypted format which is used to manage cryptocurrency.

(3) Hash value is a fixed length of secret letters that created using algorithms to protect data from hackers and fraudulent transaction.

(4) It is impossible to guess the hash when someone is trying to change the blockchain.

(5) Hash value is characterized created on the information obtainable in the block header.

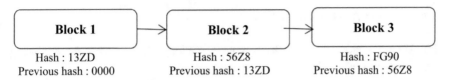

Block 1	**Block 2**	**Block 3**
Hash : 13ZD	Hash : 56Z8	Hash : FG90
Previous hash : 0000	Previous hash : 13ZD	Previous hash : 56Z8

Fig. 3 Representation of Blockchain

(6)   Block time is referred about the time taken for building the blocks. Some block may build in 5 s.

Figure 3 shows the basic architecture of the Blockchain using hash function. Hash will be determined based on the given input data.

(7)   Blockchain is a distribution decentralized system of Peer-to-Peer network where the information stored in every system network. The data is not recorded at one block as well the copy of data will be stored in each distributed system.

(8)   A Node is a device to manipulating the blockchain technology such as computers, laptop, and server.

Figure 4 represents the example of seven nodes that were connected to each other. Here the example mentioned only 7 nodes but in blockchain it may has 100 or 1000 and more nodes will be connected.

(9)   Nodes may be in online or offline mode. Online nodes can be able to receive, storing the data of latest transaction from other nodes. While it is offline, it will catch-up the data by downloading and the data will update when online comes back. This processing is called as 'Synchronization with Blockchain'.

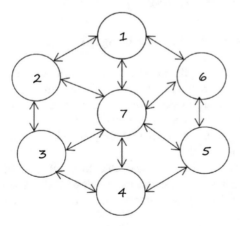

Fig. 4 7 nodes/servers/computer connected each other—Blockchain

3.3.1 Latest Blockchain Tools

Blockchain is one of the latest growing up technology where as Bitcoin is achieving huge success worldwide.

(1) Solidity
(2) Mist
(3) Solc
(4) Remix
(5) Metamask
(6) Truffle
(7) GanacheCLI
(8) Blockchain Testnet
(9) Blockchain-as-a-Service
(10) Coinbase API
(11) EtherScripter
(12) Ether.js
(13) Tierion
(14) Embark
(15) MyEtherWallet

These tools are commonly used in many developing companies to attain best expertise in building blockchain technology.

3.4 Diagnosis of Cervical Cancer Using Iot, Big Data and Blockchain Technology

3.4.1 Detection of Cervical Cancer Using IoT

Internet of Things (IoT) is updating technology in various fields. The contribution of IoT is becoming high in medical application. IoT device used to monitor the patients' health condition as well as it reports to the doctor about patient's state.

Many researchers and scientist proved that ZedScan can increase the detection of high-grade CIN (Cervical Intra-epithelial Neoplasia) in women referred about both low and high level abnormal cytopathology.

European Journal of Gynecological Oncology released that 'ZedScan' is a portable device which is used to detect the dysplasia and cancer stage of the cervix. The device helps to detect tissue changes in women cervix and able to know the abnormal pap smear test.

Duke University established **'Pocket Colposcope'** device to take self-screening test for women. The device is connected to the laptop/smart mobile where the women can able to go for screening test themselves. Another IoT technology is 'AutoPap' which is AI based diagnostic system. AutoPap is used to acquire the cervical image that the reports can be send to the pathologist to classify the presence of the tissue through smart phone.

3.4.2 Detection of Cervical Cancer Using Big Data

The number of cervical cancer patient is increasing rapidly. Many researchers and data scientist are working toward to diagnosis the cancer at early stage. Several statistics models, mathematical structure, and machine learning algorithms are using to attain the efficient cancer treatment. The use of Big Data in Healthcare is very essential to collecting, analyzing, and manipulating using machine learning algorithms for the purpose of sudden review of the patient. The main advantage of using big data is improving health outcomes and improve efficient treatment. The huge bulk of information of the patient health reports will be stored systematically.

The primary role of Big data is vast existing information, has been stored, and may help to prevent the cancer, and the doctor can be able to take better decision about the patient health. Electronic Health Record (EHR) is a digital format that the patient information will be stored electronically. This information should be protect securely using some standardized methods like HIPAA and ISO.

The key benefit of Big data in healthcare is try to diminish the death case by forecasting the disease. In machine learning, training data is helpful to identify the disease to give them accurate treatment. Cloud based storage database is accessing point by the people where anyone can manipulate the information from anywhere. Especially doctors can easily handle the patient's condition depending on the information stored in a database. Moreover, it is fast growing technology under artificial intelligence and machine learning algorithms bring the better skillfulness in healthcare field.

3.4.3 Detection of Cervical Cancer Using Blockchain Technology

Lancor Scientific has been proposed new testing methods by registering global records of the patients. It is a global cervical cancer registry where the patients can be able to own their data in blockchain platform, and it is secured by virtual currency. This method is helpful for preventing cervical cancer from existing challenges what the doctor faced. This Lancor process is a combination of quantum physics and Artificial Intelligence algorithms. Each and every record will be connected based on distributed ledger technology, this may be called as 'Lancor Blockchain Paltform'.

CEO of Lancor Scientific is 'Aamir Butt' defines that Accuracy of classification is very essential for diagnosis a cancer. In such a case, this Lancor scientific method will be very useful to decide the disease state by analyzing various patients' reports. The main aim of the blockchain technology stores the patients' reports for the purpose of pattern recognition. Blockchain is used to saving the data in memory, distributing and recovering data from biomedical database. Hyper-Ledger fabric is an intermediate device which is mainly used to transfer the data by mobile phone and also it secures the patient information. Moreover, blockchain is a transparency because of anyone can view and add the data as well as it is immutability to store the data. Blockchain is reliable technology between all connected data where structure cannot be modified by anyone.

Artificial Intelligence helps to detect the overlapped and underlying cells based on the features by using various classification algorithm. By doing so, the accuracy level will be high and could diagnosis the cervical cancer by stage wise whether it is comes under Superficial Squamous, Intermediate Squamous, Columnar Epithelial, Mild Dysplasia, Moderate Dysplasia, Severe Dysplasia, and Carcinoma in situ.

3.5 Cervical Cancer—Machine Learning Algorithms

Test samples will be taken from the women cervix to analyze that the cell is normal or abnormal. Generally, the cell contains nucleus and cytoplasm together. Those samples send to the pathologist laboratory for diagnosis the cervical cancer by using microscopic. The Machine Learning is biggest turning point which helps to detect the presence of the cancer. Three forms of machine learning algorithms are used for prediction and classification. They are given below,

(1) Supervised learning algorithm
(2) Unsupervised learning algorithm
(3) Reinforcement learning algorithm

(1) Supervised learning algorithm

Supervised learning algorithm consists of class labels which determines about the types of cancer cell. In this algorithm, it is considered two variables such as dependent variable and independent variable. Training data is taken for the input data for classification purpose. The data will be trained until the model reaches the better accuracy level.

(2) Unsupervised learning

Unsupervised learning does not follow any structure as well it does not have class labels. The example for unsupervised algorithm is K-means Clustering and Apriori algorithm. The accuracy level would be less than supervised learning algorithm while doing classification.

(3) Reinforcement learning

Reinforcement learning is multi-training model to attain the goal. The primary process of RL is taking suitable action through several trial of the machine learning models. This learning model is well suited for making decision, and the agent is act as a inter-mediator.

3.5.1 Types of Learning Algorithms

Regression based Algorithms

Regression is predictive model techniques which establish a relationship between the target and predictors. This regression model is suited for combination of two classes. For example, Rainfall prediction. The two variables are temperature and cloud cover area. Some of the regression algorithm given below,

(1) Ordinary Least Squares Regression
(2) Linear Regression
(3) Logistic Regression
(4) Stepwise Regression
(5) Ridge and Lasso Regression
(6) Polynomial Regression
(7) Multivariate Adaptive Regression Fins

Instance based Algorithms

Instance based learning is otherwise called as Memory based learning. The process of instance-based algorithm is comparing current instance with existing trained instance from the memory. It is storing instance themselves. Some classifier is working depends on Instance based learning algorithm.

Figure 5 exposes the framework of list of five Instanced based algorithms. They are KNN, SVM, LVQ, SOM, and LWL.

Regularization Learning Algorithms

Removing Over-fitting is one of techniques to improve the accuracy level. If the model is over-fitting then it will acquire less accuracy while training the model. Regularization method is used to avoid the risk of over-fitting data which makes easy implementation, and it reduces error by using fitting function.

Figure 6 lists out the four major algorithms of Regularization learning algorithms based on Ridge Regression, LASSO, Elastic net, and LWL.

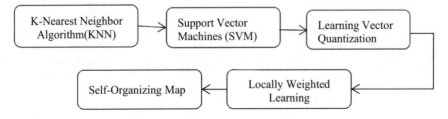

Fig. 5 List of Instance based algorithm

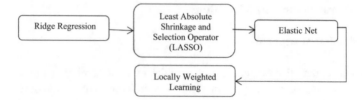

Fig. 6 List of Regularization learning algorithm

Decision Tree Classifier

Decision tree is like a tree structure form which is called as 'Predictive Modelling Approaches'. Decision tree is taken for the persistence of Regression and Classification. It contains parent node and leaf node which will take decision based on some condition in algorithm Fig. 7.

The flowchart exposing the types of Decision Tree classifier with various types of CART, CHAID, Conditional, and Stump Decision Trees.

Bayesian Algorithms

Bayes theorem is most powerful tool for calculating conditional probability. It is used to solve hypothesis probability under machine learning classifier. Bayes theorem is mostly used in the field of Data Science (Fig. 8).

Figure 9 is referring the machine learning algorithm of Bayesian Network of GNB, MNB, AODE, BN, and BBN.

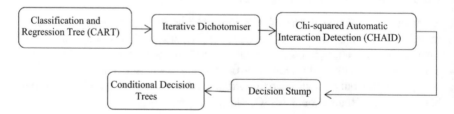

Fig. 7 List of decision tree classifier

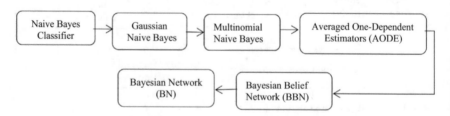

Fig. 8 List of several Bayesian classifier

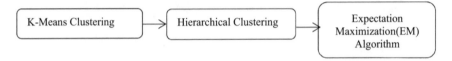

Fig. 9 Clustering based classifier

Clustering Based Algorithms

Clustering is a group of data points that each data points will be classified into a specific group. Based on the number of centroid K value, the data points will be grouped for classification.

Figure 10 displays a various kind of Cluster Based Algorithms.

Artificial Neural Network Algorithms (ANN)

Artificial Neural Network is a multiple connection of Input layer, Hidden layers, and Output layers. Input data will be loaded into an ANN layers which may divided into training set and testing set with 10 cross fold validation. Confusion matrix is calculated for finding accuracy.

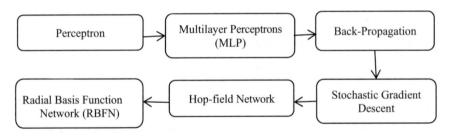

Fig. 10 List of ANN Algorithms

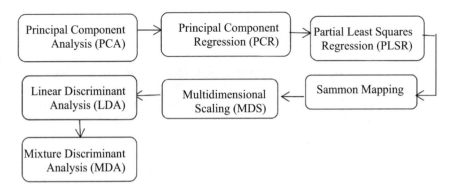

Fig. 11 List of Dimensionality Reduction Algorithm

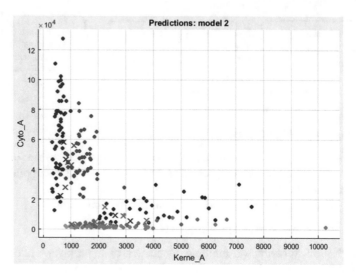

Fig. 12 Quadratic SVM result

Figure 11 represents an AI algorithms called ANN based Classifier such as Perceptron, MLP, BP, RBFN, Hop Field Network, and SGD.

Dimensionality Reduction Algorithm

Dimensionality Reduction is used reduce the size of the data. The redundancy data eliminated while using dimensionality reduction algorithm. The data should not get lose when applying dimensionality reduction algorithm because of the accuracy level might get low.

Figure 12 explains the various dimensionality reduction algorithms such as PCA, PCR, PLSR, LDA, MDS, and MDA.

4   Results and Discussion

Machine Learning algorithms have been used in medical dataset of Cervical Cancer to detect the disease. The classification phase will establish an accuracy level. In this chapter, three machine learning classification algorithms have been implemented with the tool of MATLAB R2016a.

Fig. 13 SVM confusion
matrix

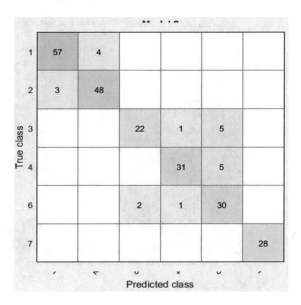

4.1 Quadratic SVM (Support Vector Machine)

Quadratic SVM is the traditional classification learning algorithm where the features
will be separated by hyper-plane. The data points have 6 class of cervical cancer that
are specified as stages of cancer such as Superficial Squamous, Intermediate Squamous, Columnar Epithelial, Mild Dysplasia, Moderate Dysplasia, Severe Dysplasia,
and Carcinoma in situ. The highest accuracy obtained in Quadratic SVM was 91.1%.

Figure 12 describes the 6 types of cervical cancer with the accuracy of 91.1%

Figure 13 shows the true class and predicted classes using fivefold cross validation.

4.2 Weighted KNN (K-Nearest Neighbor)

Weighted KNN is widely used for classification and prediction analysis which data
points are grouped based on nearest data points. Based on the selection of K value
the data will be grouped. The better accuracy attained using Cosine and Weighted
KNN Classifier with 79.3%.

Figure 14 displays the result with 79.1% with the speed of ~ 1500obs/sec.

4.3 Complex Tree

Complex tree comes under the decision tree which is used make the decision for
the complex data. It is a kind of supervised machine learning algorithms consist of

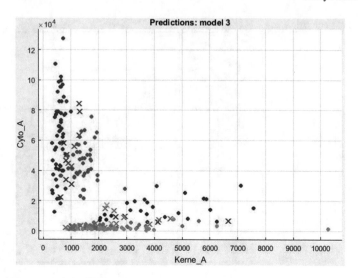

Fig. 14 Result of weighted KNN

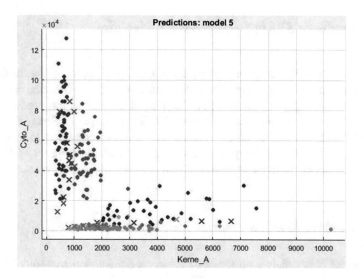

Fig. 15 Result of complex tree using 6 types of cervical cancer

nodes and leaves. It is look like tree structure as well as splitting the data based on the decision rules. The accuracy has been attained 86.1% using complex tree structure classifier with the training time of 2.538 s.

Figure 15 shows the complex tree implementation cervical cancer dataset.

4.4 Comparison of SVM, KNN, and Decision Tree

S.no	SVM	KNN	Decision tree
1	SVM can access by both linear and non-linear function by using kernel	KNN supports non-parametric function. It is based on K-value and Euclidean distance	It works to resolve the regression and classification problem
2	It handles the data points based on the hyperplane between the classes	KNN does not having any functions to train the data	It looks like tree structure where contains attributes and labels in form of leaf nodes
3	It works based on the memory	It works based on the K number of classifier value	It does not need any normalization methods
4	SVM will not give more accurate if it has a greater number of imperfect data	If more number of noise data available means, cannot attain good accuracy	Missed data never reduce the accuracy level in classification
5	It has plenty of dimensional space	It works faster than the SVM and decision tree	It takes more time to train the data. It works slower than other algorithms

4.5 Advantages of Proposed Methodology

Proposed methodology of Quadratic SVM provides good result than remaining to algorithms. Even though SVM is an old and traditional algorithm, it can able to classify a multi-class attributes from a specific dataset. This entire chapter discussed about the role of IoT and Blockchain Technology in the field of healthcare sector, especially in Cervical cancer. The dataset has been chosen here is cervical cancer dataset of pap smear images to the purpose of implementation of machine learning algorithms. To reduce the disease of cervical cancer, IoT and Blockchain technology are being important role to saving the women life by the way of wearable electronic device as well as accessing patients' database.

5 Conclusion

The contribution of IoT, Big Data, and Data Science is the most powerful mechanism, and it is used to enable enterprises to extent the digital transformation. Combining these innovative technologies would make the business to maximize their profit. In this chapter, discussed the vital role of IoT, Big Data, and Blockchain technologies toward the Challenges of diagnosis the Cervical cancer earlier in medical field. Cervical cancer is the most dangerous kind of cancer which is spread over in women cervix gradually. Thus, with the help of IoT device the women could go for screening test themselves without need of pathologist. As well, the Blockchain and Big Data are most important phase for maintaining patients database with secured manner. Machine learning and Artificial Intelligence are the grateful tool using in distinct fields, especially in medical sector it is being enormous to detect the disease with better accuracy. Thus, Quadratic SVM gives the better result while compared with KNN and Decision Tree because of SVM handles well even a unstructured data.

References

Abouelmehdi, K. (2018). Abderrahim Beni- Hessane and Hayat Khalouf, Big healthcare data: Preserving security and privacy. *Journal of Big Data*. https://doi.org/10.1186/s40537-017-0110-7.

Agbo, C. C. , Mahmoud, Q. H., & Mikael Eklund, J. (2019). Blockchain technology in healthcare: A systematic review, healthcare 2019, 7, 56. https://doi.org/10.3390/healthcare7020056.

Albesher, A. (2019). Internet of things for healthcare using effects of mobile computing: A systematic literature review. *IJCSNS International Journal of Computer Science and Network Security, 19* (2), February.

Baker, Stephanie B., xiang, Wei, & Atkinson, Ian. (2017). Internet of things for smart healthcare: Technologies, challenges, and opportunities. *IEEE Access*, vol 5. https://doi.org/10.1109/ACCESS.2017.2775180.

Dash, Sabyasachi, Shakyawar, Sushil Kumar, & Sandeep Kaushik, Mohit Sharmaand. Big data in healthcare: Management, analysis and future prospects, Dash et al. J *Big Data* 6:54. https://doi.org/10.1186/s40537-019-0217-0,(2019).

El Hakim, A. (2018). Internet of Things (IoT) System Architecture and Technologies, White Paper. *Research Gate*. https://doi.org/10.13140/RG.2.2.17046.19521

Kalipe, G. K. & Behera, R. K. (2019). Big data architectures: A detailed and application oriented review. Research Gate.

Khezr, Seyednima, Moniruzzaman, Md, Yassine, Abdulsalam, & Benlamri, Rachid. (2019). *Blockchain Technology in Healthcare: A comprehensive review and directions for future research, appl. sci.* 2019, 9, 1736. https://doi.org/10.3390/app9091736.

Manoj Kumar, Nallapaneni, & Mallick, Pradeep Kumar. (2018). Blockchain technology for security issues and challenges in IoT. *International Conference on Computational Intelligence and Data Science (ICCIDS 2018)*. https://doi.org/10.1016/j.procs.2018.05.140.

Martín, C., Soler, E., & Díaz, M. (2018). On blockchain and its integration with IoT. Challenges and opportunities, Future Generation Computer Systems. https://doi.org/10.1016/j.future.2018.05.046.

Mudholkar, Pankaj. (2020). Internet of things (IoT) and big data: A review. *International Journal of Management, Technology And Engineering*, ISSN NO: 2249–7455, vol. 8, no. XII, 5001–5007.

Nazir, Shah, Ali, Yasir, & Ullah, Naeem. (2019). Internet of things for healthcare using effects of mobile computing: A systematic literature review. *Hindawi Wireless Communications and Mobile Computing* vol. 2019, Article ID 5931315, 20 pages. https://doi.org/10.1155/2019/5931315.

Rghioui, A. & Oumnad, A. (2018). Challenges and opportunities of internet of things in healthcare, vol. 8, No. 5, October 2018, pp. 2753–2761, ISSN: 2088–8708. https://doi.org/10.11591/2018/ijece.v8i5.pp2753-2761.

Sathya, M., Madhan, S., & Jayanthi, K. (2018). Internet of things (IoT) based health monitoring system and challenges. *International Journal of Engineering &Technology, 7* (1.7), 175–178.

Tawalbeh, L., Mehmood, R., Benkhelifa, E., & Song, H. (2016). Mobile Cloud Computing Model and Big Data Analysis for Healthcare Applications. *IEEE Access*. https://doi.org/10.1109/ACCESS.2016.2613278

Tonelli, Roberto, Ortu, Marco, & Pinna, Andrea. (2020). Special issue "Advances in blockchain technology and applications 2020", Applied Scinces.

Xu, M., Chen, X., & Kou, G. (2019). A systematic review of blockchain, Xu et al. *Financial Innovation* 5:27. https://doi.org/10.1186/s40854-019-0147-z.

Remote Sensing in Public Health Environment: A Review

Puja Das, K. Martin Sagayam, Asik Rahaman Jamader, and Biswaranjan Acharya

Abstract Improvements during portable and electronic medical services are changing a contribution on behalf of together specialists along with patients during an advanced medical care structure through increasing the capacities of physiological observing gadgets. Lately there is fast exploration going in remote sensors for wireless Healthcare. These remote sensors give different functionalities in universal climate that permits sensors to associate with web anytime and anyplace. Wearable sensor frameworks which take into consideration distant or self-checking of well-being related boundaries are viewed as one intends to ease the results of segment change. Sensors assume a significant function in medical care industry. In spite of huge advancement inside the inspection tool industry, the broad reconciliation of this innovation into clinical practice stays restricted. Then again Social media has pushed forward of simply being an apparatus for young adult clients to share their own lives (data, life info) however has additionally been taken up by medical care partners to scatter health data around the world. The function of web-based media in medical services industry and effect of patient commitment has moved to focused phase and is constantly moved by quiet interest, mobile innovation, and mounting impact of the local electronic age. The movement with which the social action is developing, and it is essential to predict what affect these electronic stages are having on the recovery and result of medical care intercessions. The motivation behind this review is to sum up the turns of events and clinical utility of brilliant wearable body sensors. A review taken how far online media has been end up being powerful in spreading wellbeing data and how much advance methodologies have been useful

P. Das
Hiralal Majumdar Memorial College for Women, Kolkata, India

K. Martin Sagayam
Karunya Institute of Technology and Sciences, Coimbatore, India

A. Rahaman Jamader
Penguin School of Hotel Management, Kolkata, India

B. Acharya (✉)
KIIT Deemed to Be University, Bhubaneswar, Odisha, India
e-mail: acharya.biswa85@gmail.com

© The Author(s), under exclusive license to Springer Nature Singapore Pte Ltd. 2022
S. Biswas et al. (eds.), *Internet of Things Based Smart Healthcare*, Smart Computing and Intelligence, https://doi.org/10.1007/978-981-19-1408-9_17

in extricating related information from sheer measure of medical services information. Ultimately we additionally assessed the writing for sensor, associated gadget, trackers, telemedicine, remote innovation, and continuous home GPS tracking and their application for clinicians. So this paper presents an exhaustive investigation of the sensors that are utilized in medical services environment.

Keywords Mobile health · Sensors · Web-based platforms · Internet of things (IOTs) · E-Health · Patient education

1 Introduction

Developments in remote device and electronic medical care are reforming the contribution of both specialists along with patients into an advanced medical services structure through increasing the capacities of physiological examination gadgets (Goldman et al., 2004; Haux et al., 2010). Regarding the outcomes on behalf of the demographic modify too many societies experiences previously or should look sooner in coming days, challenges intended for the keep up an excellence of medical concern in wellbeing frameworks emerge. Extension of wellbeing information novelty and buyer e-wellbeing devices along with administrations, used for example, telemonitoring period and moveable wellbeing applications (Goldman et al., 2005), include through innovative chances used for persons toward join effectively into their medical care, along with gives a prospect for distant monitoring of clinically significant factors in nonclinical settings (Koch et al., 2009). All gadgets can be synchronized hooked on schedule contemplation of extreme and constant sicknesses along with gives fundamental information to the executives to together the medical services provider along with patients (Kam et al., 2010). Studies show so as to the all-around sophisticated patient improves individual fulfilment and patient outcome since they are bound to take an interest in sound social changes (Bloem et al., 2016; Kam et al., 2010).

Populace gauges forecast critical expansions in the outright and relative quantities of people matured 80 years or more. Changes would not just prompt a rise in the older piece of the populace and consequently to a further slope in multi-dismalness (Goldman et al., 2004), yet additionally to a reduced employees of parental figures rather than the quantity of people needing care. Machine learning is a technique which is used for data analytics to provide predicted result of healthcare diagnosis. Besides this healthcare analysis there are various societal applications interested readers can found in literature (Tripathy et al., 2019).

Data and communication skills as a rule and 'wellbeing empowering technology's' specifically are viewed as one among a few way to help the support of the significant point of value in consideration. Micro-electro-mechanical systems (MEMS) with particularly sensor based technology may assist with surveying important signs and factor that help guardians and doctors in their work (Donoghue et al., 2012). While an expansion of people experiencing at least one useful impedances is general, these people frequently have the elevated inspiration toward remain in their recognizable habitat surroundings and not in an institutional consideration office. Sensor based frameworks may uphold habitat based or portable evaluation of an individual's condition of wellbeing and the information produced might be utilized to recognize unfavorable heavenly bodies or crisis circumstances. In this way, convenient involvement and anticipation method might be engaged to keep away from additional crumbling. This individual focused, ever-present consideration situation needs innovative types of existing and care (Goldman et al., 2005; Koch et al., 2009), with alongside this another sort of data framework design with respect to wellbeing data. This engineering structure should incorporate not just the individual or home climate as an origin of applicable health information, yet in addition the parental figures and other wellbeing experts instead of current organization driven structures (Donoghue et al., 2012; Kam et al., 2010). This frameworks are known as 'sensor-improved healthinfo system (SIHIS)' (Bloem et al., 2016). Aside from their simple breadth, such frameworks should have the option to give context-needy important understandings of the information assembled, all in all individualized choice help (Donoghue et al., 2012).

Sensors are classy and complex gadget that are utilized to distinguish and react to electrical or optical signs. Sensor is a tool that estimates measure and physical amount, actual size and converts it into signal which can peruse by an eyewitness or electronic instrument. In medical services system these physical amounts incorporates temperature, pulse, heart pulsates, and so forth. Figure 1 shows the essential working of sensor, which will have in as actual amount as information and electrical sign as outcome.

The motivation behind this chapter was to calculate active wearable sensors and depict their present clinical applications. The research was performed utilizing relevant health heading terms. We explored these investigations to establish medical efficacy and advantages of sensor in health care system.

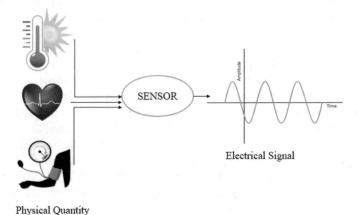

Fig. 1 Basic working principal of sensor

- Important of sensor in clinical system a case study also depicted
- To sum up the best class wearable sensors for medical services applications along with to exhibit their helpfulness by introducing more study models
- To survey sensor-upgraded wellbeing data frameworks with an attention on close to home choice emotionally supportive networks
- Different types of sensor unit define with their importance.

Outline of the paper

The organization of this paper is presented as follows.

Section 1 gives introduction and motivation and contribution. Section 2 describes about Wearable Sensors, and Sect. 3 covers the Sensor Application Areas in Healthcare. Section 4 discusses the importance of Sensor-Enhanced Health Information Systems. Section 5 defines the general discussion with benefits. Section 6 presents limitation of Mobile-based clinical applications. Section 7 covers discussion and lastly Sect. 8 represents conclusion.

2 Classification of Sensor

Sensors have become an essential piece of the implanted framework. Staring from our cell phone to security frameworks implemented at home. They are additionally getting significant for meteorological stations to foresee climate factor like temperature, weight, dampness, and some more.

To deal with any sensors microcontroller, client need to know the limit of the sensor and different sorts of sensors used in remote distinguishing, atmosphere systems, security devices, prosperity equipment, etc. But before jump into sensor and how many types sensor exists user should know the fundamental significance of the sensor and its use.

In this part we review the types of sensors presently used or being made in inaccessible recognizing. It is predictable that some new kinds of sensors will be invented in upcoming days. Detached or reactive sensors recognize the reflected or released electro-magnetic waves as of ordinary sources, although Active sensors perceive reflected responses from objects which are illuminated from speciously created energy sources, for instance, radar. Everything is segregated additional during to non-scanning and scanning structures. The sensor named a mix on behalf of reactive, non-scanning and non-imaging methodology is such the outline plotter, for illustration a microwave radiometer. Generally sensor categorized in two part, first passive, non-scanning and imaging methodology, digital camera for instance, a high exploration camera or telescope, the Russian COSMOS satellite can consider as example. Sensors categorized a blend of scanning, passive, imaging, requested additional within the picture plane checking sensors, for instance, solid state scanners, and aircraft analyzing sensors, for instance, checking microwave radiometers (Fig. 2).

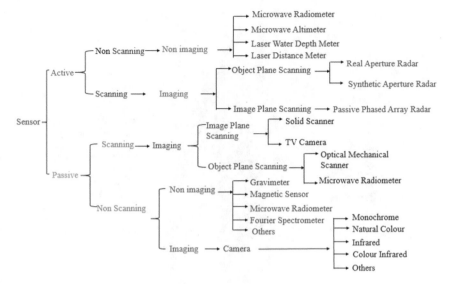

Fig. 2 Classification of different type of sensor

An illustration on behalf of the active, imaging less also non-scanning sensor is a shape plotter, for example, a laser spectrometer along with altimeter (Goldman et al., 2004; Haux et al., 2010). A functioning or vigorous, scanning along with imaging sensor is a radar, intended for instance SAR (Synthetic Aperture Radar), which preserve create elevated tenacity, symbolism, daytime or night-time, significantly below overcast coat. A generally well-known sensors utilized in RS are a camera, strong state scanner, for example, the charge joined gadget (CCD) pictures, a multi-phantom scanner and later on an aloof manufactured gap radar.

3 Wearable Sensors

The perfect sensor based structure for prosperity linked factor would be implemented at moment along with constantly quantify along with distantly report the entire prosperity related information as needed. It would not limit or impact its customer during any way along with it would need refusal help. Till date systems alike the prospected/outlined one resembles science fiction, but considering the advancement in the field of technology of the last decade, it is quite apparent that in the near upcoming systems such as viable. Some of present system are really fight with the recently referenced equipment. Major concerning issue is energy usage, surmising the need to invigorate and support the devices from time to time. This subsequently impacts the confirmation and consistence. The distance among proportions of energy so as to harvestable along with require on behalf of current sensor systems is as yet huge, yet contracting. The need to offering help to apparatuses is not just relying

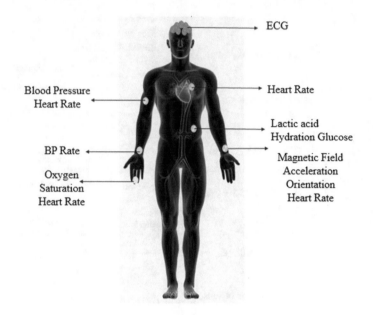

Fig. 3 Different type wearable sensor with tool

upon energy usage, but also depends upon the assessment cycle and the relationship among sensor and recognized subject as well. In (Chernew et al., 2005; Padgett et al., 2012) we arranged the couple of parameter, for example, compactness, relationship, calculated belongings and calculation progression to mastermind sensors for prosperity linked limits along with soon after enhanced the arrangement (Cook et al., 2013; Herman et al., 2011).

The resent development regarding this is summarized. The presence and accessibility of wearable sensor frameworks used for wellbeing linked factors so as to be simple to apply along with no pressure for the user is as yet one, if not the major point hamper the acceptance and foundation of wellbeing empowering innovations. The present system is developing to maintain balances in the various categorizations (Chan et al., 2012; Gómez et al., 2008). Figure 3 Different type wearable sensor with tool. This is the some major used wearable body sensor.

4   Sensor Application Areas in Healthcare

Sensor can be arranged and categorized depend upon various utilization ground, and there are different real-time applications in which sensors assume a significant job (Wang et al., 2015; Zhao et al., 2018). These different applications are medical care applications, military, fabricating, space, airplane, client hardware, and so on. In second type of category done dependent on highlights/particulars/property, there are different components that appear to be Accuracy, affectability, steadiness, ecological condition, range, adjustment, goal, cost, size, weight, repeatability, reaction time, linearity, and so on. Finally, classification done dependent on wide zone of location progressively climate that can be separated into immense and huge zones (Li et al., 2016).

Here we are essentially concentrating in on sensors those are utilized in Healthcare applications. The principle point of utilizing sensors in medical services applications is to escape the danger for client or patients. It is monetarily and socially favorable to diminish the weight of sickness therapy by upgrading or concentrating in on prevention and early recognition so we need sensors to detect different actual limitations (Table 1).

Glucose family observing

Even as numerous self-administration telephone applications have been precisely custom-made to particular wellbeing need throughout a regularly conveyed object, a large amount examination has been put resources keen on deciding glucose intensities in blood through sensors those are wearable (Fan et al., 2019). A non-intrusive consistent self-observing tool can significantly support the patient's autonomy. This system can improve the acceptability in case of diabetes (Ezimand & Kakroodi, 2019). A multi-sensor method created an arm module. In deeper level of muscles medium and long terminals are intrude. All data tracked with variation on glucose level. And lastly short terminal enters to the upper skin layer, giving information identified with different restrictions, for example, temperature and moistness (Kaplan & YigitAvdan, 2020). A new advancement, that further obliges people that are continually observing their glucose intensities, is a non-obtrusive visual glucose sensing device. Despite the fact that this innovation is as yet a work in progress, numerous organizations are making contact lances which have an incorporated demonstrative instrument that recognizes glucose intensities and sends it to an individual gadget. Sometime glucose used as an origin of energy.

Cardiopulmonary and vascular observing

The expansion in dependable observing and announcing combined through the flexibility of sensor implement has encouraged endeavors to execute SWS during medical settings (Liu & Weng, 2012; Meer et al., 2012). A large portion of the consideration regarding time has been centered scheduled circulatory strain or BP observing with home-based utilizing sensors. As per European rules for CVD avoidance suggest regular pulse observing to predict coronary infections (Padgett et al., 2012). Another non-intrusive long term circulatory strain or BP estimation gadget quantifies the BP consistently on the wrist utilizing ultrasound, a little expandable, along with an actuator (Pinter et al., 2003). For congestive cardiovascular breakdown and hypertension a ring sensor has been utilized (Suarez-Tangil et al., 2013). To measure BP organizing thru photoplethysmographic (PPG) wrist module was created (PPG) sensor. Same thing for an ECG sensor, taking into account non-stop checking. The Murata indispensable sign sensor utilizes the visual incorporation of moglobin proteins toward

Table 1 Application of sensor in different field

Use in medical system	Location	Type of sensor	Marker
Glucose Family checking	Arm rest	Multi variable	Blood glucose
	Eye	Glucose (Kovatchev et al., 2013)	Ocular glucose
	Dermatological	Glucose (Kovatchev et al., 2013)	Cell or tissue glucose
Bodily treatment and recovery	Ankle	Pedometers and accelerometer (Cook et al., 2013)	Measuring distance with foot step counts
Cardiopulmonary & vascular monitoring	Finger (ring sensor)	Heart rate (El-Amrawy & Nounou, 2015)	Heart rate and heat
		Pulse & temp(2015) "An empirical study of wearable technology acceptance in healthcare" (2015)	Heart rate and heat
	Rest or proximal segment	Heatre produce metric cardiopulmonary	HR varies since a technique to estimate stress
	Telephone connector	Single-link ECG	HR and beats
	Car seat belt	Wired like straining device	Respiration and heart rate
	Wrist	Electrocardiograph	BP and heart beat
		Ultrasound	BP
Neurological purpose observing	Garments	Inertial devices, accelerometers	Walking, progress distance, footstep calculation Throughout staircase climb and ancestry
	Hearing response ear phones	Inactivity	Walking rapidity and step distance
	Wrist or ankle	Accelerometer and gesture (Jones & Vaughan, 2010)	Removal action
Temperature checking	Body	Temperature sensors (2018) "Enabling technologies for the internet of health things" 2018)	Temperature

(continued)

Table 1 (continued)

Use in medical system	Location	Type of sensor	Marker
Identity checking	Finger	Fingerprint sensors (2015) "An empirical study of wearable technology acceptance in healthcare" 2015)	Identity
Medical diagnosis, blood pressure monitoring	…	Pressure sensors (2018) "Enabling technologies for the internet of health things" 2018)	Used in infusion pumps and sleep machines
Kidney dialysis	Kidney	Force sensors (2018) "Enabling technologies for the internet of health things" 2018)	Kidney dialysis condition

compose estimations of heartbeat plus level of oxygen in blood. It has two anodes that recognized the voltage contrasts of the heart (Wang et al., 2009).

Numerous sorts of heart checking gadgets exist. Some include careful implantation of remote gadgets that can screen and report information to an advanced cell and different gadgets can give user entry to a 24/7 h ECG through a connector which goes about as a telephone. The vast majority of the gadgets are outside and can be put on the wrist or around the chest to precisely screen heart work.

Physical treatment and recovery

The wearable wellbeing observing gadget can be coordinated into a client's garments. At a same time using this direction (those identified by sensors) which able to provide information and response to user. Lastly, it can produce warns depend on the user condition, stage of action, plus environmental situations (Tangen et al., 2014). Also, Sensors have been incorporated into pneumonic recovery. This incorporates evaluated activities, strength and adaptability preparing, collective self-administration training, and has been appeared to increase actual working with life superiority (Sibley et al., 2015). It currently viewed as a vital part of ideal consideration for individuals with extreme lung sickness. Accelerometers can quantify the verify loyalty mediation of users subsequent a pneumonic recovery process to advance actual work also exercise next project consummation.

Temperature probes

Utilized for internal heat level estimation. This assistants in giving better prescription and treatment of patients. They are called as thermometers.

Weight sensors

Utilized in infusion pumps and rest machines. In general case this sensors are coordinated with installed frameworks. They are utilized for clinical determination, pulse observing, mixture siphons, etc. **Power sensors:** Used in kidney dialysis apparatuses.

5   Importance of Sensor-Based Health Systems

With the presence of sensors for wellbeing related factors that are adequate to put together to take clinical decisions. This sensor are sufficiently modest to use in bigger accomplices, the administration of the information accumulated turns into an issue. Sources would not just be sensor frameworks delivered by clinical gadget produces and recommended by doctors (Kaplan & Avdan, 2020); however, sensors used in gadgets of regular daily existence bought and utilized on an individual premise, for example, PDAs, vehicles, brilliant homes, and so forth (Donoghue et al., 2012). While nonstop and pervasive estimation of factors potentially delivers new and significant symbolism of infections' onset. So, this way, medical usefulness on a single, customized premise, the examination of the enormous measures of various information should be achieved consequently. There are many healthcare analytics and research can found (Dash et al., 2020) using deep learning technique.

Because of the intrinsic majority of information sources, it is questionable that old style approaches produced for the administration of data frameworks of one or a couple of frequently comparative offices will be adequate for the arising sensor based health care system. The equivalent applies for the specialized system of the data framework, the same number of information may be caught for non-wellbeing related utilizations and clinical abuse may frequently be a result.

Improved Remote Device-Based Healthcare Applications

A mixture of various kinds of ease sensors (like gyrator, camera, pedometer, goniometer, fingerprint, magnetometer, accelerometer lastly pressure) implanted in cell phones have empowered these multi-functional gadgets to be pragmatic in numerous parts of upcoming medical services frameworks. Additionally, fusion of a portion of these sensors, for example, fingerprint sensors with large information has given a possibility to cell phones to massively affect the fortune of medical care frameworks. For example, a person may routinely check their cell phones hundreds times in each day. This measurement data can be utilized to empower cell phone gadgets to often get the client's facial output. Along these lines, crucial things, for example, pulse or BP can be estimated. By any chance this method is utilized over a huge populace and such biometric information is gathered in the cloud, infectious sickness episodes can be found all the more rapidly (Koch et al., 2009).

With the pervasive utilization of cell phones and the presence of fourth era of portable broadcast communications innovation that gives higher speed versatile broadband web access benefits alongside the pervasiveness of Wi-Fi innovation, medical services informatics (an interdisciplinary field consolidating medical care, software engineering, and data science) is presently ready to defeat time and area constraints. This is immensely significant explicitly in cases that a quick reaction is amazingly basic or when a patient's condition is not steady and powerfully evolving.

As opposed to meddlesome wearable gadgets that force a weight on client's day by day exercises, cell phones are less nosy, less obstructive, and less needed to follow an unwieldy utilization convention. This outcomes in lessening the conceivable ease of use difficulties.

Mobile phone do not need valuable equipment and numerous wellbeing related versatile applications are available and free which lead to a more easy to access result compared with customary wearable gadgets. Cell phones additionally can possibly supervise ongoing illnesses, for example, Alzheimer's, Hypertension, Diabetes, etc. This should be possible by regular checking of client through multipurpose applications or text updates with respect to the medication measurements data.

Case study: IoT-based remote ECG monitoring systems

An IoT-based ECG checking framework is represented in Fig. 5, which primarily comprises of three sections, i.e., the ECG detecting organization, IoT cloud, and Graphical User Interface.

The ECG detecting network is the establishment of the complete framework, which is answerable for collecting biological info from the patient body surface or skin and communicating these data to cloud via a remote channel. ECG sensor system is framed in this way that it can work with nominal effect from client or user everyday life. To continuing this process more ECG data can be collated for a specific period or even days. Using this method an ECG signal can be prepared, and it help to improve the sign excellence along with to see the fundamentals of remote communication. Electrocardiogram info collected from different sensors then it sent to cloud as particular remote convention, for example Bluetooth, Wi-Fi, Zigbee, etc.

IoT Cloud appreciates to the development of the high level if Internet of Thing strategies, Electrocardiogram information can be kept and investigated successfully and productively. Using the guideline of an IoT cloud, computation concentrated information cycle, and examination job can be done in incredible workers, which enormously facilitates the extra load of brilliant devices (Jones & Vaughan, 2010). As a rule, IoT cloud have four useful units, in ECG monitoring system i.e., information filtering, information keeping, information investigation, and illness alerting.

Graphical User Interface: The GUI is liable for information representation and the executives. It gives simple admittance to the information in the IoT cloud. Clients can sign onto the cloud to gain abstract ECG information in real time. Normally, two types of GUIs are accessible for clients to see ECG information, such as mobile applications and web pages. A portable application can give a prompt reaction to client input, while site pages are more helpful regarding upkeep and update.

For executed reason Sensor module, Controller module, Wi-Fi module; and Power module are utilized.

An ECG examination framework developed depending upon on front line IoT procedures. The design of the ECG observing framework was introduced from the

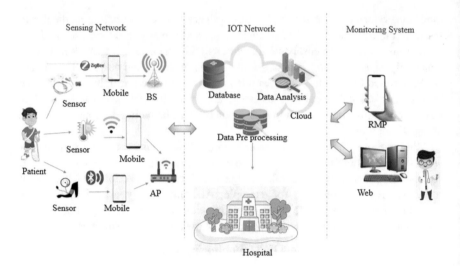

Fig. 4 A portable IoT based ECG monitoring system

start. Ordinary ECG detecting networks including Wi-Fi, Bluetooth, and Zigbee were presented and compared. In view of the proposed design, an IoT-based ECG observing framework was executed. Through a wearable checking hub with three ECG electrode, constant ECG signs can be gathered with agreeable precision. The assembled information were sent to the cloud of Internet of Thing utilizing Wi-Fi, which provided high transmission data rates plus wide zones. The IoT cloud is liable for imagining the ECG information to clients and putting away these significant information for additional investigation, which is actualized based on three servers, those are, the HTTP server, MQTT server, and capacity server. Taking out the need of portable applications, the electronic GUI gives an adaptable methods, more than ten free of any multipurpose OS platform for clients to admittance to the ECG information. Figure 4 A portable IoT based ECG monitoring system. S_n and S_f define sensitivity and specificity (Table 2).

6 Limitation of Mobile-Based Clinical Applications

A vulnerability can possible with respect to the helpfulness of infectious prevention by cell phones. In (Kaplan & YigitAvdan, 2020) reflected a cost-adequacy of using cell phone upheld self-observing of heavy breathing. It is found that self-administration via cell phones were impractical in patients. While the utilization of cell phones present extraordinary occasions to improve medical services superiority for users with ongoing situations, however there has not been a convincing methodology to transfer from preliminary research to execution in the more extensive populace (Kaplan & Avdan, 2020). Likewise, the consideration of the aged

Table 2 Comparative study between planned and earlier study

Author	Data used	Approach	Performance
Old-style ECG monitoring scheme	Leads: 12 leads beats: Every single segment	ECG observing by medical tool	Accuracy $= 100\%$
Molkentin et al., 1998)	Leads: 12 leads	Artificial NN with fuzzy system	Training $S_n = 94.2\%$ $S_f = 100\%$ Testing $S_n = 84.6\%$ $S_f = 90\%$
Proposed method	Leads: 3leads	IoT Based health care service with remote monitoring	Accuracy $= 93.59\%$ $S_n = 100\%$ $S_f = 85\%$

person cannot just depend on cell phones as older people might be visually delayed, incapable to utilize their hands viably or even, unfit to utilize the innovation.

The appropriation of RPM would not be without its difficulties, however. This article will investigate the absolute greatest boundaries to passage for RPM innovation that are yet to be survived.

Data Security

For the information communicated over any RPM stage to be sufficiently secure to satisfy the guidelines expected of medical services, it will require vigorous information with secure and strike management.

Huge areas of the information dealt with by outsiders or any third party system, which makes hazard for patients possibly having their information taken. The difficulties are no less intense for clinics, who are suffer from very danger issues to hiring an outsider framework. Because this third party system could hacked, putting their patients' security and protection in danger.

Data Accuracy

Apparently the most complicated test confronting remote health monitoring adoption when it comes for data accuracy. A lot problem comes down to perceptions between both patients and clinical parties.

Can we truly expect patients more familiar with customary medical care strategies, to believe that a little tool will give more exact information about their wellbeing than what they could give to their primary care physician themselves? So the answer will be No in most case.

Front line clinical experts will be relied upon to analyze and treat patients on the strength of the information gave. They, as well, need to believe that it is of the most important imaginable accuracy in the event that they are to take the sort of quick and conclusive activity required - particularly in the treatment of continuous and probably harmful conditions. Figure 5 Define the challenges of smartphone based healthcare system.

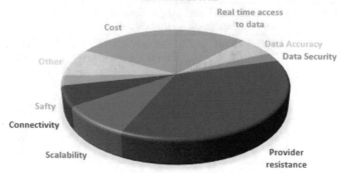

Fig. 5 Challenges of smartphone based healthcare system

Real-time Access to Data

The exchange of data needed for RPM to work is conceivably a long and confounded progression and comprises of a different exchanges (El-Amrawy & Nounou, 2015; Kouris et al., 2010).

First, information should be gathered and transferred from the patient's gadget. In any chance if this gadget is on a portable network, the information should go through that network supplier's framework and out on to the web prior to winding up in the specialist co-ops organization, possibly through different server farms and the RPM stage organization.

In any point of time any of these node is intruded, or a shutdown happens at any of the stops on this excursion, the information may be postponed in getting to its objective (Attal et al., 2015; Mougiakakou et al., 2010).

Flexible networks are not designed to be consistently accessible. This is viewed as a large enough issue in situations where remote clients cannot get to social network namely Instagram for an hour or two, however when it is truly an incomprehensibly important issue, as it very well may be for a patient, it is important that information is conveyed dependably and in an opportune way.

Cost of Devices

To attempt to reduce the threat around security and make understanding easier, clinics could decide to plan RPM gadgets themselves rather than to gather information by means of an application or outsider gadget (Mougiakakou et al., 2010).

An audit directed in the US in mid-2016 thought of a scope of expenses for turning out RPM. For battling foundations like the NHS this sort of cost is essentially unreasonable as a cross country arrangement.

7 Discussion

In 2008 researcher have expressed that unavoidable medical services as a ground of examination '…it is as yet a developing stage, with a decent arrangement of experimental exploration.' Sensor that can wearable are without question a necessary piece of the unavoidable medical care vision, and sensor innovations are, notwithstanding a few issues, for example, power utilization defendant battery life which are still to be settled, effectively progressed as to their specialized abilities. While numerous ventures have shown the advantages of utilizing sensor-based observing for explicit clinical issues, for example, cardiovascular arrhythmias, diabetes or cardiovascular breakdown, wearable sensors speak to only one bit of the riddle, since sensor information must be deciphered independently with regards to all accessible wellbeing data, such as institutional electronic wellbeing records system (Guo et al., 2019). Accordingly, the mix of sensor-based frameworks with institutional or medical also other wellbeing experts' data framework parts into a trans-institutional, sensor-upgraded wellbeing data framework is a need if complex dynamic will be encouraged. Individualized choice help has habitually been called attention to as an essential for individual wellbeing frameworks (Kam et al., 2010; Shi et al., 2019), it actually is a significant test due to the various issues that must be settled while executing sensor based medical care structures, for example, normal phrasings, semantic interoperability or the normalization of gadget boundaries, portrayal designs for medical and sensor information and choice rationale (Bloem et al., 2016). Figure 6 define a comparison between medical devices and service in present days. Figure 7 shows Comparison between different Health Analysis Parameter.

Accordingly, from the creators' perspective, wearable sensor innovations with regards to medical services ought not to be viewed as a detached field of examination yet as a component of an interdisciplinary exploration exertion where sensor information give significant extra data to be utilized for individualized choice help inside a sensor based health care system. This view in addition to further things suggests that

Fig. 6 Comparison between different health analysis parameter

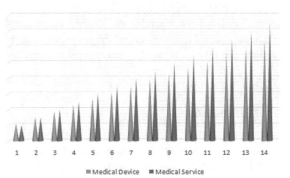

Comparison Between Different Medical Service and Device

■ Medical Device   ■ Medical Service

Comparison Between Different Health
Analysis Parameter

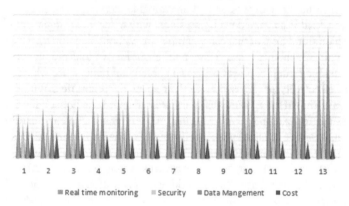

1   2   3   4   5   6   7   8   9   10   11   12   13

■ Real time monitoring   ■ Security   ■ Data Mangement   ■ Cost

Fig. 7 Comparison between different health analysis parameter

there is a requirement for rigorous approval concentrates in near cooperation with attendants, doctors, physical-therapy and other wellbeing experts demonstrating that wearable observing truly gives extra data and consequently has helpful outcomes. With respect to the inspiration to utilize wearable checking to moderate the outcomes of segment change regarding diminishing guardians' outstanding burden and of lessening medical care costs, there is as yet a requirement for such proof. Clearly constant observing of various wellbeing related boundaries is neither effective nor alluring for everybody and that organization ought to be all around considered, proof based and person. Will wearable sensors in medical services and sensor based health care system be 'every one of our days to come's and more than a 'brief flame'? Truly and no. Consistent and continuous wellbeing checking under solo, everyday life conditions as appeared in the two models above can give extra data pertinent to finding, treatment or avoidance and may even help persistent strengthening and autonomy. However it can't resolve all issues and should be practical in due thought of the favorable circumstances also downsides of this innovation.

The International Medical Informatics Association (IMIA's) employed gathering on sensor data from wearable device delivers research questions identified with the previously stated difficulties and the principal creator sincerely welcomes all people intrigued to take an interest in the collective endeavors.

8   Conclusion

Sensors adopt a significant part in medical services industry. We can utilize various sensors in various medical care applications. This will assist patients survive effectively in omnipresent or global climate. Most fundamental functionalities of human body can be inspected utilizing various types of sensors which may assist with prevention the serious difficulties in medical services. Illnesses can be effortlessly identified at beginning phase to keep away from genuine conditions. Sensors are effectively accessible and dependable gadgets. In this paper we have effectively considered sensors with its types. Also, utilization of sensor in medical services depicted. For better understanding a case study shown in ECG monitoring using IoT namely IoT-based remote ECG monitoring systems. We got good response to promote remote healthcare system. In future researcher can invest more time and thought to enhance this sensor based controlling system.

References

Attal, F., Mohammed, S., Dedabrishvili, M., Chamroukhi, F., Oukhellou, L., & Amirat, Y. (2015). Physical human activity recognition using wearable sensors. *Sensors, 15*(12), 31314–31338.

Bloem, B. R., Marinus, J., Almeida, Q., Dibble, L., Nieuwboer, A., Post, B., Ruzicka, E., Goetz, C., Stebbins, G., Martinez-Martin, P., & Schrag, A. (2016). M easurement instruments to assess posture, gait, and balance in Parkinson's disease: Critique and recommendations. *Movement Disorders, 31*(9), 1342–1355.

Chan, M., Estève, D., Fourniols, J. Y., Escriba, C., & Campo, E. (2012). Smart wearable systems: Current status and future challenges. *Artificial Intelligence in Medicine, 56*(3), 137–156.

Chernew, M. E., Goldman, D. P., Pan, F., & Shang, B. (2005). Disability and health care spending among medicare beneficiaries: Improved disability status among the elderly is unlikely to eliminate cost pressures as the number of beneficiaries continues to rise. *Health Affairs, 24*(Suppl2), W5-R42.

Cook, D. J., Thompson, J. E., Prinsen, S. K., Dearani, J. A., & Deschamps, C. (2013). Functional recovery in the elderly after major surgery: Assessment of mobility recovery using wireless technology. *The Annals of Thoracic Surgery, 96*(3), 1057–1061.

Dash, S, Acharya, B R, Mittal, M, Abraham, A., & Kelemen, A. G. (eds). (2020). Deep learning techniques for biomedical and health informatics. Cham: Springer.

Donoghue, O. A., Horgan, N. F., Savva, G. M., Cronin, H., O'Regan, C., & Kenny, R. A. (2012). Association between timed Up-and-Go and memory, executive function, and processing speed. *Journal of the American Geriatrics Society, 60*(9), 1681–1686.

El-Amrawy, F., & Nounou, M. I. (2015). Are currently available wearable devices for activity tracking and heart rate monitoring accurate, precise, and medically beneficial Healthcare informatics research, 21(4), pp.315–320.

Ezimand, K., & Kakroodi, A. A. (2019). Prediction and spatio–Temporal analysis of ozone concentration in a metropolitan area. *Ecological Indicators, 103*, 589–598.

Fan, G., Chen, F., Li, Y., Liu, B., & Fan, X. (2019). Development and testing of a new ground measurement tool to assist in forest GIS surveys. *Forests, 10*(8), 643.

Goldman, D. P., Shekelle, P. G., Bhattacharya, J., Hurd, M., & Joyce, G. F., (2004). Health status and medical treatment of the future elderly. RAND CORP SANTA MONICA CA.

Goldman, D. P., Shang, B., Bhattacharya, J., Garber, A. M., Hurd, M., Joyce, G. F., Lakdawalla, D. N., Panis, C., & Shekelle, P. G., (2005). Consequences of health trends and medical innovation for the future elderly: When demographic trends temper the optimism of biomedical advances, how will tomorrow's elderly fare health affairs, 24(Suppl2), pp.W5-R5.

Guo, L., Luo, J., Yuan, M., Huang, Y., Shen, H., & Li, T. (2019). The influence of urban planning factors on PM2. 5 pollution exposure and implications: A case study in China based on remote sensing, LBS, and GIS data. *Science of the Total Environment, 659*, 1585–1596.

Gómez, E. J., Pérez, M. E. H., Vering, T., Cros, M. R., Bott, O., García-Sáez, G., Pretschner, P., Brugués, E., Schnell, O., Patte, C., & Bergmann, J. (2008). The INCA system: A further step towards a telemedical artificial pancreas. *IEEE Transactions on Information Technology in Biomedicine, 12*(4), 470–479.

Haux, R., Hein, A., Eichelberg, M., Appell, J. E., Appelrath, H. J., Bartsch, C., Bisitz, T., Bitzer, J., Blau, M., Boll, S., & Buschermöhle, M. (2010). The Lower saxony research network design of environments for ageing: Towards interdisciplinary research on information and communication technologies in ageing societies. *Informatics for Health and Social Care, 35*(3–4), 92–103.

Herman, T., Giladi, N., & Hausdorff, J. M. (2011). Properties of the 'timed up and go'test: More than meets the eye. *Gerontology, 57*(3), 203–210.

Jones, H. G., & Vaughan, R. A. (2010). *Remote sensing of vegetation: Principles, techniques, and applications.* Oxford University Press.

Kam, H. J., Sung, J. O., & Park, R. W. (2010). Prediction of daily patient numbers for a regional emergency medical center using time series analysis. *Healthcare Informatics Research, 16*(3), 158–165.

Kaplan, G., & YigitAvdan, Z. (2020). Space-borne air pollution observation from sentinel-5p tropomi: Relationship between pollutants, geographical and demographic data. *International Journal of Engineering and Geosciences, 5*(3), pp.130–137.

Kaplan, G., & Avdan, Z. Y. (2020). COVID-19: Spaceborne nitrogen dioxide over Turkey. *Eskişehir Technical University Journal of Science and Technology A-Applied Sciences and Engineering, 21*(2), 251–255.

Koch, S., Marschollek, M., Wolf, K. H., Plischke, M., & Haux, R. (2009). On health-enabling and ambient-assistive technologies. *Methods of Information in Medicine, 48*(01), 29–37.

Kouris, I., Mougiakakou, S., Scarnato, L., Iliopoulou, D., Diem, P., Vazeou, A., & Koutsouris, D. (2010). Mobile phone technologies and advanced data analysis towards the enhancement of diabetes self-management. *International Journal of Electronic Healthcare, 5*(4), 386–402.

Kovatchev, B. P., Renard, E., Cobelli, C., Zisser, H. C., Keith-Hynes, P., Anderson, S. M., Brown, S. A., et al. (2013). Feasibility of outpatient fully integrated closed-loop control: First studies of wearable artificial pancreas. *Diabetes Care, 36*(7), 1851–1858.

Li, H., Wu, J., Gao, Y., & Shi, Y. (2016). Examining individuals' adoption of healthcare wearable devices: An empirical study from privacy calculus perspective. *International Journal of Medical Informatics, 88*, 8–17.

Liu, H., & Weng, Q. (2012). Enhancing temporal resolution of satellite imagery for public health studies: A case study of West Nile Virus outbreak in Los Angeles in 2007. *Remote Sensing of Environment, 117*, 57–71.

Molkentin, J. D., Lu, J. R., Antos, C. L., Markham, B., Richardson, J., Robbins, J., & Olson, E. N. (1998). A calcineurin-dependent transcriptional pathway for cardiac hypertrophy. *Cell, 93*(2), 215–228.

Mougiakakou, S. G., Bartsocas, C. S., Bozas, E., Chaniotakis, N., Iliopoulou, D., Kouris, I., Pavlopoulos, S., Prountzou, A., Skevofilakas, M., Tsoukalis, A., & Varotsis, K. (2010). SMART-DIAB: A communication and information technology approach for the intelligent monitoring, management and follow-up of type 1 diabetes patients. *IEEE Transactions on Information Technology in Biomedicine, 14*(3), 622–633.

Padgett, P. K., Jacobs, J. V., & Kasser, S. L. (2012). Is the BESTest at its best? A suggested brief version based on interrater reliability, validity, internal consistency, and theoretical construct. *Physical Therapy, 92*(9), 1197–1207.

Pinter, P. J. Jr., Hatfield, J. L., Schepers, J. S., Barnes, E. M., Moran, M. S., Daughtry, C. S., & Upchurch, D. R. (2003). Remote sensing for crop management. *Photogrammetric Engineering & Remote Sensing, 69*(6), 647–664.

Rodrigues, J. J. P. C., Segundo, D. B. De R., Junqueira, H. A., Sabino, M. H., Prince, R. M., Al-Muhtadi, J. & Albuquerque, V. H. C. De . (2018). Enabling technologies for the internet of health things. *IEEE Access, 6* , 13129–13141.

Shi, K., Li, Y., Chen, Y., Li, L., & Huang, C., (2019). How does the urban form-PM2. 5 concentration relationship change seasonally in Chinese cities? A comparative analysis between national and urban agglomeration scales. Journal of Cleaner Production, 239, p.118088.

Sibley, K. M., Beauchamp, M. K., Van Ooteghem, K., Straus, S. E., & Jaglal, S. B. (2015). Using the systems framework for postural control to analyze the components of balance evaluated in standardized balance measures: A scoping review. *Archives of Physical Medicine and Rehabilitation, 96*(1), 122–132.

Suarez-Tangil, G., Tapiador, J. E., Peris-Lopez, P., & Ribagorda, A. (2013). Evolution, detection and analysis of malware for smart devices. *IEEE Communications Surveys & Tutorials, 16*(2), 961–987.

Tangen, G. G., Engedal, K., Bergland, A., Moger, T. A., & Mengshoel, A. M. (2014). Relationships between balance and cognition in patients with subjective cognitive impairment, mild cognitive impairment, and Alzheimer disease. *Physical Therapy, 94*(8), 1123–1134.

Tripathy, Kumar, H, Acharya, B. R., Kumar, R., & Chatterjee, J. M. (2019). Machine learning on big data: A developmental approach on societal applications, pp. 143–165." In *Big Data Processing Using Spark in Cloud*. Springer, Singapore.

Van der Meer, F. D., Van der Werff, H. M., Van Ruitenbeek, F. J., Hecker, C. A., Bakker, W. H., Noomen, M. F., Van Der Meijde, M., Carranza, E. J. M., De Smeth, J. B., & Woldai, T. (2012). Multi-and hyperspectral geologic remote sensing: A review. *International Journal of Applied Earth Observation and Geoinformation, 14*(1), 112–128.

Wang, Y., Mitchell, B. R., Nugranad-Marzilli, J., Bonynge, G., Zhou, Y., & Shriver, G. (2009). Remote sensing of land-cover change and landscape context of the National Parks: A case study of the Northeast Temperate Network. *Remote Sensing of Environment, 113*(7), 1453–1461.

Wang, X., White, L., Chen, X., Gao, Y., Li, H., & Luo, Y., (2015a). An empirical study of wearable technology acceptance in healthcare. Industrial Management & Data Systems.

Wang, X, White, L, Chen, Xu, YiwenGao, He Li, & Luo, Y . (2015b), An empirical study of wearable technology acceptance in healthcare. Industrial Management & Data Systems.

Zhao, Y., Ni, Q., & Zhou, R. (2018). What factors influence the mobile health service adoption? A meta-analysis and the moderating role of age. *International Journal of Information Management, 43*, 342–350.

Printed in the United States
by Baker & Taylor Publisher Services